T0226588

Surgical and Medical Management of Common Oral Problems

Editor

HARRY DYM

DENTAL CLINICS OF NORTH AMERICA

www.dental.theclinics.com

April 2020 • Volume 64 • Number 2

ELSEVIER

1600 John F. Kennedy Boulevard • Suite 1800 • Philadelphia, Pennsylvania, 19103-2899

http://www.dental.theclinics.com

DENTAL CLINICS OF NORTH AMERICA Volume 64, Number 2
April 2020 ISSN 0011-8532, ISBN: 978-0-323-71336-8

Editor: John Vassallo; j.vassallo@elsevier.com
Developmental Editor: Laura Fisher

Dental Clinics of North America (ISSN 0011-8532) is published quarterly by Elsevier Inc., 360 Park Avenue South, New York, NY 10010-1710. Months of issue are January, April, July, and October. Business and Editorial Offices: 1600 John F. Kennedy Boulevard, Suite 1800, Philadelphia, PA 19103-2899. Periodicals postage paid at New York, NY and additional mailing offices. Subscription prices are $304.00 per year (domestic individuals), $633.00 per year (domestic institutions), $100.00 per year (domestic students/residents), $366.00 per year (Canadian individuals), $821.00 per year (Canadian institutions), $100.00 per year (Canadian students/residents) $424.00 per year (international individuals), $821.00 per year (international institutions), and $200.00 per year (international students/residents). International air speed delivery is included in all *Clinics* subscription prices. All prices are subject to change without notice. **POSTMASTER:** Send address changes to *Dental Clinics of North America*, Elsevier Health Sciences Division, Subscription Customer Service, 3251 Riverport Lane, Maryland Heights, MO 63043. **Customer Service (orders, claims, online, change of address): Elsevier Health Sciences Division, Subscription Customer Service, 3251 Riverport Lane, Maryland Heights, MO 63043. Tel: 1-800-654-2452 (U.S. and Canada). Fax: 314-447-8029. E-mail: journalscustomerservice-usa@elsevier.com (for print support); journalsonlinesupport-usa@elsevier.com (for online support).**

Reprints. For copies of 100 or more, of articles in this publication, please contact the Commercial Reprints Department, Elsevier Inc., 360 Park Avenue South, New York, NY 10010-1710. Tel.: 212-633-3874; Fax: 212-633-3820; E-mail: reprints@elsevier.com.

The Dental Clinics of North America is covered in *MEDLINE/PubMed (Index Medicus), Current Contents/Clinical Medicine, ISI/BIOMED* and *Clinahl*.

Contributors

EDITOR

HARRY DYM, DDS, FACS
Chairman, Department of Dentistry and Oral and Maxillofacial Surgery, Director, Oral and Maxillofacial Surgery, Residency Training Program, Chief of Oral and Maxillofacial Surgery, The Brooklyn Hospital Center, Senior Attending, Division of Oral and Maxillofacial Surgery, Woodhull Medical Center, Brooklyn, New York, USA; Clinical Professor, Oral and Maxillofacial Surgery, Columbia University College of Dental Medicine, New York, New York, USA; Fellow, The American College of Surgeons, Diplomate, American Board of Oral and Maxillofacial Surgery, Chicago, Illinois, USA

AUTHORS

DAVID R. ADAMS, DDS
Associate Professor, Clinic Chief, Oral and Maxillofacial Surgery, University of Utah School of Dentistry, Salt Lake City, Utah, USA

DAVID BARANES, DDS
Private Practice, Jerusalem, Israel

DAVID CHVARTSZAID, DDS, MSc (PROSTHO), MSc (PERIO), FRCD(C)
Graduate Program Director, Prosthodontics, Faculty of Dentistry, Assistant Professor, University of Toronto, Toronto, Ontario, Canada

EARL CLARKSON, DDS
Chairman of Dentistry, Woodhull Medical and Mental Health Center, Department of Oral and Maxillofacial Surgery, Woodhull Medical Center, Brooklyn, New York, USA

ROBERT DeFALCO, DDS
Senior Faculty, Department of Oral and Maxillofacial Surgery, St. Joseph's University Medical Center, Paterson, New Jersey, USA

DAMIAN DUDEK, DDS
Private Practice, Oral and Maxillofacial Surgeon, Artmedica Oral Surgery Department, Toruń, Poland

HARRY DYM, DDS, FACS
Chairman, Department of Dentistry and Oral and Maxillofacial Surgery, Director, Oral and Maxillofacial Surgery, Residency Training Program, Chief of Oral and Maxillofacial Surgery, The Brooklyn Hospital Center, Senior Attending, Division of Oral and Maxillofacial Surgery, Woodhull Medical Center, Brooklyn, New York, USA; Clinical Professor, Oral and Maxillofacial Surgery, Columbia University College of Dental Medicine, New York, New York, USA; Fellow, The American College of Surgeons, Diplomate, American Board of Oral and Maxillofacial Surgery, Chicago, Illinois, USA

HILLEL EPHROS, DMD, MD
Program Director and Chairman, Oral and Maxillofacial Surgery, St. Joseph's University Medical Center, Paterson, New Jersey, USA

YIJAO FAN, DDS
Resident, Division of Oral and Maxillofacial Surgery, The Brooklyn Hospital Center, Brooklyn, New York, USA

LESLIE R. HALPERN, DDS, MD, PHD, FACS, FICD
Professor, Section Head, Oral and Maxillofacial Surgery, University of Utah School of Dentistry, Salt Lake City, Utah, USA

MICHAEL KATZAP, DDS
Private Practice, General Dentist, Rego Park, New York, USA

SANG WOO KIM, DDS
Department of Oral and Maxillofacial Surgery, Nova Southeastern University College of Dental Medicine, Davie, Florida, USA; Broward Health Medical Center, Fort Lauderdale, Florida, USA

SHIWOO KIM, DMD
Resident, Department of Oral and Maxillofacial Surgery, St. Joseph's University Medical Center, Paterson, New Jersey, USA

TARUN KIRPALANI, DMD
Resident, Department of Oral and Maxillofacial Surgery, The Brooklyn Hospital Center, Brooklyn, New York, USA

GREGORI M. KURTZMAN, DDS
Private Practice, General Dentist, Silver Spring, Maryland, USA

SPENCER LIN, DMD
Intern, Division of Oral and Maxillofacial Surgery, Woodhull Medical Center, Brooklyn, New York, USA

ROMEO MINOU LUO, DMD
Resident, Department of Oral and Maxillofacial Surgery, Nova Southeastern University College of Dental Medicine, Davie, Florida, USA; Broward Health Medical Center, Fort Lauderdale, Florida, USA

NABIL TAKAHIRO MOUSSA, DDS
Resident, Department of Dentistry, Division of Oral and Maxillofacial Surgery, The Brooklyn Hospital Center, Brooklyn, New York, USA

LEVON NIKOYAN, DDS
Attending, Department of Dentistry and Oral and Maxillofacial Surgery, Woodhull Hospital, Brooklyn, New York, USA; Private Practice, Forward Oral Surgery, Floral Park, New York, USA

ORRETT E. OGLE, DDS
Former Chief/Program Director, Oral and Maxillofacial Surgery, Woodhull Hospital, Brooklyn, New York, USA; Visiting Lecturer, Mona Dental Program, University of the West Indies, Kingston, Jamaica

RINIL PATEL, DDS
Chief Resident, Department of Dentistry and Oral and Maxillofacial Surgery, Woodhull Hospital, Brooklyn, New York, USA

KARLA PEREZ, DDS
Resident, Division of Oral and Maxillofacial Surgery, The Brooklyn Hospital Center, Brooklyn, New York, USA

ROBERT PIERRE II, DMD
Chief Resident, Department of Oral and Maxillofacial Surgery, The Brooklyn Hospital Center, Brooklyn, New York, USA

JASON ELI PORTNOF, DMD, MD, FACS, FICD
Private Practice, Boca Raton, Florida, USA

JONATHAN ROSENSTEIN, DDS
Chief Resident, Department of Oral and Maxillofacial Surgery, The Brooklyn Hospital Center, Brooklyn, New York, USA

STEVEN R. SCHWARTZ, DDS
Private Practice, NY Oral and Maxillofacial Surgeon, PC, Brooklyn, New York, USA; Director of Surgical Implantology, Department of Oral and Maxillofacial Surgery, Woodhull Medical Center, Brooklyn, New York, USA

DAVID SHEEN, DDS
Department of Oral and Maxillofacial Surgery, Woodhull Medical Center, Brooklyn, New York, USA

JAYKRISHNA THAKKAR, DDS
Resident in Oral and Maxillofacial Surgery, The Brooklyn Hospital Center, Brooklyn, New York, USA

AMOS YAHAV, DMD
CEO, Augma Biomaterials, Katzir, Israel

Contents

Preface **xiii**

Harry Dym

Short Implants: An Answer to a Challenging Dilemma? **279**

Steven R. Schwartz

The purpose of this article is not to discuss the success of short dental implants versus standard/long dental implants, but to compare short dental implants with standard/long dental implants in areas that necessitated adjunctive bone grafting or augmentation procedures and as a way to avoid the need for advanced surgical procedures and their associated risks. It can be concluded that short dental implants are a viable alternative in sites that would have required additional complex and costly augmentation procedures. Short dental implants resulted in comparable survival and success rates with faster, less expensive treatment with fewer surgical complications and morbidity.

Clinical Uses of Platelet-Rich Fibrin in Oral and Maxillofacial Surgery **291**

Yijao Fan, Karla Perez, and Harry Dym

Platelet-rich fibrin (PRF) is an autogenous material that is derived from a person's own platelets and is used to enhance wound healing and tissue regeneration. Platelet concentrates have been applied in dermatology, pain management, sports medicine, plastic surgery, cardiac surgery, urology, and also dentistry. PRF has garnered significant interest in the dental community because of its proposed regenerative properties and its ability to aid in wound healing. PRF is proposed to have a direct effect on enhancing a patient's wound healing by suprasaturating the wound with growth factors that promote tissue healing. Clinically, PRF is easily produced chairside from the patient's own blood. The autologous nature of PRF makes it preferred over a variety of allografts used in dentistry today. Therefore, PRF has significant potential in being applicable to all areas of dentistry, including oral and maxillofacial surgeries.

Peri-implantitis: Evaluation and Management **305**

Hillel Ephros, Shiwoo Kim, and Robert DeFalco

With a very large number of endosseous dental implants placed by generalists and specialists, complications are to be expected. Among them are problems with the soft tissue interface and the hard tissue attachment. Peri-implant mucositis and peri-implantitis are not uncommon, but their prevalence and impact may be reduced with diagnosis and appropriate management, as can the likelihood of progression from mucositis to peri-implantitis. Successful implant dentistry does not end with integration and restoration, and both patient and professionally administered modalities are important for long-term implant maintenance.

authors present an overview of multiple treatments that would benefit from the use of this technology. From preoperative, intraoperative, to postoperative patient management, 3D technology plays a vital role in the dental practice. With the incorporation of 3D CBCT, intraoral scanners, and 3D printing, a dental provider can accurately plan and execute the treatment with greater confidence. The contemporary dentist, however, has many options for incorporating the digital workflow based on the specific practice needs.

Neuropathic Pain and Burning Mouth Syndrome: An Overview and Current Update **379**

Harry Dym, Spencer Lin, and Jaykrishna Thakkar

Burning mouth syndrome/glossodynia and trigeminal neuropathic conditions can have serious negative impact on a patient's overall quality of life. These conditions are often hard to diagnose and even harder to fully treat and manage, but it is important for dentists/oral and maxillofacial surgeons to be aware of these conditions and modalities of their treatment. Often the only method for arriving at the proper diagnosis is for patients to undergo traditional approaches for treatment of presenting signs and symptoms, and it is the unexpected failure of interventional therapies that leads ultimately to a proper diagnosis.

Zygomatic Implants: A Solution for the Atrophic Maxilla **401**

Jonathan Rosenstein and Harry Dym

Even with the great strides made in the techniques for placement of traditional endosseous dental implants, restoration of the dentition in patients with a severely resorbed or resected maxilla can prove challenging. For many decades, significant bone grafting was the mainstay of treatment for these patients. However, zygomatic implants have been shown to provide a stable and predictable alternative for the restoration of the dentition for patients with severe bone loss of the maxilla.

Treatment of the Dental Patient with Bleeding Dyscrasias: Etiologies and Management Options for Surgical Success in Practice **411**

Leslie R. Halpern, David R. Adams, and Earl Clarkson

The oral health care provider sees a significant number of patients in his or her practice who suffer from systemic diseases affecting the ability to clot. These medical issues can be acquired or inherited bleeding dyscrasias requiring pharmacologic therapy during the perioperative period. Patients with inherited or acquired bleeding disorders require careful attention with respect to the assessment of bleeding risk. This article develops algorithms to manage acquired and inherited bleeding dyscrasias. These approaches include a discussion of the epidemiology of bleeding disorders in surgical patients, mechanism of hemostasis, and strategies for patient management based on the etiology of bleeding disorder.

Soft-Tissue Grafting Solutions **435**

Romeo Minou Luo, David Chvartszaid, Sang Woo Kim, and Jason Eli Portnof

Many soft tissue grafting solutions are available for reconstruction and restoration of volume and esthetics of keratinized attached mucosa at compromised periodontal and peri-implant interfaces. Presence of healthy soft tissues is crucial for functional and esthetic implant success as well as longevity of natural dentition. The options available each provide unique characteristics with different indications. This article is intended to provide an efficient and comprehensive overview of this topic, covering the essentials of periodontal anatomy and physiology, indications for soft-tissue grafting, and keys in recipient and donor-site preparation, and exploring the available procedural arsenal in soft-tissue grafting.

Bone Regeneration: Properties and Clinical Applications of Biphasic Calcium Sulfate **453**

Amos Yahav, Gregori M. Kurtzman, Michael Katzap, Damian Dudek, and David Baranes

Dental treatment may require osseous grafting. Pathologic voids may require grafting to restore osseous anatomy. Various osseous grafting materials have been used and reported. These include autografts, allografts, xenografts, and nonbiological products. Osseous grafts act as a scaffold, maintaining volume while allowing bone formation. Calcium sulfate has been used as an osseous void filler, binder, and grafting material. It possesses many characteristics of an ideal material for bone regeneration. It provides an effective cement for maxillofacial and dental augmentation that is easy to use and cost effective, while not requiring complete soft tissue coverage or a membrane at placement.

Maxillofacial Bone Grafting Materials **473**

Nabil Takahiro Moussa and Harry Dym

The goal of bone grafting is to replace normal bone volume and structure with healthy, well-vascularized bone that will undergo normal remodeling. The ideal bone will regenerate bone and not repair it. Currently four types of grafting material are available to clinicians for regenerative use in oral and maxillofacial surgery: autologous bone, allogeneic bone, xenogenic bone, and alloplastic bone. Additionally, bioactive agents, growth factors, are now being used to stimulate osteoinductive properties of native bone for bone regeneration. This article reviews the literature and summarizes the benefits and disadvantages of each respective graft and illustrates its use in clinical practice.

DENTAL CLINICS OF NORTH AMERICA

FORTHCOMING ISSUES

July 2020
Controlled Substance Risk Mitigation in the Dental Setting
Ronald J. Kulich, David A. Keith, and Michael E. Schatman, *Editors*

October 2020
The Journey to Excellence in Esthetic Dentistry
Yair Whiteman and David Wagner, *Editors*

January 2021
Implant Surgery Update for the General Practitioner
Harry Dym, *Editor*

RECENT ISSUES

January 2020
Oral Diseases for the General Dentist
Arvind Babu Rajendra Santosh and Orrett E. Ogle, *Editors*

October 2019
Caries Management
Sandra Guzmán-Armstrong, Margherita Fontana, Marcelle M. Nascimento, and Andrea G. Ferreira Zandona, *Editors*

July 2019
Unanswered Questions in Implant Dentistry
Mohanad Al-Sabbagh, *Editor*

Preface

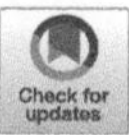

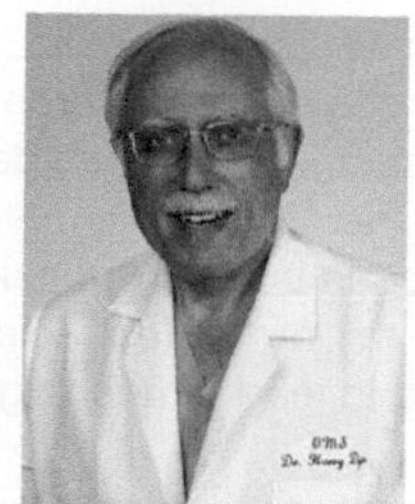

Harry Dym, DDS, FACS
Editor

As editor of this issue of *Dental Clinics of North America*, I have the duty and privilege to write a preface that is designed as an introduction to the issue, primarily stating its scope and aims, and I do so willingly now.

My vision for this text was to bring relevant and up-to-date information to our readership on a variety of different clinical areas that they would find useful and clinically relevant. The issue includes articles ranging from the use of platelet-rich fibrin to updates on soft and hard tissue grafting and reconstruction, with additional articles on the current state of short implants and 3-dimensional cone-beam reconstruction. Articles that focus on topics in oral medicine, such as surgical management of the patient on blood thinners, and a review of neuropathic pain are included as well.

In editing the finished text, I feel that my capable contributors have helped me in accomplishing this task, and I am indebted to them for their dedicated efforts and contributions. It is my hope that the readership will arrive at a similar conclusion.

Having spent my entire career, spanning over 3 decades as an attending in Oral and Maxillofacial Surgery training programs at community hospitals and involved both in direct patient care and in resident education, I feel privileged and fortunate to have had the time to be associated for many years with Elsevier and my capable editor, Mr John Vassallo, who has been the associate publisher of the *Dental Clinics of North America*. Much appreciation is owed to my assigned developmental editor, Ms Laura Fisher, and the journal manager Mrs Esther Bennitta, who worked tirelessly to assist in editing this issue, and to my executive assistant, Ms Gloria Stallings, for her loyalty and dedication.

The scope and practice of dentistry and oral and maxillofacial surgery have advanced significantly, and the current dental and oral and maxillofacial surgery office is now involved in treating patients with a variety of needs from cosmetic dentistry to facial rejuvenation, and from oral facial pain to complete prosthetic and implant rehabilitation. Elsevier, through its involvement with the *Clinics* series, along with its varied dental/medical journals and its recent Internet presence, has also played a vital role in this transformative journey.

Dent Clin N Am 64 (2020) xiii–xiv
https://doi.org/10.1016/j.cden.2020.01.001

The year 2020 marks the 175th anniversary of The Brooklyn Hospital Center (the first hospital in Brooklyn), where I have spent my entire career, and I wish to acknowledge Ms Lizanne Fontaine, Chairperson of the Board of Trustees, and Mr Gary Terrinoni for their continued support of the Department of Dentistry and Oral and Maxillofacial Surgery as a vital component of the medical team.

To my colleagues and dear friends of over 40 years, Dr Peter M. Sherman, Dr Earl Clarkson, and Dr Orrett Ogle, my sincerest appreciation for your concern, mentorship, and friendship all these many years. I am also indebted to my dear friend for decades, Dr Stan Bodner, a true kindred spirit for his insight, humor and friendship.

Oral and Maxillofacial Surgery and resident education have been both my passion and my job these past 40 years, but it is my wife Freida and my family (especially the grandchildren) who have kept me anchored and allowed me to lead a meaningful life.

I especially wish to acknowledge the oral and maxillofacial surgery residents who studied under me these past decades. They have kept me excited and passionate in the pursuit of education as I attempted to always stay ahead of them.

Harry Dym, DDS
Dentistry and Oral & Maxillofacial Surgery
The Brooklyn Hospital Center
121 DeKalb Avenue, 1st Floor
Brooklyn, NY 11201, USA

E-mail address:
hdym@tbh.org

Short Implants

An Answer to a Challenging Dilemma?

Steven R. Schwartz, DDS[a,b,*]

KEYWORDS

- Dental implants • Short dental implants • Bone grafting • Bone augmentation
- Sinus grafts • Vertical bone graft • Complications

KEY POINTS

- Short implants (<8 mm) have been promoted as a treatment option in many clinical scenarios with limited bone volume where long/standard length implants were otherwise contraindicated if not for complex, sophisticated and costly bone augmentation procedures that would have been required.
- This article reviews the efficacy of using the currently available short implants with enhanced macrosurface and microsurface technology and abutment interfaces allowing their placement in cases previously thought ill-advised.
- This allows implant treatment in a potentially faster, less expensive, less complicated manner, with decreased morbidity and comparable success rates with long/standard length implants with concomitant bone augmentation procedures.

INTRODUCTION

Mankind's desire for teeth to be able to chew and smile precedes all recorded dissertations on dentistry. Human mandibles with seashells carved into tooth shapes and placed into extraction sockets date back as far 600 AD.[1] But, at what cost, physically, financially, and emotionally to our patients? Decreasing bone quantity and quality has traditionally necessitated increasing surgical complexity, cost, and potential complications. Is there anything we can do to mitigate these potential road blocks to successful implant treatment? Maybe short implants can be part of the solution.

WHAT ARE SHORT IMPLANTS?

There is still no generally accepted length to classify implants as standard or long, short, and ultrashort. Various authors have defined implant lengths less than 11 mm,[2] 10 mm,[3] 8 mm,[4] and 7 mm[5] as short implants. When this author first wrote about this topic in

[a] Private Practice: NY Oral & Maxillofacial Surgeon, PC, 2844 Ocean Parkway, Brooklyn, NY 11235, USA; [b] Department of Oral & Maxillofacial Surgery, Woodhull Medical Center, 760 Broadway 2c320, Brooklyn, NY 11206, USA
* Department of Oral & Maxillofacial Surgery, Woodhull Medical Center, 760 Broadway 2c320, Brooklyn, NY 11206.
E-mail address: nyomsdds@gmail.com

Dent Clin N Am 64 (2020) 279–290
https://doi.org/10.1016/j.cden.2019.11.001
0011-8532/20/

2015, 10 mm was used as the cut off for short dental implants versus long dental implants.[6] Over the ensuing years, multiple studies have been published using an intrabony implant length of 8 mm or less as the definition of a short dental implant and has been gaining acceptance worldwide. Therefore, 8 mm or less will be used as the definition of a short dental implant[7] for the purposes of this discussion.

WHY DID WE FAVOR LONG OVER SHORT IMPLANTS?

Initially, it was thought that the longer the implant the more stable and long lasting it would be because the occlusal forces would be dissipated over a greater surface area.[8] This would prevent overloading the bone to implant interface. Implants ranged in length from as short as 7 mm to an enormous 20 mm.[9] Evidence to support this theory that short implants (<10 mm) had inferior success and survival rates than long implants (≥10 mm) came from multiple early (1991–2005) studies done by Herrmann and colleagues,[10] Friberg and colleagues,[5] Wyatt and Zarb,[11] Bahat,[12] Attard and Zarb,[13] and Weng and colleagues.[14] Cumulatively, these studies showed failure rates of short dental implants ranging from a low of 15% to a high of 26%.[10–14]

This notion that longer is better is also probably rooted in our dental experience of longer roots being stronger than short-rooted teeth. Perhaps this concept came from Ante's law of fixed prosthodontics, which stated that the total periodontal membrane area of the abutment teeth must equal or exceed that of the teeth to be replaced.[15] Additionally, it was believed that a reduced crown-to-implant ratio was an important factor in decreasing marginal bone loss and improving long-term survivability.[16,17] Implant diameter was not considered a critical factor at this time.[9] To allow for the placement of these longer implants, there had to be adequate vertical bone height (quantity) and preferably sufficient density (quality).[18]

Restorative biomechanical forces also have to be taken into consideration when planning an implant borne restoration. The posterior occlusion, closer to the temporomandibular joint acts as a class II lever exerting considerably more force (200–250 PSI) than is encountered anteriorly (25–50 PSI) where the jaw functions as a class III lever.[19] This serves to highlight the need for increased bone to implant contact in the posterior mandible and especially the posterior maxilla where both quality and quantity are decreased.[4,8,20,21]

What is preventing us from placing our preferred long implants wherever we want? The answer lies primarily with anatomic limitations. There are a multitude of clinical scenarios where the placement of a long implant is not possible owing to anatomic deficiencies. In the maxilla, posteriorly the pneumatized maxillary sinus and/or resorbed posterior alveolar ridge and anteriorly the nasal floor, nasopalatine canal, and/or resorbed ridge can thwart long implant placement. In the posterior mandible, the position of the inferior alveolar nerve and canal and mental nerve foramen in relation to the mandibular crest are the determining factor. These anatomic difficulties relate to the quantity or volume of the bone. The quality or density of the bone in the posterior mandible and in particular the posterior maxilla is inferior as compared with the anterior region.[4,8]

If the posterior aspect of the mandible or maxilla is atrophied from tooth loss or trauma and there is not enough bone height to place the long implants that we would traditionally choose, what are the choices?

WHAT ARE THE SURGICAL SOLUTIONS TO INSUFFICIENT BONE HEIGHT AND MASS?

What are we to do if satisfactory bone does not exist? The answer was bone regeneration, augmentation, or nerve transposition. To deal with these bone deficits successfully to allow for long implants in adequate numbers many different advanced bone regeneration, augmentation, grafting, and transposition procedures have been developed and upgraded over the years.

Maxillary Sinus Grafts

In the posterior maxilla, inadequate bone volume is often encountered owing to progressive sinus pneumatization coupled with typical postextraction alveolar bone atrophy. To magnify the problem, the posterior maxilla has poor bone quality, typically type IV bone.[22]

When Boyne and James[23] first reported on grafting of the maxillary sinus floor with autogenous bone and marrow the problem of vertical height deficiency preventing the placement of standard/long implants was overcome. Since then, the technique has been refined and studied using various autogenous, allografts, xenografts, and alloplasts alone or in combination with or without membranes, both resorbable and nonresorbable.[24] This advanced surgical procedure, maxillary sinus floor grafting (both laterally and crestally), has been well-documented and found to be equal to conventionally placed implants without grafting.[25–27]

Guided Bone Regeneration

Guided bone regeneration techniques have been used for alveolar defects, socket grafts, and lateral augmentation as well as vertical ridge augmentation.[25] There are various protocols using a variety of grafting materials, including autogenous bone, xenografts, allografts, alloplasts, or a combination thereof. The procedure includes a cell occlusive membrane with or without tacks or miniscrews or sutures to aid in membrane stabilization to promote bone healing by space maintenance while excluding gingival cell invagination. The membranes can be resorbable or nonresorbable membranes. Nonresorbable membranes that include internal titanium struts to help maintain the underlying space and their shape[28] and/or long screws used as tent poles[29] to support the membrane are often used in vertical augmentations. These techniques do require advanced training and skills. Guided bone regeneration techniques also seem to yield comparable and favorable results as compared with implant placement in healed nonaugmented bone.[25–27]

Block Grafts

Block grafts for onlay or inlay/interpositional grafting involves either harvesting blocks of bone from an intraoral sites such as the chin, external oblique ridge, ramus,[25,30] and palate[31] or from extraoral sites such as the iliac crest or calvaria.[32] The intraoral donor sites can be accomplished as in office procedures, whereas the extraoral sites require general anesthesia in an operating room setting. The advantages of block grafts include vertical and/or horizontal bone augmentation and decreased frequency of inferior alveolar nerve injuries with the onlay technique. The inlay/interpositional graft technique improves graft revascularization with more of the graft bone block in contact with vascularized host bone at time of graft placement and less resorption compared with onlay block grafts. Implant survival and marginal bone levels were comparable with block grafted bone and ungrafted bone.[30]

Distraction Osteogenesis

Distraction osteogenesis involves a technique of osteotomies and a distractor device that in a controlled fashion distracts or stretches the bone by repeatedly pulling the osteotomy line apart, allowing new bone to continually form in the newly created gap. During the active phase of treatment, the device is actuated twice a day to slowly elongate the osteotomized segment until the desired dimension is achieved. Then the device is left for an additional 90 to 120 days until the newly formed bone has healed sufficiently.[33]

Distraction osteogenesis showed the greatest gain in vertical height, an average of 8.04 mm compared with guided bone regeneration and onlay blocks.[25] Additional advantages included no donor site morbidity, less postoperative bone resorption, and gains in soft tissue along with the increased vertical bone height.[33]

Inferior Alveolar Nerve Transposition

Inferior alveolar nerve repositioning can be carried out to increase useable vertical alveolar height and bone mass in an effort to place long dental implants.[32,34,35] The stated advantages of this procedure included shorter surgical treatment time because the implants are always placed at the same operative procedure as the nerve transposition and autogenous bone grafts are superfluous; therefore, no donor site morbidity and minimal allogenic or xenograft materials are needed.[34]

WHY REINVESTIGATE THE CONCEPT OF SHORT IMPLANTS?

With the ability to augment and regenerate bone as noted above all of the negative results in so many early studies why did clinicians and researchers continue to pursue the idea of short dental implants? First, the disadvantages and potential complications associated with these complex and invasive grafting procedures became apparent over the years. Some of these methods are extremely technique sensitive, time consuming, costly, require advanced skills and training, and increased surgical morbidity and complications.[8,34,36–38] Second, it must be remembered that all of the previously cited early studies done by Herrmann and colleagues,[10] Friberg and colleagues,[5] Wyatt and Zarb,[11] Bahat,[12] Attard and Zarb,[13] and Weng and colleagues[14] were based on the original externally hexed, turned/machine surface Brånemark implants that were placed using the generally accepted drilling protocols of that era. Last, our understanding of dental implant configuration, prosthesis design, biomechanics, and surgical protocols have evolved.

COMPLICATIONS OF ADVANCED BONE GRAFTING TECHNIQUES

With every surgical technique there are inherent risks and complications that must be considered when planning a course of treatment. Bone augmentation and related procedures are no different.

Maxillary Sinus Grafts

The complication most commonly seen with maxillary sinus elevation from both a lateral or crestal/transalveolar approach is Schneiderian membrane perforation (18%). Additional complications include postoperative bleeding (14.5%), infections (1%), pain (0.6%), abscess formation (0.2%), sinusitis (0.2%),[25] and partial or total graft loss (0.1%).[27]

Guided Bone Regeneration

The most common complication associated with guided bone regeneration is premature membrane exposure or membrane loss, which can cause the bone graft to become infected, leading to partial or total graft loss. This complication can occur with either resorbable membranes or nonresorbable membranes, which have the inconvenience of requiring removal as a secondary procedure. Nonresorbable membranes, polytetrafluoroethylene, and titanium mesh have higher incidences of exposure than resorbable membranes.[25,27,30] Nonrigid resorbable membranes with insufficient support beneath them can collapse leading to inadequate volume of augmentation requiring supplemental grafting. A disadvantage of all of these membranes is that they can be expensive.[30]

Block Grafts

Block grafts are technique-sensitive procedures that demand a complete knowledge of the anatomy of the donor area. Donor site morbidity, protracted treatment time in part owing to the need for 2 operative sites and soft tissue complications, such as recipient site wound dehiscence and graft resorption and failure, make this an advanced procedure.[25,27,30] Inlay or interpositional grafts in the posterior edentulous mandible have a high rate of inferior alveolar nerve temporary hypoesthesia. Additionally, there is a risk of mandibular fracture and an inability to achieve the desired vertical augmentation owing to soft tissue tension.[30] Intraorally, the symphysis donor region has a high incidence of temporary neurosensory deficits as opposed to the ramus, which is much lower.[27] Iliac crest grafts have their own set of potential complications, including perforation of the peritoneum or bowel, infection, ilial fracture, and gait disturbances.[39] Calvarial bone graft minor complications include incision line alopecia and hematomas. Major complications could include cerebrospinal fluid leak, extradural hematoma, and direct intracerebral trauma if the inner table of the diploë is violated during the graft harvest.[39]

Distraction Osteogenesis

Potential complications, both minor and major, associated with distraction osteogenesis are numerous. It is paramount that the surgeon knows how to manage these problems as much as they know how to perform the actual procedure. Mazzonetto and colleagues[33] divided complications into minor and major categories. Minor complications were defined as those complications that had "no effect on final result, but immediate intervention required" and major complications as "lead[ing] to technique failure."[33] Minor complications included tilting of the transport segment (secondary to in-elastic palatal mucosa or muscle pull), soft tissue dehiscence or perforation, infection, and lack of patient cooperation. Major complications included distractor failure, transport fragment resorption, mandibular fracture, bony nonunion, neurosensory disturbances, and insufficient bone distraction.[33]

Inferior Alveolar Nerve Transposition

The most common complication of inferior alveolar nerve transposition is neurosensory disturbance, including hypoesthesia (decreased sensitivity to all stimuli except for special senses), paresthesia (abnormal sensation even spontaneously or for no reason), and hyperesthesia (hypersensitivity to all stimuli except for special senses). These injuries are caused by mechanical trauma to the nerve and impairment of the microvascular network by direct injury and stretching of the microvascular circulation in the mesoneurium.[34,35] Putting aside the fact that surgical technique itself is technique sensitive, sophisticated, and requires general anesthesia in an operating room setting,[35] even the postoperative care is protracted and complex. Follow-up for monitoring the return of normal neurosensory function, excluding cases that required microneurosurgical repair, can take weeks to 6 months, and has been reported to take up to 1 year. There is a percentage of cases with permanent neurosensory loss.[34,35] Additionally, low-level laser therapy, using a GaA1As laser, starting immediately postoperatively 4 times a week for 40 treatments has been advocated to hasten paresthesia recovery.[34,35] Because of the ubiquitous nature of nerve injuries, some researchers believe that sensory deviations should not be considered a complication, but a normal outcome associated with this procedure.[34]

Implant Configuration and Biomechanics

Advances in the design of dental implants both externally, thread design, macrosurface, and microsurface topography and internally, the implant to abutment connection and have been dramatically transformed. All of these changes have led to enhanced implant survivability.

The implants studied in the earlier articles by Herrmann and colleagues,[10] Friberg and colleagues,[5] Wyatt and Zarb,[11] Bahat,[12] Attard and Zarb,[13] and Weng and colleagues[14] did show poor survival rates compared with their long counter parts. However, these were the results for turned/machine surface (smooth), externally hexed implants. A meta-analysis of observational studies by Pommer and colleagues[8] in 2011 separated rough surface implants from smooth surface implants and "suggested that rough surfaced implants with a minimum length of 7 mm represent no risk factor for implant failure." Annibali and colleagues[40] in their systematic review found that a rough surface on short implants yielded superior cumulative survival rates of 99.2% as compared with machine-surfaced implants at 94.6%. They concluded there were high survival rates with low rates of biological and biomechanical complications and "rough-surfaced implants preferred."[40] Nisand and Renouard[41] also concluded that rough surface implants improve bone-to-implant contact.

Changes in the abutment to implant connection have been studied since the original flat to flat, external hex interface was first used. Multiple connection configurations, including internal hexes, splines, octagons, triangular shapes, and Morse tapers or cones to list but a few, have been scrutinized. Morse taper connections have been shown to induce less marginal bone loss as compared with the external abutment connection and also can promote bone growth over the top of implant shoulder contacting the abutment surface. The lack of meaningful micromotion between the abutment and the implant, a well-documented benefit of the Morse taper connection is probably responsible.[42] Furthermore, platform switching maintains the crestal marginal bone levels as opposed to abutment–implant platform matched components.[43]

Finite element analyses have shown that increasing the implant diameter is more efficient than increasing implant length for reduction of stresses at the bone to implant interface,[44,45] because the greatest concentration of stress is found at the bony crest and much lower forces are found at the implant apex. Therefore, although longer implants might improve primary mechanical stability, wider implants could improve both primary stability and long-term bone-to-implant stress reduction, and result in less crestal marginal bone loss.[46,47]

The greater crown-to-implant ratio has been a topic of concern for clinicians and researchers particularly when discussing short implants. This concern is most likely in part fueled by our prior belief in Ante's law. However, implants are not teeth and do not have a periodontal membrane. Additionally, Ante's law was subsequently disproven by Lulic and associates.[48] Some early studies correlated an increase in biomechanical complications associated the greater crown-to-implant ratios. These elongated clinical crown lengths were considered vertical cantilevers, which caused greater marginal bone stresses, leading to marginal bone loss or implant loss[49] or technical complications, including prosthetic component failure.[50] Nevertheless, more recent studies concluded that the crown-to-implant ratio is not a reliable predictor of marginal bone loss or implant survival. The Study by Blane,[16] which included machined surface, solid implants, and rough surface hollow cylinder and solid implants, concluded that crown to implant ratio did not affect the degree of peri-implant marginal bone loss. Nedir and colleagues[51] conducted a 7-year life table analysis of rough surface long and short implants with varying crown-to-implant ratios and found a cumulative success rate of 99.4% and that short implants did not fail more than longer ones despite the greater crown to implant ratios with the short implants. Schulte and colleagues[52] retrospectively determined the crown-to-root ratio of 889 implants that ranged from 0.5:1 to 3:1, and found that the guidelines of crown to root ratios of natural tooth single crown restorations have no relationship with crown to implant ratios of single implant restorations. Meijer and colleagues[53] found that, with crown-to-implant ratios ranging from 0.9 to 2.2, there was not a high incidence of biological or technical complications.

Modified Surgical Protocols

Many of the early failures of short implants were seen primarily in areas of poor quality, low-density bone, predominantly the posterior maxilla. These studies, although primarily using turned/machined surface implants, were also done using the standard drilling protocols of the era. There was no generally accepted differentiation in site preparation for soft versus normal bone.[5,10–14]

The development and adoption of modified or adapted surgical protocols, sometimes referred to as soft bone drilling protocols, allow for improved primary mechanical stability and have been advocated by several researchers including, Tawil and Younan,[20] Fugazzotto and colleagues,[54] Renouard and Nisand,[4] and Nisand and Renouard.[41] The concept is to enhance primary mechanical stability specifically in poor quality bone by either finishing the osteotomy with a drill that is narrower than the standard final diameter drill, or eliminating a countersink or bone tap or any combination of these techniques.[6] Many implant companies themselves have adopted and promote this idea by actually manufacturing specific narrow final drills and publishing modified or soft bone drilling protocol guidelines.[6]

Studies Comparing Short Implants versus Long Implants with Grafting

Numerous papers, including systematic reviews, meta-analyses, randomized controlled trials, and retrospective and observational studies, have been published comparing short implants with long or standard implants in grafted, augmented, or modified sites.

Posterior maxilla

Thoma and colleagues[55] in a randomlzed in a randomized controlled multicenter study comparing 6-mm implants with 11- to 15-mm implants with sinus graft procedures found equal success at 1-year after loading. However, the 6-mm implant group had a substantially shorter surgical time and cost less than 50% as the long implant plus graft group.

Hadzik and colleagues[56] published a similar study in 2018 using the same 6-mm (short) and 11- to 13-mm (long) implants. They came to the same conclusion that short implants can be used successfully in the posterior maxilla and that they decrease the need for complicated adjunctive procedures, thereby decreasing patient postoperative pain and morbidity.

The European Academy of Osseointegration Consensus Conference[7] found predictably high implant survival for both short implants and long implants with their corresponding sinus grafting procedures. However, given the added number of biological complications, and the increased cost, surgical time, and morbidity associated with longer implants in grafted sinuses, "shorter implants may represent the preferred alternative."

Fan and coworkers[57] in their systematic review concluded that there was no difference in the survival rate between short (5–8 mm) implants and long (>8 mm) implants with simultaneous lateral window sinus grafts. Complication rates, cost and operating time were all less with short implants. They also suggested additional studies to confirm their findings.

Nielsen and colleagues[58] in their systematic review of 3 randomized controlled trials comparing short (≤8 mm) with long (>8 mm) implants with lateral window maxillary sinus grafts with follow-up periods for at least 3 years found no significant difference between the 2 techniques in regards to implant survival, marginal bone loss and patient satisfaction. "Short implants seem to be a suitable alternative to standard length implants in conjunction with maxillary sinus floor augmentation." However, they also recommended additional studies with more patients and observation times of more than 3 years to determine the superiority of one technique over the other.

Posterior mandible

Nisand and colleagues[59] undertook a systematic review that included 4 articles comparing long implants placed in vertically augmented bone with short implants in native nonaugmented sites. They concluded that the implant and prosthetic survival rates were comparable for both techniques. Nonetheless vertical augmentation using interpositional inlay block grafts is costlier, lengthens treatment time and increases complications. They also suggested additional studies using different methods of vertical grafting, larger sample size and longer follow-ups.

Dias and coworkers[60] performed a meta-analysis using 4 studies evaluating long (>8 mm) implants with various vertical augmentation techniques with short (≤8 mm) dental implants in ungrafted bone with at least 1 year of follow-up after final prosthesis insertion. They found a 97% versus 92.6% implant survival rate for short and long implants with grafting, respectively. Moreover, there was an increased trend of complications with bone augmentation procedures and long implants. They determined, owing to the decreased incidence of surgical complications, that short implants should be preferred when adequate bone is present.

Pieri and colleagues[61] conducted a 5-year retrospective study comparing clinical and radiographic findings comparing short (6 mm) and standard (≥9 mm) length implants that were placed after vertical ridge augmentation with autogenous bone blocks. Although there were no statistically significant differences in the number of implant or prostheses failures, prosthetic or biological complications, the number of surgical complications was greater in the standard length implants with augmentation. Plus, the short implants had statistically significant less marginal bone loss than the long implants.

Felice and colleagues[62] completed a randomized controlled trial comparing 5-mm length (short) implants with 10-mm length (standard) implants placed in sites augmented with anorganic bovine xenograft bone blocks using the interpositional vertical grafting technique. They found no statistically significant differences in implant or prosthetic failures or biological or prosthetic complications. There was a statistically significant difference in marginal bone loss over the 5-year study, with short implants loosing less bone than the standard length implants. They concluded that both techniques provided acceptable results up to 5 years, but that treatment with short implants less costly and quicker.

SUMMARY

The purpose of this article is not to discuss the success of short dental implants versus standard/long dental implants, but rather to compare short dental implants with standard/long dental implants in areas that necessitated adjunctive bone grafting or augmentation procedures and as a way to avoid the need for advanced surgical procedures and their associated risks. Therefore, it can be concluded that, in a multitude of clinical scenarios, short dental implants are a viable alternative to long implants in sites that would otherwise have required additional complex and costly augmentation procedures. Overall, short dental implants resulted in comparable survival and success rates with faster and less expensive treatment with fewer surgical complications and morbidity.

DISCLOSURE

The author has nothing to disclose.

REFERENCES

1. Ring ME. Dentistry: an illustrated history. New York: Harry N Abrams; 1985.
2. Neves FD, Fones D, Bernardes SR, et al. Short implants—an analysis of longitudinal studies. Int J Oral Maxillofac Implants 2006;21:86–93.
3. Morand M, Irinakis T. The challenge of implant therapy in the posterior maxilla: providing a rationale for the use of short implants. J Oral Implantol 2007;33(5):257–66.
4. Renouard F, Nisand D. Impact of implant length and diameter on survival rates. Clin Oral Implants Res 2006;17(Suppl 2):35–51.
5. Friberg B, Jemt T, Lekholm U. Early failures in 4,641 consecutively placed Bra°nemark dental implants: a study from stage 1 surgery to the connection of completed prostheses. Int J Oral Maxillofac Implants 1991;6:142–6.
6. Schwartz SR. Short implant are they a viable option in implant dentistry? Dent Clin North Am 2015;59:317–28.
7. Thoma DS, Zeltner M, Hüsler J, et al. EAO Supplement Working Group 4 – EAO CC 2015 short implants versus sinus lifting with longer implants to restore the posterior maxilla: a systematic review. Clin Oral Implants Res 2015;26(Suppl 11):154–69.
8. Pommer B, Frantal S, Willer J, et al. Impact of dental implant length on early failure rates: a meta-analysis of observational studies. J Clin Periodontol 2011;38:856–63.
9. Lee JH, Frias V, Lee KW, et al. Effect of implant size and shape on implant success rates: a literature review. J Prosthet Dent 2005;94:377–81.
10. Herrmann I, Lekholm U, Holm S, et al. Evaluation of patient and implant characteristics as potential prognostic factors for oral implant failures. Int J Oral Maxillofac Implants 2005;20:220–30.
11. Wyatt CC, Zarb GA. Treatment outcomes of patients with implant-supported fixed partial prostheses. Int J Oral Maxillofac Implants 1998;13:204–11.
12. Bahat O. Bra°nemark system implants in the posterior maxilla: clinical study of 660 implants followed for 5 to 12 years. Int J Oral Maxillofac Implants 2000;15:646–53.
13. Attard NJ, Zarb GA. Implant prosthodontic management of partially edentulous patients missing posterior teeth: the Toronto experience. J Prosthet Dent 2003;89:352–9.
14. Weng D, Jacobson Z, Tarnow D, et al. A prospective multicenter clinical trial of 3i machined-surface implants: results after 6 years of follow-up. Int J Oral Maxillofac Implants 2003;18:417–23.

15. Ante IH. The fundamental principles of abutments. Mich State Dent Society Bulletin 1926;8:14–23.
16. Blanes RJ. To what extent does the crown-implant ratio affect survival and complications of implant-supported reconstructions? A systematic review. Clin Oral Implants Res 2009;20(Suppl 4):67–72.
17. Rossi F, Lang NP, Ricci E, et al. Long-term follow-up of single crowns supported by short, moderately rough implants—A prospective 10-year cohort study. Clin Oral Implants Res 2018;29:1212–9.
18. Thoma DS, Cha JK, Jung UW. Treatment concepts for the posterior maxilla and mandible: short implants versus long implants in augmented bone. J Periodontal Implant Sci 2017;47(1):2–12.
19. Misch CE. Occlusal considerations for implant-supported prostheses: implant-protective occlusion, dental implant prosthetics. Chapter 31. 2nd edition. St. Louis (MO): Mosby; 2015. p. 874–912.
20. Tawil G, Younan R. Clinical evaluation of short, machined-surface implants followed for 12 to 92 months. Int J Oral Maxillofac Implants 2003;18:894–901.
21. McAllister BS, Haghigat K. Bone augmentation techniques. J Periodontol 2007; 78(3):377–96.
22. Truhlar RS, Orenstein IH, Morris HF, et al. Distribution of bone quality in patients receiving endosseous dental implants. J Oral Maxillofac Surg 1997;55:38–45, 63.
23. Boyne PJ, James RA. Grafting of the maxillary sinus floor with autogenous marrow and bone. J Oral Surg 1980;38:613–6.
24. Wallace SS, Froum SJ, Cho SC, et al. Sinus augmentation utilizing anorganic bovine bone (Bio-Oss) with absorbable and nonabsorbable membranes placed over the lateral window: histomorphometric and clinical analyses. Int J Periodontics Restorative Dent 2005;25:551–9.
25. Jepsen S, Schwarz F, Cordaro L, et al. Regeneration of alveolar ridge defects. Consensus report of group 4 of the 15th European Workshop on Periodontology on Bone Regeneration. J Clin Periodontol 2019;46(Suppl. 21):277–86.
26. Aghaloo TL, Moy PK. Which hard tissue augmentation techniques are the most successful in furnishing bony support for implant placement? Int J Oral Maxillofac Implants 2007;22(Suppl):49–73.
27. Chiapasco M, Zaniboni M, Boisco M. Augmentation procedures for the rehabilitation of deficient edentulous ridges with oral implants. Clin Oral Implants Res 2006;17(Suppl 2):136–59.
28. Urban IA, Lozada JL, Jovanovic SA, et al. Vertical ridge augmentation with titanium-reinforced, dense-PTFE membranes and a combination of particulated autogenous bone and anorganic bovine bone-derived mineral: a prospective case series in 19 patients. Int J Oral Maxillofac Implants 2014;29(1):185–93.
29. Le B, Rohrer MD, Prassad HS. Screw "tent-pole" grafting technique for reconstruction of large vertical alveolar ridge defects using human mineralized allograft for implant site preparation. J Oral Maxillofac Surg 2010;68:428–35.
30. Louis PJ, Sittitavornwong S. Managing bone grafts for the mandible. Oral Maxillofacial Surg Clin N Am 2019;31:317–30.
31. Hernández-Alfaro F, Pages CM, García E, et al. Palatal core graft for alveolar reconstruction: a new donor site. Int J Oral Maxillofac Implants 2005;20(5): 777–83.
32. Carinci F, Farina A, Zanetti U, et al. Alveolar ridge augmentation: a comparative longitudinal study between calvaria and iliac crest bone grafts. J Oral Implantol 2005;31(1):39–45.

33. Mazzonetto R, Allais M, Maurette PE, et al. A retrospective study of the potential complications during alveolar distraction osteogenesis in 55 patients. Int J Oral Maxillofac Surg 2007;36:6–10.
34. Hassani A, Motamedi M, Saadat S. Inferior alveolar nerve transpositioning for implant placement, a textbook of advanced oral and maxillofacial surgery. Rijeka (Croatia): InTech Publishing; 2013. p. 659–93.
35. Chrcanovic BR, Neto Custodio AL. Inferior alveolar nerve lateral transposition. Oral Maxillofac Surg 2009;13:213–9.
36. Kotsovilis S, Fourmousis I, Karoussis I, et al. A systematic review and meta-analysis on the effect of implant length on the survival of rough-surface dental implants. J Periodontol 2009;80:1700–18.
37. Esposito M, Grusovin M, Felice P, et al. The efficacy of horizontal and vertical bone augmentation procedures for dental implants–a Cochrane systematic review. Eur J Oral Implantol 2009;2(3):167–84.
38. Milinkovic I, Cordaro L. Are there specific indications for the different alveolar bone augmentation procedures for implant placement? A systematic review. Int J Oral Maxillofac Surg 2014;43:606–25.
39. Tolstunov L, Hamrick JFE, Broumand V, et al. Bone augmentation techniques for horizontal and vertical alveolar ridge deficiency in oral implantology. Oral Maxillofacial Surg Clin N Am 2019;31:163–91.
40. Annibali S, Cristalli MP, Dell'Aquila D, et al. Short dental implants: a systematic review. J Dent Res 2012;91(1):25–32.
41. Nisand D, Renouard F. Short implant in limited bone volume. Periodontol 2000 2014;66:72–96.
42. de Castro D, de Araujo M, Benfatti C, et al. Comparative histological and histomorphometrical evaluation of marginal bone resorption around external hexagon and Morse cone implants: an experimental study in dogs. Implant Dent 2014;23: 270–6.
43. Atieh MA, Ibrahim HM, Atieh AH. Platform switching for marginal bone preservation around dental implants: a systematic review and meta-analysis. J Periodontol 2010;10:1350–66.
44. Eazhill R, Swaminathan SV, Gunaseelan M, et al. Impact of implant diameter on stress distribution in osseointegrated implants: a 3D FEA study. J Int Soc Prev Community Dent 2016;6(6):590–6.
45. Anitua E, Tapia R, Luzuriaga F, et al. Influence of implant length, diameter, and geometry on stree distribution: a finite element analysis. Int J Periodontics Restorative Dent 2010;30(1):89–95.
46. Himmlova L, Dostalova T, Kacovsky A, et al. Influence of implant length and diameter on stress distribution: a finite element analysis. J Prosthet Dent 2004; 91:20–5.
47. Baggi L, Cappelloni I, Di Girolamo M, et al. The influence of implant diameter and length on stress distribution of osseointegrated implants related to crestal bone geometry: a three dimensional finite element analysis. J Prosthet Dent 2008; 100:422–31.
48. Lulic M, Bragger U, Lang NP, et al. Ante's (1926) law revisited: a systematic review on survival rates and complications of fixed dental prostheses (FDPs) on severely reduced periodontal tissue support. Clin Oral Implants Res 2007; 18(Suppl 3):63–72.
49. Misch CE, Suzuki JB, Misch-Dietsh FM, et al. A positive correlation between occlusal trauma and peri-implant bone loss: literature support. Implant Dent 2005;14(2):108–16.

50. Rangert B, Krogh PHJ, Langer B, et al. Bending overload and implant fracture: a retrospective clinical analysis. Int J Oral Maxillofac Implants 1995;10:326–34.
51. Nedir R, Bischof M, Briaux JM, et al. A 7-year life table analysis from a prospective study on ITI implants with special emphasis on the use of short implants. Results from a private practice. Clin Oral Implants Res 2004;15:150–7.
52. Schulte J, Flores AM, Weed M. Crown-to-implant ratios of single tooth implant-supported restorations. J Prosthet Dent 2007;98:1–5.
53. Meijer H, Boven C, Delli K, et al. Is there an effect of crown-to-implant ratio on implant treatment outcomes? A systematic review. Clin Oral Implants Res 2018; 29(Suppl. 18):243–52.
54. Fugazzotto P, Beagle J, Ganeles J, et al. Success and failure rates of 9 mm or shorter implants in the replacement of missing maxillary molars when restored with individual crowns: preliminary results 0 to 84 months in function. A retrospective study. J Periodontol 2004;75:327–32.
55. Thoma DS, Haas R, Tutak M, et al. Randomized controlled multicentre study comparing short dental implants (6 mm) versus longer dental implants (11–15 mm) in combination with sinus floor elevation procedures. Part 1: demographics and patient-reported outcomes at 1 year of loading. J Clin Periodontol 2015;42:72–80.
56. Hadzik J, Krawiec M, Kubasiewicz-Ross P, et al. Short implants and conventional implants in the residual maxillary alveolar ridge: a 36 month follow-up observation. Med Sci Monit 2018;24:5645–52.
57. Fan T, Li Y, Deng WW, et al. Short implants (5 to 8 mm) versus longer implants (>8 mm) with sinus lifting in atrophic posterior maxilla: a meta-analysis of RCTs. Clin Implant Dent Relat Res 2017;19(1):207–15.
58. Nielsen HB, Schou S, Isidor F, et al. Short implants (<8 mm) compared to standard length implants (>8 mm) in conjunction with maxillary sinus floor augmentation: a systematic review and meta-analysis. Int J Oral Maxillofac Surg 2019;48: 239–49.
59. Nisand D, Picard N, Rocchietta I. Short implants compared to implants in vertically augmented bone: a systematic review (EAO). Clin Oral Implants Res 2015;26(Suppl 11):170–9.
60. de Dias FJ, Pecorari VGA, Martins CB, et al. Short implants versus bone augmentation in combination with standard-length implants in posterior atrophic partially edentulous mandibles: systematic review and meta-analysis with the Bayesian approach. Int J Oral Maxillofac Surg 2019;48:90–6.
61. Pieri F, Forlivesi C, Caselli E, et al. Short implants (6 mm) vs. vertical bone augmentation and standard-length implants (>9 mm) in atrophic posterior mandibles: a 5-year retrospective study. Int J Oral Maxillofac Surg 2017;46:1607–14.
62. Felice P, Barausse C, Pistilli R, et al. Five-year results from a randomized controlled trial comparing prostheses supported by 5-mm long implants or by longer implants in augmented bone in posterior atrophic edentulous jaws. Int J Oral Implantol 2019;12(1):25–37.

Clinical Uses of Platelet-Rich Fibrin in Oral and Maxillofacial Surgery

Yijao Fan, DDS[a], Karla Perez, DDS[a], Harry Dym, DDS[b,*]

KEYWORDS

• Platelet-rich fibrin • Platelet-rich plasma • Blood collection

KEY POINTS

- Platelet-rich fibrin (PRF) is an autogenous material that is derived from a person's own platelets and is used to enhance wound healing and tissue regeneration.
- PRF has garnered significant interest in the dental community because of its proposed regenerative properties and its ability to aid in wound healing.
- PRF is proposed to have a direct effect on enhancing a patient's wound healing by supra-saturating the wound with growth factors that promote tissue healing.
- Clinically, PRF is easily produced chairside from the patient's own blood.
- Because the autologous nature of PRF makes it preferred over a variety of allografts used in dentistry today, PRF has significant potential in being applicable to all areas of dentistry, including oral and maxillofacial surgeries.
- PRF can be utilized in various surgical procedures performed by both dentists and oral surgeons in their private offices.

PLATELET-RICH PLASMA AND PLATELET-RICH FIBRIN

Platelet-rich fibrin (PRF) is actually a second-generation technology. It is anteceded by platelet-rich plasma (PRP), which is whole blood centrifuged to remove red blood cells, leaving behind a suspension rich in white blood cells and plasma components that are thought to be important in promoting wound healing. Both PRF and PRP use autologous blood. Both PRF and PRP aim to use blood growth factors to promote the body's own healing process. PRF builds on PRP by preserving the growth factors in a fibrin matrix and can exert its effects days or weeks after the surgery. As opposed to PRP, PRF is prepared without the use of anticoagulation factors, which are known

[a] Division of Oral and Maxillofacial Surgery, The Brooklyn Hospital Center, 121 DeKalb Avenue, Brooklyn, NY 11201, USA; [b] Department of Dentistry and Oral & Maxillofacial Surgery, The Brooklyn Hospital Center, Outpatient Care Building–1st Floor, 121 DeKalb Avenue, Brooklyn, NY 11201, USA
* Corresponding author.
E-mail address: hdym@tbh.org

Dent Clin N Am 64 (2020) 291–303
https://doi.org/10.1016/j.cden.2019.12.012

to inhibit wound healing. In comparison to PRP, PRF preparations tend to have higher leukocyte count because of centrifuge technique improvements, a fibrin matrix that promotes healing and allows growth factors to be slowly released over time, and comes in moldable forms that improve workability.

A BRIEF HISTORY OF PLATELET-RICH FIBRIN

As early as the 1950s, Kingsley[1] used the term PRP to describe a thrombocyte concentrate used for patients with thrombocytopenia. Hematologists started to widely use the term in the 1970s.[2]

The study of PRP took off in varying directions in the following decades with varying investigators proposing different protocols and different applications in medicine.[2–4] These early ways to prepare PRP were sometimes lengthy, and anticoagulants such as bovine thrombin or $CaCl_2$ were part of the preparation to prevent clotting and to keep the concentrate in a liquid form.[3]

In the 1970s, Matras[5] studied skin healing in rats. He proposed the use of what he called "fibrin glue" in various preparations to enhance healing in rats. The stickier fibrin glue had less anticoagulant effects, and he was unable to achieve consistent results. After that, there was a growing number of reports of platelet concentrates in "glue" or "gelatin" in general surgery, neurosurgery, and ophthalmology.[4]

Interest in use of platelet concentrates in oral and maxillofacial surgery was elevated when in 1998 Marx[6] showed that bone grafts grew more (74% vs 55% control) when infused with supraconcentrated platelet solution.

In 2000, Choukroun[4,7] finally coined the term PRF by using a form of platelet-rich concentrate that was firmer in consistency. This form of platelet concentration is widely accepted as the second-generation platelet concentration and is the focus of this article. In the 2 decades that followed, the original preparation was built upon to produce the PRF variants available today, including sticky bone (autologous fibrin glue mixed with bone graft) by Sohn, advanced PRF (A-PRF) by Choukroun, and injectable PRF (I-PRF) by Muorao.[3,4]

MECHANISM OF ACTION

When the body tries to repair itself, it will undergo 3 phases: inflammatory phase, proliferative phase, and the remodeling phase. The first, inflammatory phase, is an acute inflammation reaction to injury. Blood is the vector that brings these inflammatory cells to the site of the injury. In addition to phagocytes that clean the wound, white blood cells and platelets release important cellular mediators that begin the healing process. Important growth factors that are released include TGFB1, PDGF, VEGF, IGF1, which mediate cell migration, proliferation, and differentiation. Platelets also secrete coagulation factors that ensure initial hemostasis. After 24 to 48 hours, the proliferative phase takes over by virtue of the presence of the inflammatory mixture of cellular signals created during the inflammatory phase. There can now be proliferation of fibroblasts, leukocytes, macrophages, and mesenchymal stem cells, which begin to lay the first foundations of the new tissue. Depending on the extent of the defect along with the immune capabilities of the body, the site will transition to the remodeling phase of healing when there is stability in the first tissues laid.

PRF is formed by dividing autologous blood into components that promote the wound-healing process and components that do not. Components that promote wound healing are suspended in a fibrin matrix for preservation and slow release as the wound heals. The red blood cells ideally are spun out during the centrifuge process, and what are kept are the white blood cells, platelets, and fibrin. Per volume, these ingredients for wound healing are found at much higher than physiologic levels. Refinement of PRF preparation techniques aims to preserve as much of the white blood cells and platelets and exclude as much of the red blood cells as possible.

The fibrin matrix is the main advantage PRF has over PRP. It acts as a 3-dimensional scaffold for the leukocytes and platelets and their release products. The matrix allows for delayed release of its contents so that the beneficial wound-healing effects are present for a longer time period. The matrix is also thought to trap more leukocytes within its network, although this is hard to prove because the slow centrifuge preparations can also have this effect. The mass effect of the fibrin clot is also advantageous in that it can take up space where PRP cannot. Peripherally proliferating cells can use the scaffold to penetrate the wounded site, which is not possible with the pure liquid preparation of PRP. The scaffold nature of PRF is especially true because the fibrin clot is workable and can be adapted to many tissue defect forms.

TYPES OF PLATELET-RICH FIBRIN

Broadly speaking, there are 2 types of PRF: a solid and a liquid. The solid PRF is the initial form of PRF made by Choukroun and colleagues.[7,8] As previously discussed, it improves on PRP by preparing the platelet concentrate without anticoagulation, thus producing a solid medium capable of allowing for a slow release of growth factors. Choukroun[9] used a high centrifugal force (708*g*) in glass tubes to separate his blood products. This type of PRF had a dense fibrin structure. He would improve his technique in 2014 with Ghanaati[10] by using a reduced centrifugal force (208*g*) and plastic tubes that are less likely to activate a clotting cascade to produce with he called A-PRF. This dense nature of the clot is the main form of solid PRF used today. A-PRF has a higher concentration of retained leukocytes because of its slow centrifugation and a more porous fibrin matrix, allowing for greater release of its contents. The greater porosity also allows for more blood vessel penetration during angiogenesis. These solid forms of PRF are malleable and can be shaped into pellets or cut into smaller pieces for bone grafting or pressed flat and be used as a membrane. I-PRF builds on this slow centrifugal force concept by being prepared at 60*g* centrifugation force (at higher rpm but for less time) (**Fig. 1**). The result is a suspension without anticoagulation that can be manipulated like PRP but retains the ability to form a slow release matrix once applied to tissue.[3,4,11] This form of PRF can be injected into

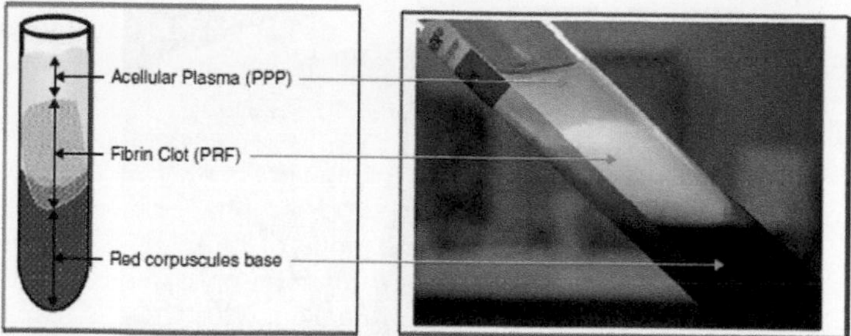

Fig. 1. Solid PRF after centrifugation. The bottom layer is predominantly red blood cells and is discarded. The solid middle layer is clotted solid PRF. The top layer is unclotted plasma. Both the middle and the top layers have useable growth factors. In I-PRF, the clotting is not allowed during centrifugation, resulting in a liquid top and middle layer that is indistinguishable. PPP, Platelet Poor Plasma.

deep tissue spaces, onto open wounds, and mixed with other graft materials, such as bone-grafting particles, to produce "sticky bone," which has a puttylike consistency.

PLATELET-RICH FIBRIN PREPARATION

Blood Collection

Venipuncture must be performed (**Fig. 2**). Blood needs to be collected in 10-cc cylinders. The ratio of recommended blood needed per volume of defect varies from protocol to protocol. Typically, 10 to 100 cc of blood is needed. Plastic containers activate clotting factors less compared with glass containers. Again, choice will depend on the protocol being followed.

Centrifuge

Transfer the blood to the centrifuge immediately (**Fig. 3**). Transport times greater than 60 seconds are associated with premature clotting before there is adequate separation of the blood constituents. Use the protocol for the intended purpose. Some common preparations of PRF are listed in **Table 1**.

After the centrifuge is finished, remove the supernatant or coagulated top layer from the spun-down red blood cells. Solid PRF can be pressed, cut, or shaped into the form of the defect (**Figs. 4–6**). I-PRF should be used immediately before clotting can occur.

APPLICATIONS OF PLATELET-RICH FIBRIN IN ORAL AND MAXILLOFACIAL SURGERY

Implantology

PRF has several applications in implantology. As I-PRF, it can be mixed with other grafts to bestow slow-releasing osteoinductive properties to the graft. As solid PRF, it can wholly substitute grafted bone entirely. As shaped solid PRF, it can act as membranes that are useful in guided bone regeneration, maxillary sinus membrane grafting, or aid in healing in connective tissue grafting.

Platelet-Rich Fibrin in Bone Grafting

Bone grafting has become a mainstay of many oral maxillofacial surgeons, especially with the increase in implant reconstruction (**Figs. 7** and **8**). Traditionally, grafts can either be autologous or nonautologous. Autogenous grafts are the gold standard but have the disadvantage of donor site morbidity. PRF is an autogenous source of growth factors that provide a noninvasive medium between the two. Marx and

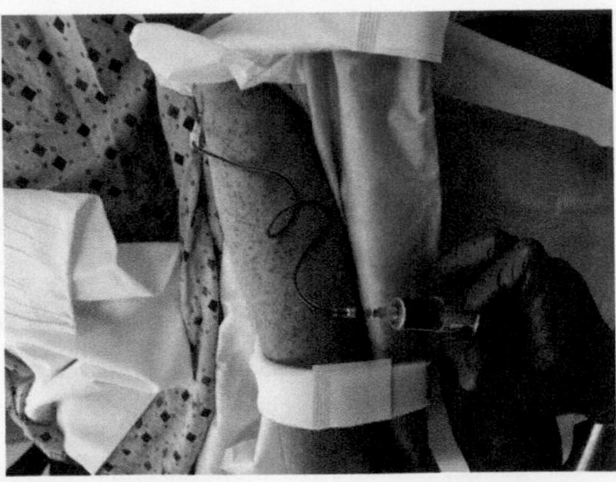

Fig. 2. Obtaining blood from the patient chairside after venipuncture.

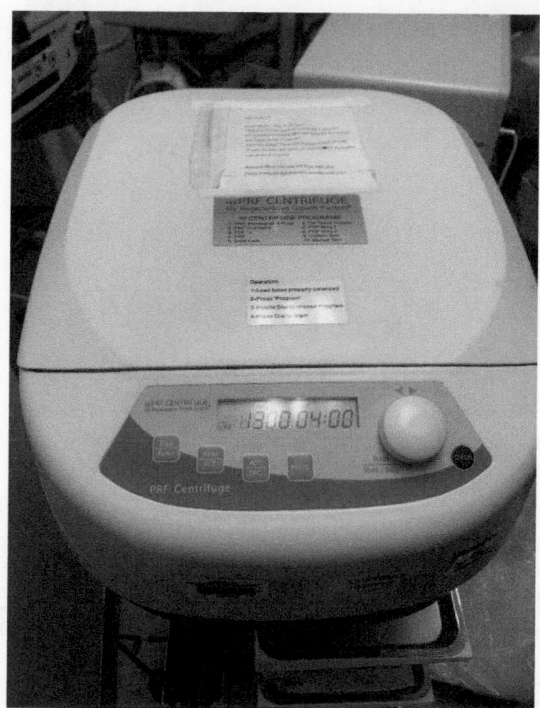

Fig. 3. PRF machine. This is essentially a centrifuge with preprogrammed spin cycles. There are slots for manufacturer-provided plastic or glass tubes for holding the blood obtained from the patient. Arrange them circumferentially in a balanced manner. This machine also provides weights one can place into intervening empty tubes for balance.

colleagues[12] in 1998 showed that PRP can be an osteoinductive force by retaining a high concentration of PDGF and TGFbeta, which act to promote mitogenesis of stem cells nearby and chemotaxis incoming inflammatory cells. These actions produce an almost 2-fold increase in bone density in their surgeries. PRF can also be mixed with a bone graft material. I-PRF in particular can be used exactly the same way as PRP but results in a higher concentrate of leukocytes and a prolonged beneficial effect. Much of the evidence since Marx has come from the periodontologists who are using PRF to grow bone in infrabony defects around dentition. Seventeen random clinical trials on this topic from 2011 to 2016 have shown clinically significant osseous growth using PRF in intrabony defects.[3] Sohn's sticky bone, a combination of I-PRF and particulate graft, allows the bone graft to be easily molded and handled. The sticky bone was also noted to retain much of its shape during the healing process. Sohn[13] showed that this

Table 1
Common preparations of platelet-rich fibrin

	rpm	Centrifuge Force, *g*	Time, min
L-PRF (2000)	2700	708	12
A-PRF	1500	208	14
I-PRF	3300	60	2

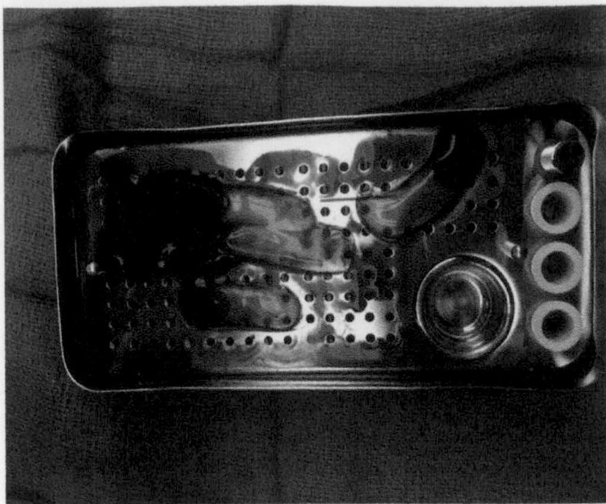

Fig. 4. The contents of the tube are removed after centrifugation. The PRF can be prepared and shaped at this stage depending on intended use.

technique can be successful in alveolar ridge and sinus augmentations. Fennis and colleagues[14] showed that PRF scaffolds can be used in reconstructing mandibular continuity defects in animal models. Garg[15] and Kim and colleagues[16] showed that PRF can successfully be used to bone graft around implants. PRF can also be used with or without a bone graft material because it is inherently already a scaffold for osteoblastic conduction. Del Corso and colleagues[17] showed that PRF was used in the liquid PRF (L-PRF) form during immediate implant placement of a maxillary central incisor with good healing and good esthetics. In ridge-preservation procedures, a PRF graft shaped as a plug to fit into an extraction socket showed minimal ridge width loss of 7.38% and ridge height loss of 7.13% versus 11.59% and 17.79%, respectively, in groups whereby only a bone graft with a collagen membrane was used.[18]

PRF alone or in conjunction with autogenous or allogenous bone can be used to reconstruct large bony defects after enucleation of cystic lesions of the jaws. The goal after removal of any large cystic lesion is to promote bone regeneration to fill the defect (**Fig. 9**). In a case report, Dhote and colleagues[19] reported the successful treatment of radicular cyst associated with primary second molar in a 10-year-old patient. The cyst was enucleated, tooth extracted, and remaining cavity was filled with

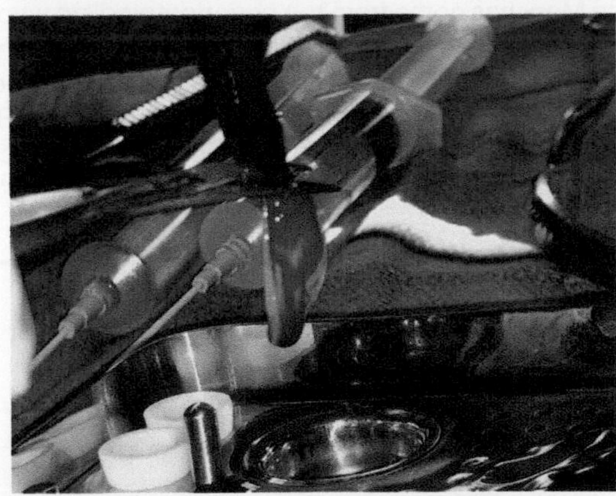

Fig. 5. The biologically inactive cellular portions are excised.

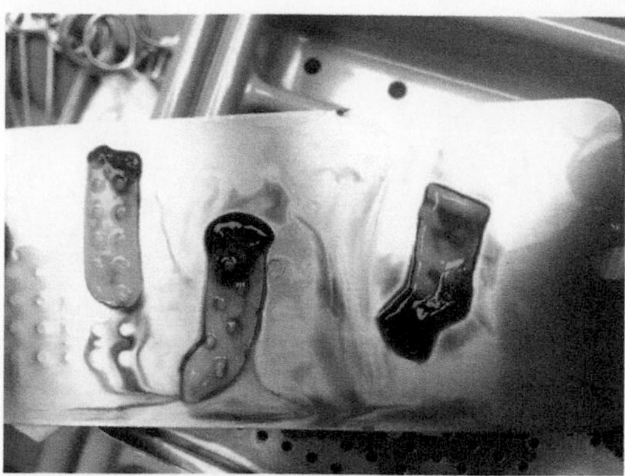

Fig. 6. The most versatile preparation of PRF is solid PRF pressed flat. The manufacturer-provided handling tray is designed to detach into 2 layers that can be used to press the PRF. The resultant thickened PRF material can be used as membranes or divided further and mixed with an array of graft materials.

only PRF. Two-year follow-up showed fill of bony defect as well as eruption of displaced second premolar.

Platelet-Rich Fibrin in Exodontia

Following exodontia, there is an inevitable resorption of bone at the extraction site. Although there are a plethora of allogenic, xenogeneic, and synthetic materials as well as surgical techniques involving autogenous bone available to reduce resorption, there are none that can prevent resorption.[3] PRF can improve wound healing and support ridge preservation by introducing angiogenic cytokines, positive inflammatory cytokines, and growth factors, which will stimulate healing in the extraction socket. Studies have shown that PRF improves the preservation of the alveolar ridge and

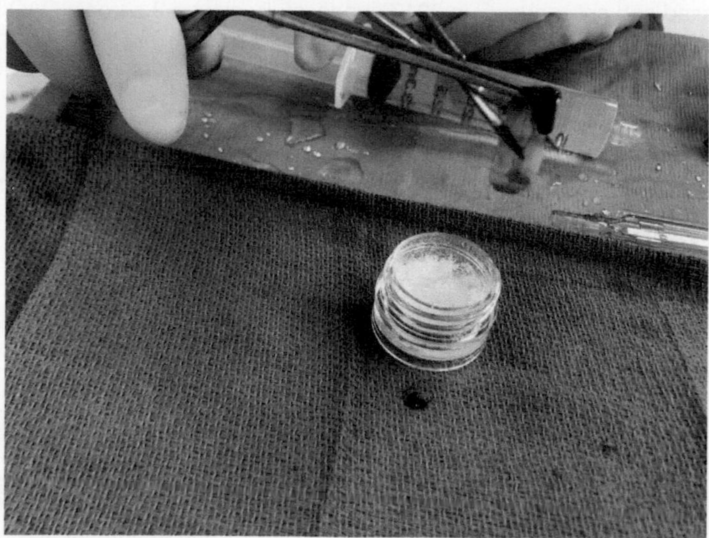

Fig. 7. L-PRF is being sectioned and can be mixed with particulate allograft.

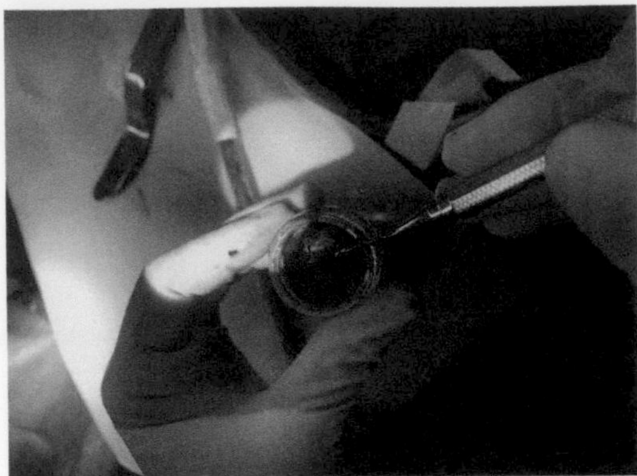

Fig. 8. I-PRF is often mixed with stock bone. The stock bone is bathed in an environment of slow releasing growth factors.

results in less bone resorption when compared with control groups with no filling material or graft without PRF.[20] Another study found no statistical difference but did note faster bone healing when compared with control.[21] PRF improves bone fill, vertical gain of oral cortical plate, and alveolar ridge contour when compared with control groups without PRF. In addition, implants that are placed in sockets filled with PRF are more stable and experience less resorption than implants placed in nontreated bone.[10]

PRF placed at third-molar extraction sites have been shown to reduce the incidence of alveolar osteitis and postoperative pain when compared with natural alveolar healing.[20]

Platelet-Rich Fibrin in Oroantral Communications Closure

Oral-Antral Communications (OAC) are often encountered with extraction of posterior maxillary teeth. Current techniques for closure include buccal fat pad advancement, buccal mucosal flap advancement, bone, palatal flaps, or any combination of these. PRF offers another alternative alone or in conjunction with these established techniques. Assad and colleagues[22] in 2017 successfully closed 2 chronic OAC because of extraction of the maxillary first molar. OAC was closed with 2 PRFs, 1 clot inside the socket and then an additional PRF membrane sutured to the gingiva. They reported successful closure of both OACs with an 8-week follow-up.

In a modification to the 3-layer closure of OAC described by Weinstock and colleagues[23] in 2014, PRF was added to obtain a 4-layer closure of a chronic OAC. Combination of bone, which was mortised into the defect, followed by coverage with buccal fat pad, PRF, and buccal mucosa, was used to successfully close a chronic OAC (**Fig. 10**).

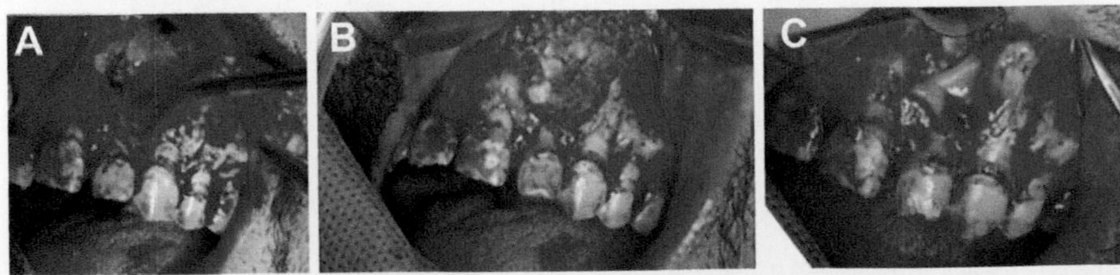

Fig. 9. Maxillary cyst status post enucleation (*A*), reconstruction by anterior iliac crest bone graft with interposed PRF fragments (*B*), and covered by a PRF membrane (*C*).

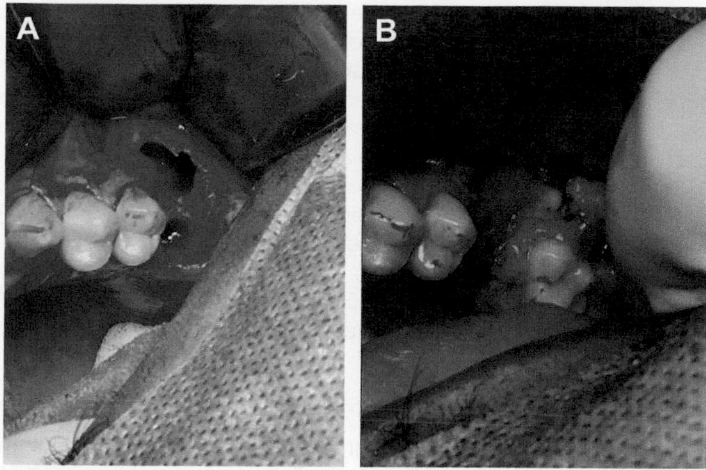

Fig. 10. Before (*A*) and after (*B*) an OAC was closed by bone, buccal fat, PRF, and mucosa.

Platelet-Rich Fibrin in Soft Tissue Grafting

When solid PRF is flattened, it can also be used as a membrane in bone-grafting applications (**Fig. 11**).[3] In guided bone regeneration, not only does the membrane act as a barrier against penetrating epithelial cells but also the membrane slowly releases growth factors that enhance the activities of the incoming osteoblasts. The caveat is that the porosity of the PRF membrane to optimize bone healing versus epithelial infiltration is not well understood and can vary depending on the protocol used. In addition, PRF's regenerative properties can also be used in combination with keratinized tissue or mesenchymal tissue grafting. Multiple sources have demonstrated that PRF used alone with a coronally positioned gingival flap can achieve connective tissue growth without the use of a donor site.[24–26] Possibilities for keratinized tissue regeneration around implants is the logical next step.

Platelet-Rich Fibrin in Sinus Augmentation

Sinus augmentation is a unique application of PRF in implantology where one can take advantage of PRF's promise in soft and hard tissue grafting. There have been many reports of PRF being used as the sole material or in conjunction with bone to augment the maxillary sinus floor for implants. Mazor[27] showed that PRF shaped into

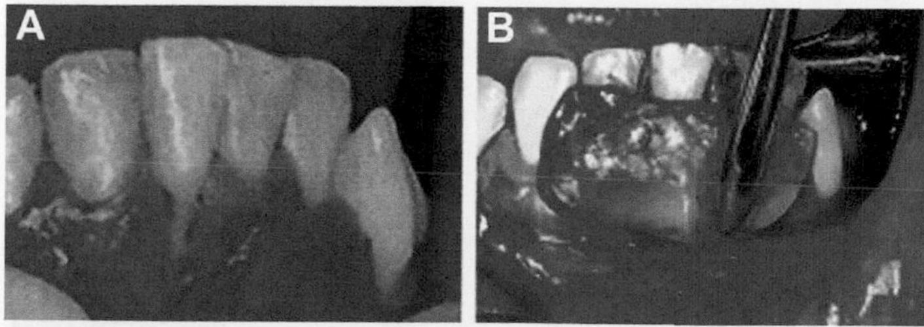

Fig. 11. (*A*) Localized vertical mucogingival defect labial to tooth no. 26 (lower right lateral incisor). (*B*) A flattened PRF membrane used to graft the defect instead of a palatal connective tissue harvest.

membranes, grafted to the sinus membrane by lateral window approach with implant placement, showed an average of 7-mm bone growth at 6 months.[27] Simonpieri and colleagues[28] repeated Mazur's positive results with a longer-term follow-up. They also grafted PRF into the sinus as the sole graft material with implant placement. They found that an average of 10 mm of bone was gained, and the bone level was always to the level of the apical extent of the implant. No implant was lost after 6 years of follow-up. Choukroun and colleagues[29] also experimented with mixing demineralized freeze-dried bone allograft with PRF fragments. They found that with their PRF protocol, the same amount of bone can be seen radiographically in 4 months versus 8 months. Finally, although controversial, some investigators advocate for using PRF for membrane perforations less than 5 mm during sinus lift surgeries.[3] Greater perforations than 5mm the same investigations advocate to about the procedure and re-attempt after 3 months.

Platelet-Rich Fibrin in Cleft Patient Reconstruction

PRF in conjunction with autogenous bone graft showed significantly higher mean percentage of newly formed bone in comparison with autogenous bone graft alone. The case control study by Shawky and Seifeldin[30] consisted of 24 patients with unilateral maxillary clefts. One group was grafted with PRF and autogenous Anterior Iliac Crest Bone Graft (AICBG), and the control group was grafted using only autogenous AICBG. The PRF group was noted to have a statistically significant increase in the percentage of newly formed bone.[30]

Platelet-Rich Fibrin in Osteonecrosis of the Jaw

Osteonecrosis of the jaw (ONJ) is most often found in patients who have had high doses of radiation to the head and neck or high doses of bisphosphonates resulting in exposed necrotic bone. Limited vascularization is commonly associated with ONJ, and the goal is often to attain reepithelization and vascularization of bone. PRF has angiogenic properties that can enhance new blood vessel formation and promote angiogenesis.[3] Studies have reported statistically significant improvement in

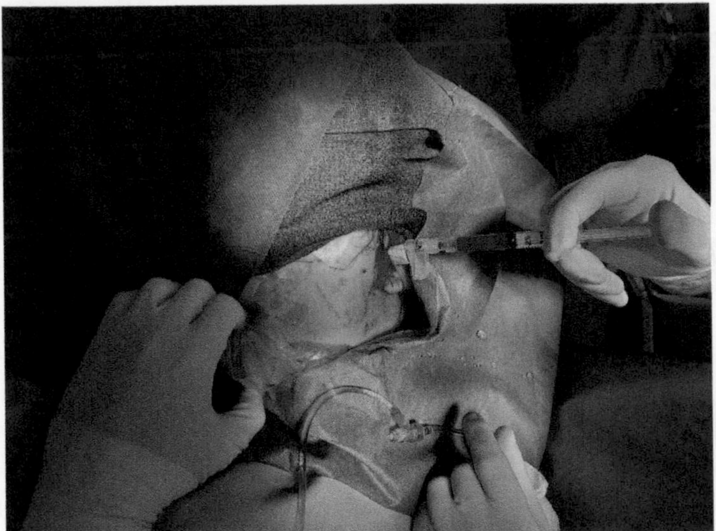

Fig. 12. I-PRF intracapsular TMJ injection.

wound healing in Medication Related Osteo Necrosis of the Jaws (MRONJ) with PRF when compared with the control group. Reepithelialization was observed faster in the PRF group than in the control group (2–4 weeks vs 2–8 weeks).[10]

Platelet-Rich Fibrin as Intracapsular Injection

L-PRF, developed by adjusting the relative centrifuge force and the centrifuge time, has a higher concentration of immune cells, platelets, and growth factors (**Fig. 12**). Albilia and colleagues[31] evaluated pain and dysfunction in patients with painful temporomandibular joint (TMJ) internal derangement undergoing liquid PRF injections. Thirty-seven patients with a total of 48 TMJ internal derangements were included in the study and were classified with Wilkes' classification I to V. A total of 2 cc of L-PRF was injected per TMJ into the superior joint space (1.5 cc) and retrodiscal tissue (0.5 cc). Thirty-three TMJs (69%) showed improvement to liquid PRF with statistically significant reduction in pain. Also, a decrease in dysfunction and an increase in Maximum incisal opening were noted. The best response to liquid PRF was patients with Wilkes' IV and V.[31]

SUMMARY

There is abundant literature and case studies discussing the benefits of PRF, and most studies favor the usage of PRF versus the control group. There is currently no standard PRF protocol, but there are many uses in dentistry and maxillofacial surgery all showing promising results. Standard protocols are needed to establish and more randomized controlled trials needed to confirm surgical indications.

DISCLOSURE

The authors have nothing to disclose.

REFERENCES

1. Kingsley CS. Blood coagulation; evidence of an antagonist to factor VI in platelet-rich human plasma. Nature 1954;173:723–4.
2. Alves R, Grimalt R. A review of platelet-rich plasma: history, biology, mechanism of action, and classification. Skin Appendage Disord 2018;4(1):18–24.
3. Miron R, Choukroun J, editors. Platelet rich fibrin in regenerative dentistry: biological background and clinical indications. Hoboken (NJ): John Wiley & Sons; 2017.
4. Agrawal AA. Evolution, current status and advances in application of platelet concentrate in periodontics and implantology. World J Clin Cases 2017;5(5):159–71.
5. Matras H. Effect of various fibrin preparations on reimplantations in the rat skin. Osterr Z Stomatol 1970;67:338–59.
6. Knighton DR, Ciresi KF, Fiegel VD, et al. Classification and treatment of chronic nonhealing wounds. Successful treatment with autologous platelet-derived wound healing factors (PDWHF). Ann Surg 1986;204(3):322–30.
7. Choukroun J, Adda F, Schoeffer C, et al. PRF: an opportunity in perioimplantology. Implantodontie 2000;42:55–62.
8. Kobayashi E, Fluckiger L, Fujioka-Kobayashi M, et al. Comparative release of growth factors from PRP, PRF, and advanced-PRF. Clin Oral Investig 2016;20:2353.
9. Choukroun J, Ghanaati S. Reduction of relative centrifugation force within injectable platelet-rich-fibrin (PRF) concentrates advances patients' own inflammatory cells, platelets and growth factors: the first introduction to the low speed centrifugation concept. Eur J Trauma Emerg Surg 2018;44(1):87–95.

10. Ghanaati S, Herrera-Vizcaino C, Al-Maawi S, et al. Fifteen years of platelet-rich fibrin in dentistry and oromaxillofacial surgery: how high is the level of scientific evidence? J Oral Implantol 2018;44(6):471–92.
11. Mourão CF, Valiense H, Melo ER, et al. Obtention of injectable platelets rich-fibrin (i-PRF) and its polymerization with bone graft: technical note. Rev Col Bras Cir 2015;42:421–3.
12. Marx RE, Carlson ER, Eichstaedt RM, et al. Platelet-rich plasma: growth factor enhancement for bone grafts. Oral Surg Oral Med Oral Pathol Oral Radiol Endod 1998;85:638–46.
13. Sohn DS. Lecture titled with sinus and ridge augmentation with CGF and AFG. In Symposium on CGF and AFG. Tokyo, June, 2010.
14. Fennis JP, Stoelinga PJ, Jansen JA. Mandibular reconstruction: a clinical and radiographic animal study on the use of autogenous scaffolds and platelet-rich plasma. Int J Oral Maxillofac Surg 2002;31:281–6.
15. Garg AK. The use of platelet-rich plasma to enhance the success of bone grafts around dental implants. Dent Implantol Update 2000;11:17–21.
16. Kim SG, Chung CH, Kim YK, et al. Use of particulate dentin-plaster of Paris combination with/without platelet-rich plasma in the treatment of bone defects around implants. Int J Oral Maxillofac Implants 2002;17:86–94.
17. Del Corso M, Mazor Z, Rutkowski JL, et al. The use of leukocyte- and platelet-rich fibrin during immediate postextractive implantation and loading for the esthetic replacement of a fractured maxillary central incisor. J Oral Implantol 2012;38:181–7.
18. Tanaskovic N. Use of platelet-rich fibrin in maxillofacial surgery. Contemp Mater 2016;7:1, 45-50.
19. Dhote V, Thosar N, Baliga S, et al. Surgical management of large radicular cyst associated with mandibular deciduous molar using platelet-rich fibrin augmentation: a rare case report. Contemp Clin Dent 2017;8(4):647.
20. Canellas J, Medeiros P, Figueredo C, et al. Platelet-rich fibrin in oral surgical procedures: a systematic review and meta-analysis. Int J Oral Maxillofac Surg 2019; 48(3):395–414.
21. Suttapreyasri S, Leepong N. Influence of platelet-rich fibrin on alveolar ridge preservation. J Craniofac Surg 2013;24(4):1088–94.
22. Assad M, Bitar W, Alhajj MN. Closure of oroantral communication using platelet-rich fibrin: a report of two cases. Ann Maxillofac Surg 2017;7(1):117–9.
23. Weinstock RJ, Nikoyan L, Dym H. Composite three-layer closure of oral antral communication with 10 months follow-up—a case study. J Oral Maxillofac Surg 2014;72(2):266.e1-7.
24. Aroca S, Keglevich T, Barbieri B, et al. Clinical evaluation of a modified coronally advanced flap alone or in combination with a platelet-rich fibrin membrane for the treatment of adjacent multiple gingival recessions: a 6-month study. J Periodontol 2009;80:244–52.
25. Jankovic S, Aleksic Z, Klokkevold P, et al. Use of platelet-rich fibrin membrane following treatment of gingival recession: a randomized clinical trial. Int J Periodontics Restorative Dent 2012;32:41–50.
26. Kumar G, Murthy K. A comparative evaluation of subepithelial connective tissue graft (SCTG) versus platelet concentrate graft (PCG) in the treatment of gingival recession using coronally advanced flap technique: a 12-month study. J Indian Soc Periodontol 2013;17:771–6.
27. Mazor Z, Horowitz RA, Del Corso M, et al. Sinus floor augmentation with simultaneous implant placement using Choukroun's platelet-rich fibrin as the sole

grafting material: a radiologic and histologic study at 6 months. J Periodontol 2009;80:2056–64.
28. Simonpieri A, Choukroun J, Del Corso M, et al. Simultaneous sinus-lift and implantation using microthreaded implants and leukocyte- and platelet-rich fibrin as sole grafting material: a six-year experience. Implant Dent 2011;20:2–12.
29. Choukroun J, Diss A, Simonpieri A, et al. Platelet-rich fibrin (PRF): a second-generation platelet concentrate. Part V: histologic evaluations of PRF effects on bone allograft maturation in sinus lift. Oral Surg Oral Med Oral Pathol Oral Radiol Endod 2006;101:299–303.
30. Shawky H, Seifeldin SA. Does platelet-rich fibrin enhance bone quality and quantity of alveolar cleft reconstruction? Cleft Palate Craniofac J 2016;53(5):597–606.
31. Albilia JB, Vizcaíno CH-, Weisleder H, et al. Liquid platelet-rich fibrin injections as a treatment adjunct for painful temporomandibular joints: preliminary results. Cranio 2018;1–13.

Peri-implantitis

Evaluation and Management

Hillel Ephros, DMD, MD, Shiwoo Kim, DMD*, Robert DeFalco, DDS

KEYWORDS

- Dental implants • Mucositis • Peri-implantitis

KEY POINTS

- Because of their prevalence and potential impact on outcome, peri-implant mucositis and peri-implantitis are important complications of implant placement.
- Clinicians placing and/or restoring implants must be familiar with the diagnostic features of these conditions and monitor their patients carefully.
- Management strategies should take into account local and systemic factors and should be as evidence-based as allowed by available data.

INTRODUCTION

As do our natural teeth, endosseous implants emerge from the bone through oral soft tissues into a cavity that harbors a vast array of microorganisms.[1] The mucosal barrier is heavily colonized and also subjected to repeated trauma from normal functions.[2,3] Placement of implants requires not only adequate bony anatomy, but a favorable soft tissue covering and a healthy oral environment. Maintenance is critical to the long-term success of implant-borne restorations just as it is to natural teeth and conventional prosthetic devices. Having a clear understanding of the techniques used for maintenance is essential to implant health as is patient selection.

Foundational to understanding, preventing, and managing diseases affecting implant attachment is a review of the ways that hard and soft tissues interface with implants and how those differ from teeth. Clinicians are quite famlilar with the concept of osseointegration, the direct structural and functional connection between host bone and the implant surface. This resembles ankylosis, as there is no intervening tissue between the bone and the integrated surfaces of an endosseous fixture. Many technical aspects of implant placement contribute to successful osseointegration, from site selection to surgical technique to the need for

Department of Oral and Maxillofacial Surgery, St. Joseph's University Medical Center, 703 Main Street, Paterson, NJ 07503, USA
* Corresponding author.
E-mail address: R_Kims@sjhmc.org

Dent Clin N Am 64 (2020) 305–313
https://doi.org/10.1016/j.cden.2019.11.002
0011-8532/20/Published by Elsevier Inc.

undisturbed healing. The long-term success of implant-borne restorations depends not only on osseointegration, but on the soft tissue interface that exists where the implant and associated hardware emerge into the oral cavity. Teeth and implants share the same basic structures at the mucosal barrier: a sulcus, junctional epithelium, and a connective interface. However, implants have a weaker implant connective interface as the orientation of collagen fibers is different than for teeth with Sharpey's fibers providing a tight seal between the bone and cementum. In addition, blood supply to peri-implant soft tissues may not be as robust as in the natural periodontium due to the absence of a periodontal ligament and surgical manipulation during implant placement. The integrity of the mucosal barrier is established by appropriate implant placement in an environment that is suitable, or in a site that has been developed for that purpose, allowing for well-designed prosthetic connections that support the soft tissue interface. Maintenance of this important barrier over time is a shared responsibility involving the patient as well as clinician-administered modalities.

Peri-implant complications may be limited to soft tissue inflammation or can lead to bone loss. Similar to gingivitis, peri-implant mucositis (**Fig. 1**) is the term applied to soft tissue inflammation alone. This inflammatory response is strictly limited to the soft tissue, with no evidence of progressive bone loss subsequent to the initial remodeling after implant placement, and is known to be reversible.[3–5] Peri-implantitis, such as periodontitis, involves hard tissue loss, most importantly, the supporting bone around the implant beyond biological bone remodeling (**Fig. 2**).[3,5] In retrograde peri-implantitis (RPI), a symptomatic periapical lesion is associated with a coronally osseointegrated fixture. RPI is thought to be caused by bacteria that are retained in the extraction socket and may remain in that site for up to a year after the tooth is removed. Some authors divide cases of RPI into 2 groups: (1) those that occur at the time of implant placement, including contaminated surgical sites, excessive heat or compression at the time of implant placement, large osteotomies, presence of a foreign body, and premature loading causing microfractures of the bone, and (2) those associated with preexisting diseases, including a pulpoperiapical pathological condition in the extraction site, retained root tips, underlying bone disease, periapical radiolucencies in adjacent teeth, and remnant cells from cysts or granulomas. Symptoms of pain and swelling can manifest as early as 1 week after implant placement and have been reported to occur as late as 4 years after the procedure. Because RPI is related to microorganisms similar to those found in chronic periodontitis, its treatment is the same as other forms of peri-implantitis, which include the removal of the biofilm and bacteria that are the source of the infection.[6]

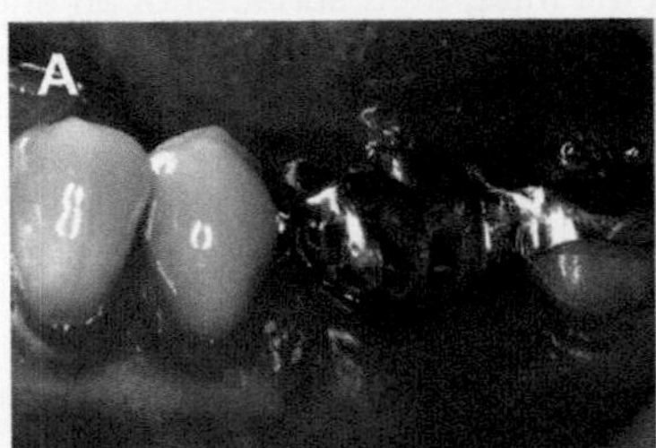

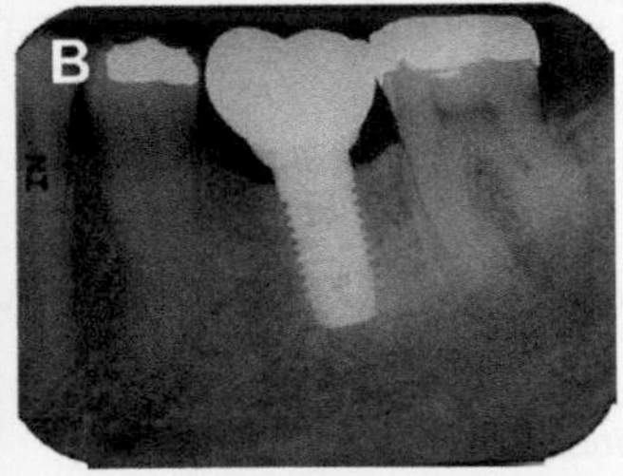

Fig. 1. (*A*) Example of soft tissue peri-implant mucositis. (*B*) Radigraphic view of peri-implant mucositis. (*From* Fu JH, Wang HL. Can periimplantitis be treated? Dent Clin North Am. 215;59(4):952; with permission.)

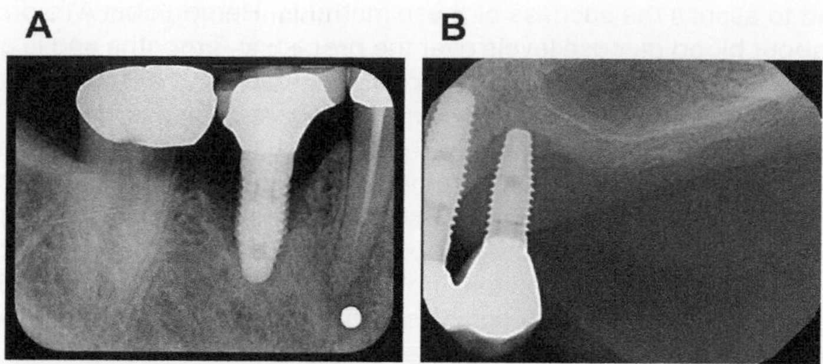

Fig. 2. (*A*) Example of peri-implantitis. (*B*) Example of severe peri-implantitis.

PREVALENCE

Data on the prevalence of peri-implant disease are inconsistent and vary greatly among published studies. Lee and colleagues[7] conducted a systematic review and meta-analysis published in 2017 that estimated the mean prevalence of implant-based and subject-based peri-implantitis. They found it to be 9.25% and 19.83%, respectively, and the estimated implant-based and subject-based peri-implant mucositis prevalence was 29.48% and 46.83%, respectively.[6] In an earlier meta-analysis published in 2013, Atieh and colleagues found the estimated prevalence of implant-based and subject-based peri-implantitis to be 9.6% and 18.8%, respectively. The estimated prevalence of implant-based and subject-based peri-implant mucositis in this review was 30.7% and 63.4%, respectively.[8] Although not perfectly aligned, the results of these 2 analyses demonstrate that the process of providing patients with implants does not end with successful integration and restoration. It seems that about half of our patients, perhaps more, will develop peri-implant mucosal inflammation and a smaller, but significant number will lose bone.

Prevalence data may be affected by many factors, including the duration of follow-up after implant placement—the longer the follow-up period the higher the prevalence of peri-implantitis and the number of fixtures placed per patient—higher numbers are associated with an increased risk of peri-implantitis.[8–11] Other associations with an increased risk of peri-implant disease are: poor oral hygiene, dental cement from the implant restoration, history of periodontal disease, certain systemic diseases, and cigarette smoking. Among these, a history of periodontal disease is most compelling, as that is often the reason for tooth loss and the need for implants. However, patients who have a history of periodontal disease may have a 5-fold increase of the risk of peri-implantitis.[12] All of factors listed above may contribute to individual risk for developing peri-implant disease and point to the need for careful patient selection, a strong emphasis on patient education and a commitment to professionally guided and monitored long-term maintenance. Critical risk factors are discussed later.

RISK FACTORS

The likelihood of developing peri-implantitis may be increased in patients with unfavorable medical and/or social histories. Before undertaking any surgical procedure, a thorough medical history and physical examination must be done. For diabetics, it is essential to explore the methods used to achieve control of blood glucose and to assess the success of these methods. Hemoglobin A1c provides information about blood glucose levels over the preceding 3 months and is a valuable tool in determining how well controlled a particular patient is over time. The established associations between diabetes and periodontal disease should increase concerns about peri-implant disease in this population because bacteria responsible for periodontal disease are the same as those found in peri-implantitis.[13,14] Patients with poor control of blood glucose have periods of sustained hyperglycemia, decreased white blood cell chemotaxis, a negative impact on wound healing, and a potentially adverse effect on the implant-bone attachment (**Fig. 3**). Similar effects may be anticipated at the implant-soft tissue interface. Smokers should be urged to discontinue the habit as studies have demonstrated greater marginal bone loss around the implants of smokers.[13] The negative effects of smoking are well documented and the oral cavity is not spared. Smoking impairs wound healing, including bone consolidation by reducing the inflammatory chemotactic response, migration, and bacteriocidal mechanisms. These and other smoking-related defects may contribute to peri- implantitis and eventual implant failure. Another concern is a history of periodontal disease before implant placement. Alterations in the normal oral flora associated with periodontal disease include an increase in the total bacterial load as well as selective increases in potentially pathogenic organisms that may then impact on the integrity of the peri-implant soft tissue interface and ultimately on the bony attachment. *Aggregatibacter actinomycetemcomitans* and *Porphyromonas gingivalis*, which are normally present in small quantities in healthy implant biofilms, may become the predominant pathogens responsible for peri-implant mucositis and progression to peri-implantitis. Other risk factors include inadequate attached gingiva, occlusal overload, residual cement from crown restoration, and poor hygiene. Compliance with supportive therapy in patients has been shown to significantly decrease the likelihood of progression to peri-implantitis.[15,16]

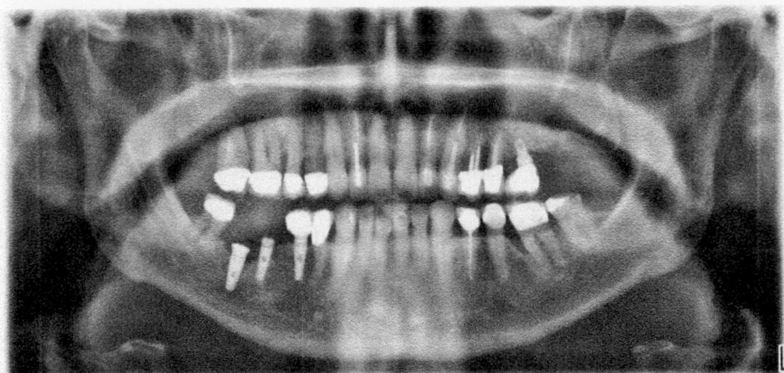

Fig. 3. Radiographic and clinical presentation of multiple failing implants in a patient with a history of diabetes.

DIAGNOSIS

Peri-implant mucositis is diagnosed by bleeding during probing, a clinical technique that demonstrates gingival soft tissue inflammation.[4] Peri-implantitis presents with bleeding as well, but in addition probing depths will reflect progressive bone loss indicating that the disease progress is irreversible (**Fig. 4**).[12] Various studies suggest a range of thresholds for peri-implantitis, but a consensus seems to exist around a probing depth of equal to or greater than 4 or 5 mm.[3] When probing, light pressure (about 0.25 N) has been advocated to accurately judge depth without causing damage to the peri-implant tissue.[17] Several authors emphasize the need to record baseline probing depths as soon as the prosthesis has been completed. They suggest that baselines be measured on all 6 surfaces of each implant to have an accurate reference point for monitoring. Bleeding that occurs on light probing is an indicator of loss of peri-implant attachments and supporting tissue.[18,19] Another key tool for diagnosis of peri-implant disease is radiographic imaging. Periapical radiographs should be taken to help evaluate the bone margins around the implant. A 2-mm vertical bone loss from the estimated baseline bone level is considered the threshold for diagnosis of peri-implantitis.[20] Galindo-Moreno and colleagues[21] found that a marginal bone loss of more than 0.44 mm per year is an indicator of progressive peri-implantitis. When used along with probing depths, radiographs contribute to the monitoring of bone levels and accurate documentation of potential progression of hard tissue loss.

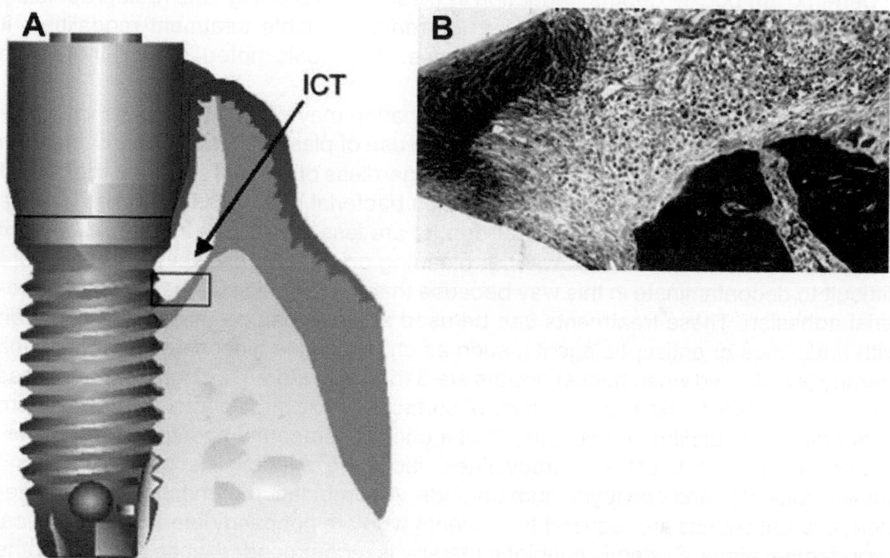

Fig. 4. (*A*) Illustration of a peri-implantitis lesion where there is inflammatory cell infiltrate (ICT) progression apically. (*B*) Histologic section of peri-implantitis with noted ICT and osteoclasts on the bone surface.

PREVENTION AND MANAGEMENT

The development of peri-implantitis has been studied in both animals and humans, and microorganisms have been shown to play a major role.[2,22] The available literature does not yet validate plaque removal for primary prevention of peri-implant disease as it does for primary prevention of gingivitis. Nonetheless, patients should be advised to maintain a strict hygiene program at home, particularly around implants, and any necessary instructions and hygiene aids should be provided. Reduction of inflammation has been demonstrated with the use of patient-administered plaque control modalities.[16] Consistent follow-up appointments with the dentist and/or hygienist should include clinical examination with recording of probing depths and radiographs when indicated. Professionally administered plaque removal modalities have also been shown to reduce inflammation, but resolution of bleeding on probing was not achieved. Adjunctive techniques, including antiseptics, local and systemic antibiotics and abrasive devices did not impact on reduction of inflammation.[2,12]

Questions raised about the efficacy of perioperative antibiotic administration have been addressed by many authors; however, only a small number of studies have been included in meta analyses and the evidence supporting even a single pre-incision dose is marginal. Nonetheless, there is a suggestion that a single dose of systemic antibiotic before implant placement may be associated with a slightly better outcome, although no impact on the likelihood of infection was noted.[23]

TREATMENT

For patients with disease that has progressed to peri-implantitis there are nonsurgical as well as surgical interventions available. The goals of treatment are clinical reduction of peri-implant pocket depths, reduction in bleeding on probing, and radiographically demonstrated bone consolidation. With currently available treatment modalities, it may only be possible to arrest the disease. The goals noted above should be tempered by reasonable expectations.

Nonsurgical methods of implant decontamination may be effective in the management of peri-implant mucositis and include the use of plastic, carbon fiber, or titanium hand instruments, ultrasonic tips, or lasers. Regardless of the tool selected, the goal of debridement is to effectively remove as much bacterial buildup as possible.[11] These treatments are indicated when pocket depths are less than 3 mm in the presence of plaque and/or calculus, with or without bleeding on probing. However, implants are difficult to decontaminate in this way because their roughened surfaces promote bacterial adhesion. These treatments can be used alone or can be used in combination with antibiotics or antiseptic agents, such as chlorhexidine gluconate.[24,25] Antiseptic therapy is indicated when pocket depths are 3 to 5 mm without radiographic bone loss around the implant. There are a variety of surface-detoxifying agents, all of which aim to decrease the biofilm on implants. These chemotherapeutic agents include supersaturated citric acid, EDTA, tetracyclines, including minocycline and doxycycline applied topically, and cetylpyridinum chloride. A combination of mechanical debridement and antiseptics are required for patients who are not candidates for mechanical debridement alone. Systemic antibiotic therapy is recommended when pocket depths are greater than 5 mm and there is bleeding on probing with radiographic bone loss. Multimodal approaches, including mechanical debridement, antiseptic therapy, and systemic antibiotic therapy may be necessary to reduce the colonization of bacteria and progression of bone loss in such cases.[17]

A combination of surgical, open debridement, and antimicrobial treatment has been advocated for treatment of peri-implantitis.[17,24] Surgical intervention is required once a patient has bleeding on probing, greater than 5 mm of probing depth, and severe bone loss beyond that expected with remodeling. Access flaps require full thickness elevation of the mucoperiosteum facilitating debridement and decontamination of the implant surface via hand instruments, ultrasonic tips, or lasers.[17,26,27] When necessary, surgical procedures may be used in conjunction with detoxification of the implant surface by mechanical devices, such as high-pressure air powder abrasion or laser. Resective procedures, such as implantoplasty, have been described and may be selected when there is horizontal bone loss. This approach involves smoothing the implant surface and the implant threads with a high-speed diamond or carbide burr to create a polished implant surface with the goal of limiting plaque retention.[17,27] One study suggested that implantoplasty may be associated with higher implant survival rate than was noted when comparably affected fixtures were treated with an apically positioned flap.[27]

Lasers have been used for decontamination of the implant surface by causing cellular necrosis via thermal damage. Lasers used include: Nd:YAG, Er:YAG, diode, and CO_2 lasers. Nd:YAG and Er:YAG have high bactericidal potential on implant surfaces, and of these the Er:YAG laser is known to be more effective at removing calculus.[17,25] Recent studies have reported that the ER:YAG laser can remove the bacterial-contaminated titanium oxide layer, promoting reosseointegration and healthy soft tissue adaptation around the compromised implant.[26] Lasers do have limitations and have not been shown to be more effective than other methods of decontamination. Lasers are potentially effective adjuncts to previously described treatments.

Procedures should be undertaken only if their potential outcome is retention of an implant that can be functional and maintainable. Implant removal must be considered along with procedures designed to prolong the life of implants with peri-implantitis. Depending on the status of the fixture and its attachment, as well as any relevant host factors, a case-specific risk/benefit analysis should be formulated and shared with the patient. Patients with implants that have increasing bone loss with mobility, those who are committed to smoking, or have a history of aggressive periodontal disease, and patients who have poor oral hygiene are not likely to have good salvage outcomes and should be treated more definitively. A balanced presentation outlining potential risks and benefits of the reasonable treatment options allows the patient to make an appropriate, informed decision. When implant retention is chosen, clinician experience and preference must play a role as data are lacking at this time for fully evidence-based procedure selection.

SUMMARY

With a very large number of endosseous dental implants placed by generalists and specialists, complications are to be expected. Among them are problems with the soft tissue interface and the hard tissue attachment. Peri-implant mucositis and peri-implantitis are not uncommon, but their prevalence and impact may be reduced with diagnosis and appropriate management as can the likelihood of progression from mucositis to peri-implantitis. Successful implant dentistry does not end with integration and restoration and both patient and professionally administered modalities are important for long-term implant maintenance.

DISCLOSURE

The authors have nothing to disclose.

REFERENCES

1. Wang WC, Lagoudis M, Yeh CW, et al. Management of peri-implantitis—a contemporary synopsis. Singapore Dent J 2017;38:8–16.
2. Klinge B, Hultin M, Berglundh T. Peri-implantitis. Dent Clin North Am 2005;49:661–76.
3. Belibasakis GN. Microbiological and immune-pathological aspects of peri-implant diseases. Arch Oral Biol 2014;59:66–72.
4. Rosen P, Clem D, Cochran D, et al. Peri-implant mucositis and peri-implantitis: a current understanding of their diagnoses and clinical implications. J Periodontol 2013;84(4):436–43.

5. Ramanauskaite A, Juodzbalys G, Tözüm TF. Apical/retrograde periimplantitis/implant periapical lesion: etiology, risk factors, and treatment options: a systematic review. Implant Dent 2016;25:684–97.
6. Soldatos N, Romanos GE, Michelle M, et al. Management of retrograde peri-implantitis using an air-abrasive device, Er,Cr:YSGG laser, and guided bone regeneration. Case Rep Dent 2018;2018:1–9.
7. Lee CT, Huang YW, Zhu L, et al. Prevalences of peri-implantitis and peri-implant mucositis: systematic review and meta-analysis. J Dent 2017;62:1–12.
8. Atieh MA, Alsabeeha NH, Faggion CM Jr, et al. The frequency of peri-implant diseases: a systematic review and meta-analysis. J Periodontol 2013;84:436–43.
9. Zitzmann NU, Berglundh T. Definition and prevalence of peri-implant diseases. J Clin Periodontol 2008;35:286–91.
10. Derks J, Tomasi C. Peri-implant health and disease. A systemic review of current epidemiology. J Clin Periodontol 2015;42:S158–71.
11. Renvert S, Polyzois I. Risk indicators for peri-implant mucositis: a systematic literature review. J Clin Periodontol 2015;42:S172–86.
12. Algraffee H, Borumandi F, Cascarini L. Review: peri-implantitis. Br J Oral Maxillofac Surg 2012;50:689–94.
13. Carlsson GE, Lindquist L, Jemt T. Long-term marginal periimplant bone loss in edentulous patients. Int J Prosthodont 2000;13:295–302.
14. Sorensen LT. Wound healing and infection in surgery (the clinical impact of smoking and smoking cessation: a systematic review and meta-analysis). Arch Srug 2012;147:373.
15. Jepsen S, Berglundh T, Genco R, et al. Primary prevention of peri-implantitis: managing peri-implant mucositis. J Clin Periodontol 2015;42:S152–7.
16. Albrektsson T, Isidor F. Consensus report: implant therapy. In: Lang NP, Karring T, editors. Proceedings of the 1st European workshop on periodontology. Berlin: Quintessence; 1994. p. 265–369.
17. Fu JH, Wang HL. Can periimplantitis be treated? Dent Clin North Am 2015;59: 951–80.
18. Heitz-mayfield LJ. Peri-implant diseases: diagnosis and risk indicators. J Clin Periodontol 2008;35:292–304.
19. Nogueira-Filho G, Iacopino AM, Tenenbaum HC. Prognosis in implant dentistry: a system for classifying the degree of peri-implant mucosal inflammation. J Can Dent Assoc 2011;77:535–40.
20. Sanz M, Chapple IL, Working Group 4 of the VIII European Workshop on Periodontology. Clinical research on peri-implant disease: consensus report of Working Group 4. J Clin Periodontol 2012;39:202–6.
21. Galindo-Moreno P, León-Cano A, Ortega-Oller I, et al. Marginal bone loss as success criterion in implant dentistry: beyond 2 mm. Clin Oral Implants Res 2015;26: 28–34.
22. Pontoriero R, Tonelli MP, Carneval G, et al. Experimentally induced peri-implant mucositis. A clinical study in humans. Clin Oral Implants Res 1994;5:254–9.
23. Balvei B. Patients who received preoperative antibiotics showed fewer early implant failures. J Am Dent Assoc 2014;145:1068–70.
24. Natto ZS, Aladmawy M, Levi PA Jr, et al. Comparison of the efficacy of different types of lasers for the treatment of peri-implantitis: a systematic review. Int J Oral Maxillofac Implants 2015;2:338–45.
25. Mailoa J, Lin GH, Chan HL, et al. Clinical outcomes of using lasers for peri-implantitis surface detoxification: a systematic review and meta-analysis. J Periodontol 2014;85:1194–202.

26. Nevin M, Nevins ML, Yamamoto A, et al. Use of Er:YAG laser to decontaminate infected dental implant surface in preparation for reestablishment of bone-to-implant contact. Int J Periodontics Restorative Dent 2014;24:461–6.
27. Romeo E, Ghisolfi M, Murgolo N, et al. Therapy of peri-implantitis with respective surgery. A 3-year clinical trial on rough screw-shaped oral implants. Part I: clinical outcomes. Clin Oral Implants Res 2005;16:9–18.

New Approaches to Pain Management

Orrett E. Ogle, DDS[a,b,*]

KEYWORDS

- Acute pain management • NSAIDs • Dental pain • Adjunctive pain management
- Postoperative pain

KEY POINTS

- Approaches to reduce the use of opioids for pain control in the dental patient.
- Transdermal, transmucosal and other agents that can be used in the safe management of dental pain.
- Pharmacology, dosages and principles of using NSAIDs to control dental pain.

Opioid addiction has reached epidemic proportions in the United States. It is thought that the problem started with the prescription for legal pain medications by health care professionals, particularly for treating patients who had undergone surgery. Since 2018, there has been an increased effort by the US Justice Department to identify and prosecute physicians involved in overprescribing opioids. Several states have passed legislation limiting opioid prescriptions. In New York State a practitioner may not initially prescribe more than a 7-day supply of an opioid medication for acute pain. There is also a mandatory online course on pain management for all licensed health care professionals in New York, with the emphasis on decreasing opioid prescription. The opioid addiction situation and new laws have led to a paradigm shift in the management of pain, particularly acute pain. This article presents strategies for pain management for dentists that will de-emphasize the reliance on opioids.

PAIN

The International Association for the Study of Pain defines pain as an unpleasant sensory and emotional experience associated with actual or potential tissue damage.[1] In reality, it is a complex neurologic condition that can be both psychologically and physically debilitating to the patient. Dental problems, from whatever cause, is commonly associated with pain that will have a significant effect on the oral health quality of life.

[a] Oral and Maxillofacial Surgery, Woodhull Hospital, Brooklyn, NY, USA; [b] Mona Dental Program, University of the West Indies, Kingston, Jamaica
* 4974 Golf Valley Court, Douglasville, GA 30135.
E-mail address: oeogle@aol.com

Dent Clin N Am 64 (2020) 315–324
https://doi.org/10.1016/j.cden.2019.12.001
0011-8532/20/ dental.theclinics.com

One study reported that dental pain is the most common type of orofacial pain.[2] Toothache appears high on many different listings of the most excruciating painful conditions experienced by humans. The fact that dental pain is intense and constant is believed to be the main reason why toothache is considered one of the worst pains a human has to endure.

MOLECULAR BASES OF DENTAL PAIN

Dental pain is associated with inflammatory reactions that involve different molecular mechanisms. Peripheral pain mechanisms associated with odontogenic painful conditions are similar to the mechanisms observed in all other body parts. These similarities include the type of sensory neurons involved as well as the different molecules that play a role in these processes.[3] The pain signal is transmitted via thin fibers of unmyelinated C fibers and myelinated A fibers of primary sensory neurons to secondary order neurons in the spinal cord and finally to the S1 and S2 areas of the cortex via a relay in the thalamus.[4] The A fibers transmit pain directly to the thalamus, generating a fast, sharp pain that can be easily localized. The C fibers reach the thalamus slower and result in a slow pain that is generally characterized as dull and aching.

Evidence shows that neuropeptides are considerably involved in the molecular mechanisms underlying dental pain.[5] One such neuropeptide that plays a significant role in dental pain and inflammation is substance P (SP), which is found in large concentrations in the fibers that innervate the dental pulp and dentin.[5] SP is released from C fiber nerve terminals and is involved both in inflammation and in pain. Nearly all pathologic conditions that affect oral tissues increase the production and release of SP and it plays a major role in the development and maintenance of dental pain and inflammation. In fact, extracellular levels of SP are increased in symptomatic pulp tissue diagnosed as irreversible pulpitis. The 2 key components of pulpal inflammation are microcirculation and the activation of nerve fibers. The excitation of the A∂ fibers seems to have an insignificant effect on the pulp blood flow, whereas the activation of the C fibers enhances the blood flow and causes pain by the action of neurokinins, especially SP.[6] The dental pulp is encased within a hard firm structure and cannot expand, therefore the inflammation increases the intrapulpal pressure significantly, lowering the pain threshold of nerve endings in the pulp.

Although SP plays a major role in pulpal pain it is not the only inflammatory mediator involved in the pain mechanism. Tissue injury results in the release of inflammatory mediators from damaged cells, including ions (K^+, H^+), bradykinin, histamine, 5-hydroxytryptamine, adenosine triphosphate, and nitric oxide. Activation of the arachidonic acid pathway leads to the production of prostanoids and leukotrienes.[7] Prostaglandins are important mediators of inflammation, fever, and pain. In some situations prostaglandins contribute to pain by directly activating nociceptors, but they are generally considered to be sensitizing agents. Prostaglandins increase levels of cyclic adenosine monophosphate and may enhance nociceptor sensitization by reducing the activation threshold for tetrodotoxin resistance sodium channels via a protein kinase A pathway. They sensitize primary afferent neurons to bradykinin and other mediators and are likely to be involved at multiple sites along the nociceptive pathway.[7]

The anxiety of having to see the dentist and the fear of dentistry can activate the pituitary-adrenal axis, leading to an increased experience of pain.

CAUSES OF DENTAL PAIN

The dental pulp, when stimulated, has only one response, which is pain. The sensory nerve fibers within the dental pulp are afferent endings of the trigeminal nerve. These nerve fibers transmit only pain. The fibers are divided into 2 categories—A∂ (myelinated) and C (unmyelinated)—based on their diameter, conduction velocity, and function. The myelinated A∂ fibers have a fast conduction speed and low stimulation threshold, are located at the dentinopulpal junction, transmit pain directly to the thalamus, and generate a sharp and stabbing pain that is easily localized. They are the first nerve fibers to transmit the pain impulse from the tooth. C fibers are unmyelinated and have a smaller diameter, slower conduction velocity, a higher threshold, and are located within the core of the pulp.

Tooth pain is caused by exposed dentinal tubules following bacterial (caries), chemical, or mechanical erosion of enamel and/or gingival recession. External stimuli causes dentinal fluid movements that transfers the stimulation to the underlying dental pulp via odontoblasts through their apical extension into the dentinal fluid running in the tubules; or via a dense network of trigeminal sensory axons intimately related to the odontoblasts.[8] Bacterial, chemical, or mechanical stimuli can cause inflammation within the pulp. A variety of endogenous chemical mediators have been associated with inflammation and pain; these include histamine, bradykinin, 5-hydroxytryptamine, prostaglandins,[8] and neuropeptides.[5] These chemical mediators will cause irreversible pulpitis, pulp necrosis, and possibly periapical inflammation/infection.

Chronic periodontitis is also associated with orofacial pain. The inflammation associated with periodontitis is related to a lowered pain threshold. Periodontal pockets are a source of subgingival biofilm and function as a reservoir of periopathogenic gram-negative bacteria. The biofilm is the source of proinflammatory mediators that can lead to dull, throbbing, and persistent pain.

Like periodontal disease, pericoronitis will also present with local inflammation associated with food impaction and persistent pain.

TREATMENT OF DENTAL PAIN

The treatment of dental pain will always require a dental or oral surgical procedure, and pharmaceutical intervention will be an adjunct. Even the strongest pain medication will not produce optimal and continuous pain relief to the patient if the underlying cause of pain is not removed. The underlying cause of dental pain is the inflammatory response, which activates the pain-producing mediators (**Table 1**). If the patient comes to the dentist with pain, there will be existing inflammation and the cause has to be removed or controlled. Generally, procedures on hard tooth structures that do not involve the pulp create little or no inflammatory response, but, when soft tissues are traumatized, a pain response can be expected[9]

Apart from myofascial pain, the vast majority of dental pain will be acute pain; therefore, the management of pain in the average dental patient is not likely to be affected by central neurophysiological plasticity as it would be in the chronic pain situation. Although dental pain is usually acute pain, it is important, however, for the dentist to screen the patient for chronic pain elsewhere in the body, for example, arthritis, back pain, migraine. The patient with chronic pain problems may not respond to the treatment of dental pain as would the pain-free patient and may require adjustments to routine analgesics.

PHARMACOLOGIC TREATMENT

A 2011 systematic review of treatment of acute pain in adults with moderate to severe pain after oral surgery in which single-dose therapy of a single drug has been published.[10] Several drug/dose combinations were found to reduce the postsurgical pain by over 50% (pain of 8 on the visual analog scale going to 4). Drugs and doses

Table 1
Causes of dental pain and suggested treatment

Pathologic Condition	Treatment
Irreversible pulpitis	Endodontic treatment or exodontia, analgesics
Periapical infection	Endodontic treatment or exodontia, analgesics
Infection involving fascial spaces	Remove the source of infection, incision and drainage if fluctuance is present, Antibiotics and analgesics
Periodontitis	Root planning and scaling, adjunctive periodontal treatment, analgesics
Dental trauma	Tooth repositioning/reimplantation, endodontics, restoration of fractured tooth, analgesics
Facial trauma	Close soft tissue wounds, reduction and fixation of facial bone fractures, analgesics, antibiotics for compound fractures
Temporo-mandibular joint/ myofascial pain	Diagnosis, analgesics, anti-inflammatory agents, muscle relaxants, dental splint, physical therapy
Acute necrotizing ulcerative gingivitis	Superficial debridement, antibiotics (metronidazole), chlorhexidine mouthwashes, nutritional support
Dry socket	Local anesthesia, irrigation, dry socket dressing, analgesics

were: ibuprofen 400 mg, diclofenac 50 mg, etoricoxib 120 mg, acetaminophen 1000 mg plus codeine 60 mg, celecoxib 400 mg, and naproxen 500/550 mg. The longest duration of action (≥8 hours) was found to occur with etoricoxib 120 mg, diflunisal 500 mg, acetaminophen (paracetamol) 650 mg plus oxycodone 10 mg, naproxen 500/550 mg, and celecoxib 400 mg.[10] It should be noted that all the effective drugs were NSAIDs (**Table 2**).

Opioids should never be the first drug of choice for dental pain. In fact, NSAIDs are more effective for musculoskeletal pain than are conventional doses of opioids (dental pain is considered as musculoskeletal pain).[11] The Centers for Disease Control and Prevention issued an advisory to dentists and physicians against prescribing opioid-based pain killers to women of childbearing age. The advisory stated that, because half of all pregnancies are unplanned, women may be prescribed opioid-based pain medications before they or their health care providers know they are pregnant. The use of opioids may increase the risk for serious birth defects of the baby's brain, spine, and heart, as well as preterm birth when taken during pregnancy.[12]

Nearly all dental pain has an inflammatory component. For this reason, NSAIDs are the most rational first-line agents. Studies have repeatedly found that NSAIDs are generally superior to opioids at conventional dosages.[13,14] NSAIDs reduce the

Table 2
Nonsteroidal anti-inflammatory drugs and acetaminophen most commonly used for pain by dentists

NSAID Analgesic	Dosage
Ibuoprofen (Motrin)	400–800 mg tid/qid
Naproxen sodium (Anaprox)	550 mg bid
Diclofenac potassium (Cataflam)	50–100 mg loading dose, then 50 mg tid
Diflunisal (Dolobid)	1000 mg loading dose, then 500 mg q8–q12 h
Acetaminophen (Tylenol)	500–1000 mg q8 or q6 h

synthesis of prostaglandins, which is implicated in pain, fever, and inflammation. All NSAIDs have similar analgesic effects and none is more effective than the other. The choice is up to the practitioner. Ibuprofen and naproxen (Naprosyn) are good, first-line NSAIDs for mild to moderate acute pain based on effectiveness, adverse effect profile, cost, and over-the-counter availability.[15] The safest NSAID is ibuprofen in doses of 400 mg. Although NSAIDs all have a similar mechanism of action, some individuals may not respond to 1 NSAID but may respond to another. The reason for this is unclear. If one particular NSAID is not effective, the dentist should, therefore, not assume that NSAIDs will not alleviate the pain, but should try a different one.

Because NSAIDs block or reduce the synthesis of prostaglandins it is more beneficial to have the patient take the NSAID doses at regular "clock-based" time intervals rather than on an as-needed basis. NSAIDs have an analgesic ceiling above which no additional analgesia is obtained. Their analgesic dose is lower than their anti-inflammatory dose, but it is not unreasonable to prescribe the higher doses for most cases of dental pain to derive benefit from their anti-inflammatory property and it may even offer somewhat greater analgesia despite the ceiling effect.

NSAIDs are contraindicated for patients who have a current history of nephropathy, erosive or ulcerative conditions of the gastrointestinal (GI) mucosa, anticoagulant therapy, hemorrhagic disorders, or intolerance or allergy to any NSAID. They also should be avoided during pregnancy because prostaglandins maintain patency of the ductus arteriosus during fetal development. Although this concern is most relevant during the third trimester, NSAIDs generally should be avoided throughout pregnancy.[16] Acetaminophen can be prescribed any time during pregnancy.

In all cases where NSAIDs are contraindicated, acetaminophen is the usual nonopioid alternative. NSAIDs give better pain relief than acetaminophen, which does not suppress inflammation and suppress pain by blocking synthesis of prostaglandins in the central nervous system.[17] As an analgesic, acetaminophen is equal in potency and efficacy to aspirin and it is thought to be somewhat inferior to ibuprofen and other NSAIDs.[16] Hepatotoxicity is the most significant adverse effect of acetaminophen.

ADJUNCTS

Transmucosal Analgesic

The administration of a drug by a transmucosal route offers the advantage of being a relatively painless administration and has the potential to maintain a steady drug concentration for a long period of time. The oral transmucosal delivery, especially the buccal and sublingual routes, have been used successfully for many drugs. The transmucosal membranes are relatively permeable, have a rich blood flow, and hence allow the rapid uptake of a drug into systemic circulation to avoid first-pass metabolism.[18] A pain-management approach that has demonstrated efficacy in reducing pain following dental extraction is the use of a buccoadhesive film in combination with an oral NSAID. Ketorolac tromethamine (KT), a NSAID, is incorporated into an adhesive film that is applied to the oral mucosa. The concentration of KT in the oral cavity will be maintained at therapeutic levels for at least 6 hours.[19] The buccal KT film is well tolerated by patients and no complaints of GI side effects have been reported. In clinical studies, it was shown that an adhesive film containing 30 mg of KT was effective in controlling postsurgical pain with no observable gastrointestinal effects.[19,20]

Benzydamine Rinse

Benzydamine a locally acting NSAID with local anesthetic and analgesic properties. It can be used as a topical rinse after third molar surgery. By itself, however, it will not be adequate for pain relief following mandibular third molar surgery and must be used in combination with an oral NSAID. The combination of benzydamine and an oral NSAID will improve the pain relief since the benzydamine is working locally and the oral NSAID is working systemically.

Combination Therapy

Combinations of analgesic drugs can produce better pain relief in cases in which a single drug has not been very effective. The purpose of combining 2 or more drugs with different mechanisms of action is to achieve a synergistic interaction.[21] Acetaminophen is a familiar drug that can serve as an efficient complement to the NSAIDs. Combining these individual agents that have different mechanisms or location of action can produce excellent control of mild to moderate pain in the outpatient setting. Acetaminophen works in the central nervous system, whereas the site of action for the NSAID is peripheral, where the inflammation is present. Effective pain relief is achieved by attacking the pain at 2 different sites—centrally and peripherally. In the clinical scenario, the patient could be started on the NSAID at a fixed time interval (eg, every 4 hours) and acetaminophen added if there is pain before the next dose of NSAID is scheduled or if the NSAID is not adequately effective.

ORAL SURGICAL CONSIDERATIONS

Oral surgical procedures will always produce postoperative pain whether it is performed on an outpatient or inpatient basis. Because it is known that the patient will experience postoperative pain, the oral and maxillofacial surgeon should develop a plan before surgery as to how intraoperative and postoperative pain will be addressed. Perioperative pain management refers to actions before, during, and after a surgical procedure that are intended to reduce or eliminate postoperative pain before the patient is discharged after the procedure.[22] The best approach for perioperative pain control would be preemptive analgesia and a multimodal therapy to eliminate the need for opioids. Multimodal analgesia uses several agents, each acting at different sites of the pain pathway. This approach reduces the dependence on a single medication and mechanism.[22]

Preemptive Analgesia

This refers to analgesia that is administered preoperatively in an attempt to reduce subsequent pain or analgesic requirements. Preemptive analgesia with oral analgesics may be beneficial in ambulatory cases. Blocking prostaglandins at different times during the surgical procedure may reduce surgical inflammation and postoperative pain. Ketorolac (Toradol), a potent nonsteroidal anti-inflammatory drug indicated for treatment of moderate to severe pain in adults, has been suggested as an NSAID for preemptive analgesia. The benefits of preemptive analgesia, however, is controversial. A meta-analysis of 20 trials studying various odontological, abdominal, and orthopedic procedures using NSAIDs for preemptive analgesia showed improvements in postoperative pain in 4 of the 20 trials, but no improvements were demonstrated in the remaining 16 trials. This meta-analysis concluded that there is no analgesic benefit for preemptive compared with postincisional administration of NSAIDs.[23]

In general anesthesia cases, infiltration or nerve block with local anesthetics is effective as preemptive analgesia. To relieve postoperative pain, surgeons will frequently inject local anesthetic preemptively at the incision site.

Intraoperative Analgesia

Whether the surgery is performed solely with local anesthesia, intravenous (IV) sedation, or general anesthesia, better pain control is achieved if local anesthesia is used. Local anesthesia includes infiltration and nerve blocks. With IV sedation, profound local anesthesia will decrease the amount of drugs necessary to sedate the patient and increase the level of safety. Injection of local anesthesia at the surgical site a few minutes before the incision and at the end of the procedure will produce a significant reduction in postoperative pain.

Other intraoperative factors that contribute to postoperative swelling and pain, including length of incision, tissue manipulation, cutting of bone and length of surgery. Postoperative swelling, and pain, are significantly lower following a smaller incision,[24,25] because of less tissue manipulation and shorter surgical time. Corticosteroids are the most effective method for dealing with pain because of these factors; they can directly reduce pain, as well as having other beneficial symptomatic effects outside of pain relief. Glucocorticoids reduce pain by inhibiting prostaglandin synthesis.[26] Dexamethasone in doses of 4 to 8 mg IV or intraorally is the most commonly used corticosteroid for pain in oral and maxillofacial surgery. It can be injected at third molar sites or given IV for trauma or orthognathic surgery.

Postoperative Analgesia

The major factor with regard to managing postoperative pain is to start the use of analgesics before the effects of the local anesthetic has worn off. Transdermal patches are an effective way to control postoperative pain. They offer the following benefits. (1) Direct-to-bloodstream delivery while bypassing the liver's metabolic activity. A patient's body heat activates a patch, prompting it to begin releasing medication through the skin and into the bloodstream. (2) The medication is supplied gradually and constantly achieving steadier blood levels, rather than in a large, single dose. (3) It bypasses the acidic environment found in the GI tract. (4) It is easy to apply and will not irritate the stomach. Ketorolac and diclofenac are available for postoperative pain. Transdermal systems for delivery of NSAIDs can replace oral and other traditional forms of drug administration. The drug contained in the transdermal patch enters the body through the skin and ultimately diffuses into capillaries for systemic delivery. The steady permeation of the drug across the skin allows for more consistent serum drug levels[27] and decreasing of the analgesic gaps, which is often a goal of therapy. Both diclofenac and ketorolac patches are applied twice a day, once every 12 hours, and will have therapeutically effective levels for a period of 12 hours or more. The patches should be used in conjunction with oral NSAIDs or acetaminophen.

NEW APPROACHES TO THE MANAGEMENT OF PAIN

Recent approaches to the management of acute perioperative pain focus on ways to improve the risk/benefit profile of various analgesics, enhance the consistency of pain control, address interpatient differences in responses to pain and treatments, and avoid periods of ineffective pain relief—the so-called analgesic gaps.[28] The timing of analgesic interventions is important in controlling pain. Pain medication should be taken as soon as there is awareness of pain. It is easier to treat pain of 5/10 on the pain scale than to treat it at 8/10, and the reduction of pain will be better with early intervention. It takes a lot more drugs to control pain after it has started as opposed to treating it in its incipient stages. If the patient is in between the time schedule for redosing a rescue medication should be available. Maximizing pain control with preemptive analgesia and multimodal therapy, and the availability of transdermal NSAIDs, has expanded the armamentarium of effective options for perioperative pain control.

NONPHARMACOLOGIC TREATMENT

This section focuses on nonpharmacological methods for treating acute pain.

Treating pain with heat and cold can be effective. After oral surgery, ice can be used for the acute pain and inflammation. The cold will reduce blood flow to the surgical site, which will tend to reduce the inflammation that causes pain. It may also temporarily reduce nerve activity, which can also relieve pain.

Salt water rinses can help reduce inflammation by reverse osmosis. Edema fluid comes out of the cells because the salt concentration in the saline solution is of a higher concentration than that in the cells.

Clove has been used to treat toothaches throughout history, because clove oil can effectively numb pain and reduce inflammation. It contains eugenol in concentrations of 80% to 90% in the clove bud. Clove applied to the gums at the extraction site can help to relieve the pain following a tooth extraction. To use this approach, place a small amount of clove oil onto a cotton swab and apply it to the affected area. It takes about 10 minutes for pain relief to be noticeable. If clove oil is not available, then blend 1 teaspoon of whole cloves with 1 tablespoon of olive oil. Clove gel is as effective as the topical ester anesthetic benzocaine gel.[29] Eugenol-containing compounds need to be used in small amounts because they can cause local irritation, some cytotoxic effects, and hypersensitivity reactions.

Black tea bags can be used to treat dry socket (localized osteitis) pain. Black tea contains tannic acid, which can reduce both swelling and pain. Immerse the tea bag in a cup of boiling water for about 5 minutes, and then allow it to cool. Gently bite down on the tea bag and keep it in place for about 15 minutes. This does not have a pleasant taste and may cause nausea.

SUMMARY

The United States faces a very serious problem with the current crisis of opioid misuse, addiction, and overdosing. Medical prescriptions for opioids are thought to be the genesis of the crisis. There are now trends through law enforcement and international agreements to attempt to remove nonmedical street opioids from society. There is also a push by training and State legislations to decrease the number of opioid prescriptions written by doctors. This general effort to reduce opioid usage in pain management has produced a new paradigm in how to manage postsurgical pain.

The understanding of the molecular bases of acute pain is vital to be able to appreciate the current concepts of pain management and what will come in the future as the reliance on opioids decrease. NSAIDs now play a greater role in pain control, but because the NSAIDs that are widely used are mainly for mild to moderate pain, a multimodal analgesia approach becomes necessary. Multimodal analgesia is the administration of 2 or more drugs that act by different mechanisms to provide analgesia. These drugs may be administered via the same route or by different routes. In this article, NSAIDs were widely discussed along with adjunctive agents for pain control. Synergistic drug usage, NSAID rinses, and transdermal patches for postoperative pain have expanded the methods that the dentist can use to manage pain without relying on opioids.

DISCLOSURE

The author has nothing to disclose.

REFERENCE

1. IASP terminology. 2017. Available at: https://www.iasp-pain.org/Education/Content.aspx?ItemNumber=1698#backtotop. Accessed July 17, 2019.
2. Lipton JA, Ship JA, Larach-Robinson D. Estimated prevalence and distribution of reported orofacial pain in the United States. J Am Dent Assoc 1993;124(10):115–21.
3. Sacerdote P, Levrini L. Peripheral mechanisms of dental pain: the role of substance P. Mediators Inflamm 2012;2012:951920.
4. Coutaux A, Adam F, Willer JC, et al. Hyperalgesia and allodynia: peripheral mechanisms. Joint Bone Spine 2005;72(5):359–71.
5. Caviedes-Bucheli J, Muñoz HR, Azuero-Holguín MM, et al. Neuropeptides in dental pulp: the silent protagonists. J Endodontics 2008;34(7):773–88.
6. Hargreaves KM, Swift JQ, Roszkowski MT, et al. Pharmacology of peripheral neuropeptide and inflammatory mediator release. Oral Surg Oral Med Oral Pathol 1994;78(4):503–10.
7. Kidd BL, Urban LA. Mechanisms of inflammatory pain. Br J Anaesth 2001;87(1):3–11.
8. Jain N, Gupta A, Meena N. An insight into neurophysiology of pulpal pain: facts and hypotheses. Korean J Pain 2013;26(4):347–55.
9. Pozzi A, Gallelli L. Pain management for dentists: the role of ibuprofen. Ann Stomatol (Roma) 2011;2(3–4 Suppl):3–24.
10. Moore RA, Derry S, McQuay HJ, et al. Single dose oral analgesics for acute postoperative pain in adults. Cochrane Database Syst Rev 2011;(9):CD008659 (ISSN: 1469-493X).
11. Moore PA, Ziegler KM, Ruth D, et al. Benefits and harms associated with analgesic medications used in the management of acute dental pain. J Am Dent Assoc 2018;149(4):256–65.
12. CDC advisory to health care providers regarding opioid based painkillers in women of childbearing age. Prescription painkillers, widely used by childbearing age women, double birth defects risk. Available at: http://www.cdc.gov/mmwr/preview/mmwrhtml/mm6402a1.htm?s_cid=mm6402a1_w. Accessed July 20, 2019.
13. Forbes JA, Kehm CJ, Grodin CD, et al. Evaluation of ketorolac, ibuprofen, acetaminophen, and an acetaminophen-codeine combination in postoperative oral surgery pain. Pharmacotherapy 1990;10(6 (Pt 2)):94–105.
14. Fricke JR Jr, Angelocci D, Fox K, et al. Comparison of the efficacy and safety of ketorolac and meperidine in the relief of dental pain. J Clin Pharmacol 1992;32(4):376–84.
15. Marjoribanks J, Proctor M, Farquhar C, et al. Nonsteroidal anti-inflammatory drugs for dysmenorrhoea. Cochrane Database Syst Rev 2010;1:CD001751.
16. Becker DE. Pain management: part 1: managing acute and postoperative dental pain. Anesth Prog 2010;57(2):67–79.
17. Piletta P, Porchet HC, Dayer P. Central analgesic effect of acetaminophen but not aspirin. Clin Pharmacol Ther 1991;49(4):350–4.
18. Abhang P, Momin M, Inamdar M, et al. Transmucosal drug delivery—an overview Drug Deliv Lett 2014;4(1):26–37.

19. Alsarra IA, Alanazi FK, Mahrous GM, et al. Clinical evaluation of novel buccoadhesive film containing ketorolac in dental and post-oral surgery pain management. Pharmazie 2007;(10):773–8.
20. Al-Hezaimi K, Al-Askar M, Selamhe Z, et al. Evaluation of novel adhesive film containing ketorolac for post-surgery pain control: a safety and efficacy study. J Periodontol 2011;82(7):963–8.
21. Tallarida RJ. Drug synergism: its detection and applications. J Pharmacol Exp Ther 2001;298(3):865–72.
22. American Society of Anesthesiologists. Task force on acute pain management. Practice guidelines for acute pain management in the perioperative setting: an updated report by the American Society of Anesthesiologists Task Force on Acute Pain Management. Anesthesiology 2004;100(6):1573–81.
23. Møiniche S, Kehlet H, Dahl JB. A qualitative and quantitative systematic review of preemptive analgesia for postoperative pain relief—the role of timing of analgesia. Anesthesiology 2002;96(3):725–41.
24. Shevel E, Koepp WG, Butow KW. A subjective assessment of pain and swelling following the surgical removal of impacted third molar teeth using different surgical techniques. SADJ 2001;56(5):238–41.
25. Kim K, Brar P, Jakubowski J, et al. The use of corticosteroids and nonsteroidal anti-inflammatory medication for the management of pain and inflammation after third molar surgery: a review of the literature. Oral Surg Oral Med Oral Pathol Oral Radiol Endod 2009;107(5):630–40.
26. Vyvey M. Steroids as pain relief adjuvants. Can Fam Physician 2010;56(12): 1295–7.
27. Tracy H. Breaking barriers in transdermal drug delivery. JAMA 2005;293(17): 2083.
28. Polomano RC, Rathmell JP, Krenzischek DA, et al. Emerging trends and new approaches to acute pain management. J Perianesth Nurs 2008;23(1 Suppl): S43–53.
29. Alqareer A, Alyahya A, Andersson L. The effect of clove and benzocaine versus placebo as topical anesthetics. J Dent 2006;34(10):747–50.

Botox and Dermal Fillers

Review and Its Role in the Dental Office

David Sheen, DDS*, Earl Clarkson, DDS

KEYWORDS

• Botox • Botulinum • Toxin • Dermal • Filler • Dentist • Oral • Face

KEY POINTS

- For the general dentist, the use of BTA and dermal fillers confers the ability to exert control over the soft tissues surrounding the mouth to better create a harmonious smile.
- The injection of BTA and fillers into the facial musculature and dermis requires a level of finesse to achieve the desired outcomes.
- A sound understanding of the mechanisms of action and the ability to manage potential complications are also necessary, as the dentist administering BTA and dermal fillers must be competent to the same level as other providers who have traditionally been the gatekeepers of such agents.

BOTULINUM TOXIN A

Neuromodulators, or neurotoxins, have long been used by medical specialists—namely plastic surgeons and ophthalmologists. These medications alter the relationship between nerve and muscle fiber conduction. The most well-known neuromodulator, botulinum toxin type A or Botox, has only recently been added to the armamentarium of general dentists. Although numerous abbreviations exist to represent botulinum toxin type A, it is referred to as BTA throughout this article.

History

Before the application of BTA for therapeutic purposes, it was recognized as a lethal toxin responsible for botulism poisoning. Justinus Kerner, a German physician, was the first to report on BTA in 1817. Kerner realized that an outbreak of food poisoning was attributed to rotten sausage—hence the name "botulism," from the Latin word *botulus*, meaning sausage. In 1897, Emile van Ermengem, a Belgian microbiologist, isolated the toxin from a patient who contracted botulism and named it *Bacillus botulinus*, a spore-forming obligate anaerobic bacterium. In 1922 the pathogen was renamed *Clostridium botulinum*.

Department of Oral & Maxillofacial Surgery, Woodhull Medical Center, 760 Broadway, Brooklyn, NY 11206, USA
* Corresponding author.
E-mail address: dsheen16@gmail.com

Dent Clin N Am 64 (2020) 325–339
https://doi.org/10.1016/j.cden.2019.12.002

In the late 1970s, Alan Scott, an ophthalmologist, was granted approval by the US Food and Drug Administration (FDA) to begin clinical trials of BTA for the treatment of strabismus. After many successful trials proved the efficacy of BTA, the FDA finally approved pharmaceutical preparations of BTA in 1989 for the treatment of strabismus and blepharospasm. Subsequently, Jean Carruthers, an oculoplastic surgeon, discovered that one of her patients had a decrease in glabellar wrinkles—in addition to being treated successfully for blepharospasm with BTA.

After extensive studies and investigations, the FDA approved BTA for additional therapeutic uses, including cervical dystonia in 2000, glabellar rhytids in 2002, and axillary hyperhidrosis in 2004.

Mechanism of Action

Thus far, 8 serologic types of botulinum toxin have been identified (designated A–H).[1] Although the molecular configuration and function of the 8 serotypes are similar, BTA is the most potent and has the longest-lasting effect. Botulinum toxin causes paralysis at the neuromuscular junction by preventing communication between the nerve and muscle.

The toxin is composed of a 2-chain protein, consisting of a light chain polypeptide bound to a heavy chain polypeptide via a disulfide bond. The active part of the toxin is the light chain and the heavy chain mediates binding to the presynaptic nerve terminal. Through the mechanism of endocytosis, the toxin enters the nerve once it is bound to the nerve terminal. Ordinarily, a complex of SNARE proteins mediates the fusion of acetylcholine vesicles to the nerve cell membrane and the subsequent release of the neurotransmitter acetylcholine into the synaptic cleft. However, once inside the nerve cell cytoplasm, the light chain of the toxin cleaves the SNARE protein, SNAP-25, thus preventing fusion of acetylcholine vesicles to the cell membrane. With the nerve cell unable to release the neurotransmitter acetylcholine, nerve signaling is blocked, which leads to weakness or flaccid paralysis. Because of the storage vesicles of acetylcholine already in the synaptic cleft, the effect of the toxin is not manifested until the stores are depleted, which takes approximately 24 to 48 hours.[2] The paralytic effect of the toxin lasts for 2 to 6 months—the length of time required for the generation of new axonal sprouts that restore the function of the neuromuscular junction (**Fig. 1**).

Preparation

In the United States, there are 3 FDA-approved BTA neuromodulators: Botox (onabotulinum toxin A), Dysport (abobotulinum toxin A), and Xeomin (incobotulinum toxin A). Although the 3 neuromodulators share the same therapeutic indications, they differ with respect to potency per unit and the nonprotein constituents that emerge from various manufacturing practices.[3] To allow for convenience of dosing for the practitioner, the commercially available vials of these neuromodulators contain a certain amount of biologically active units. The literature demonstrates that Botox and Xeomin are equivalent in potency with respect to units, whereas the potency of 1 unit of Botox is equivalent to approximately 2.5 to 3 units of Dysport.[4] The variance in potency is caused by the purification method, the strain from which BTA is isolated, and the diverse methods for measuring potency.[5] Throughout this article, all doses refer to Botox units for the sake of consistency, with the comprehension that an equivalent dose of Xeomin or Dysport is as effective.

Botox that is unreconstituted may be stored at 2°C to 8°C for a period of 24 months in a standard refrigerator. Only 4.8 ng of BTA is contained in a standard 100-unit vial of Botox. Because the amount is so small, BTA is transported in empty glass vials

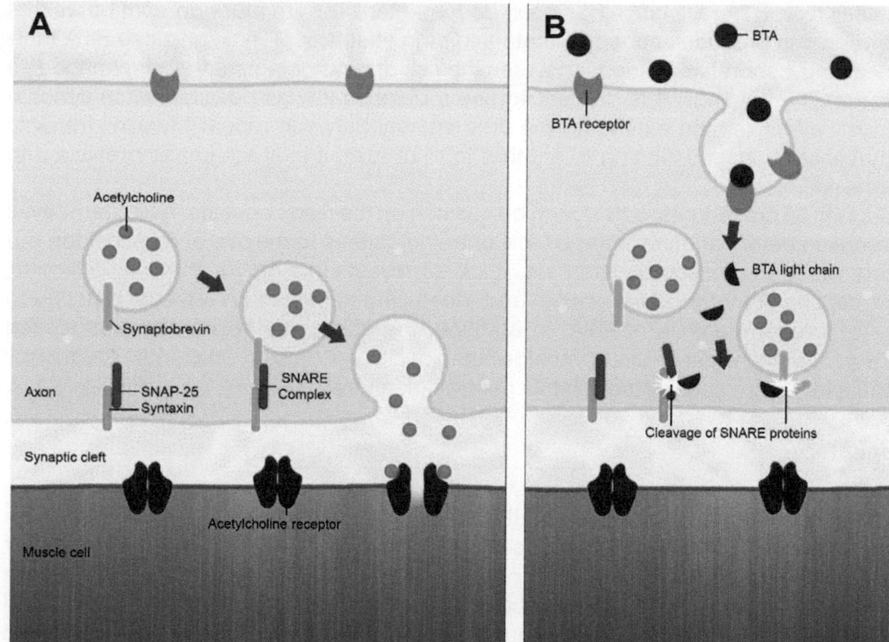

Fig. 1. Diagram depicting the action of botulinum toxin at the neuromuscular junction. (*A*) Normal acetylcholine release. Synaptobrevin and VAMP-2 (not shown) on the surface of the vesicle containing acetylcholine joins with SNAP-25 and syntaxin on the internal axonal surface. This forms a complex that allows fusion of the vesicle with the membrane to release acetylcholine into the synaptic cleft. Acetylcholine binds to its receptor on the surface of the muscle cell, opening voltage-gated sodium channels that result in membrane depolarization. (*B*) Action of botulinum toxin. BTA is internalized by the axon when bound by its receptor on the cell surface. The light chain of the toxin is taken up and cleaves the SNARE proteins before the acetylcholine vesicles can bind. The result is a lack of acetylcholine release into the synaptic cleft, and subsequent paralysis of the muscle.

consisting of a thin layer of precipitate. To maintain proper temperature, Botox is shipped on dry ice. After reconstitution with 2.5 mL preservative-free 0.9% sodium chloride for injection, it is stored under refrigeration and should be used within 24 hours.[6] This dilution ratio allows for aspiration into 5 syringes (1 mL), each containing 0.5 mL solution of 20 units of Botox.[7] Dilution with 2 or 4 mL of preservative-free saline may also be used depending on practitioner preference.

General Considerations

It is paramount to inform patients receiving BTA injections that the therapy varies in efficacy from one patient to another. After approximately 3 months from the time of BTA treatment, motor function is restored due to resprouting of nerve axons. A salient point to keep in mind is that this time frame is highly inconsistent. Some patients may require touch-up injections in just several weeks, whereas for other patients, the effects of the toxin may persist much longer than 3 months. Consistent BTA therapy causes muscular atrophy due to extended immobility, which decreases the ability of muscles to produce deep wrinkles.[8] For patients who regularly present for follow-up repeat therapy, the treatment interval can typically be prolonged once the muscles begin to atrophy.

Albeit rare, BTA resistance has been documented. The literature demonstrates that the toxin can produce antibodies that inhibit the effects of BTA. High-dose BTA therapy during a short time period increases the risk of developing neutralizing antibodies against BTA.[9,10] Thus, it is prudent to use a dose as low as possible while simultaneously effective, and extending the time interval between repeat therapy. Patients may benefit from substituting to another form of toxin if they are immunoresistant to a specific form.

As with all procedures, a thorough discussion on the risks, benefits, and alternatives is required before administering BTA. Contraindications to the use of BTA include patients with neuromuscular disorders, such as myasthenia gravis, multiple sclerosis, and peripheral motor neuropathies, and those who have had an adverse reaction to any of the components of BTA. In addition, the effect of BTA can be potentiated with concomitant use aminoglycoside antibiotics and muscle relaxants. Pregnancy and lactation are considered relative contraindications.

Upper Face

Frontalis

The frontalis is a thin, paired muscle that moves vertically, producing horizontal wrinkles in the skin of the forehead. The fibers of the frontalis insert into the brow depressor muscles: the procerus, the corrugator supercilii, and the orbicularis oculi. The frontalis is the only forehead elevator, where contraction of the muscle raises the upper eyelid and eyebrows. Therefore, simultaneous treatment of the brow depressors is indicated to prevent an unwanted eyebrow shape and height.

Multiple low-dose BTA injections are needed for the treatment of frontalis rhytids because of the large surface area and thin muscle mass of the frontalis. Injection points are typically spaced 20 to 30 mm apart because the diffusion of BTA from the site of injection is approximately 10 to 15 mm. Two to 5 units of Botox are administered at each injection point, with the upper end of this range being reserved for patients with larger muscle mass. If patients desire to maintain some mimetic function of the frontalis then a lower amount of Botox may be used (2–3 units), which will still soften wrinkles and permit animation. Based on patient's desired result, a total of 10 to 30 units of Botox may be administered across the forehead. To determine the ideal location of needle placement, the practitioner should use his or her nondominant hand to stabilize the patient's forehead during animation (**Fig. 2**).

Patients with dermatochalasis have a subconscious habit of continually elevating their brows with the hope of masking the excess upper eyelid skin. These patients need special consideration because excess Botox for the treatment of their frontal rhytids may prevent them from retaining their usual brow position. Therefore, all patients pursuing frontalis treatment need a careful preoperative assessment to determine if they posture their brows; and, if so, the practitioner has to discuss this possibility before initiating treatment.

Glabellar region

The brow depressors are the procerus, corrugator supercilii, and medial orbicularis oculi. These paired muscles overlap in the glabellar region and are responsible for the frown lines—commonly referred to as the 11 because they present as 2 vertical lines between the eyebrows (patients may also present with 1 or 3 lines). The procerus originates from the nasal bone and cartilage, extends laterally as its fibers run superiorly, and inserts into the skin of the forehead. The skin in this region develops rhytids through movement of the procerus. The corrugator supercilii originates from the medial aspect of the superior orbital rim, runs laterally nearly following the boundary

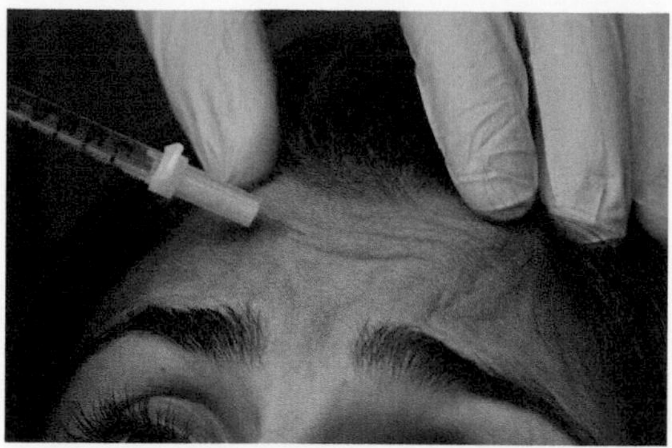

Fig. 2. Frontalis treatment with multiple diffuse injections. Care is taken to include rhytids near the hairline.

of the rim, and inserts into the skin of the mid-brow. This muscle pulls the brow in an inferior and medial direction, which contributes to brow furrowing. The procerus and corrugator supercilii, along with the medial orbicularis oculi are primarily targeted when treating frown lines (**Fig. 3**).

For the ordinary presentation of the 11, a centrally placed injection into the procerus with 5 units of Botox is adequate. Subsequently, 5 units are injected into each corrugator supercilii and each superior orbicularis oculi (**Fig. 4**). If several ridges are present in the glabellar region or if the rhytids in the procerus are diverse then the central 5-unit injection is spread uniformly across them. For most patients, 20 to 30 units of Botox

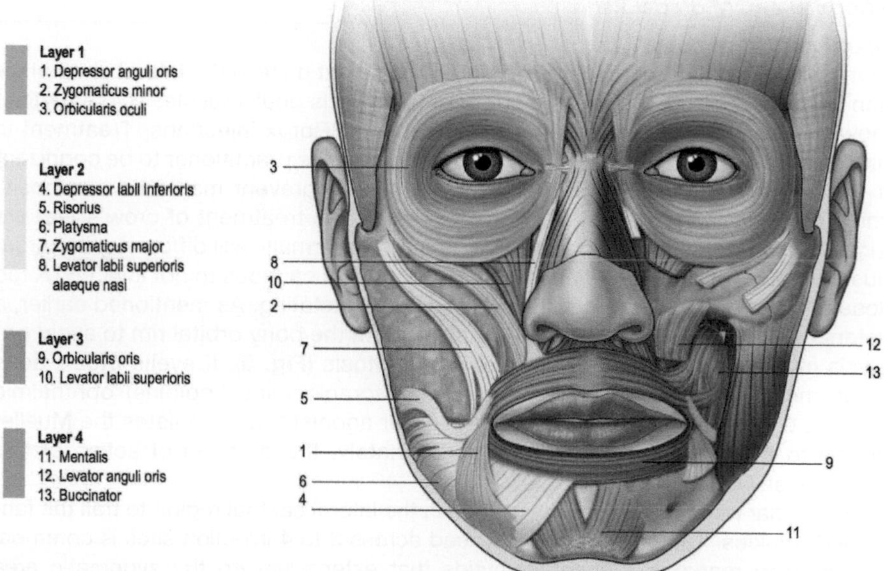

Fig. 3. Muscles of facial expression, color coded to indicate relative depths. (*From* Afifi AM, Sanchez RJ, Djohan RS. Anatomy of the head and neck. In: Rodriguez ED, Losee JE, Neligan PC, editors. Plastic surgery: Volume 3: craniofacial, head and neck surgery and pediatric plastic surgery, 4th edition. Philadelphia" Elsevier; 2018. p. 14; with permission.)

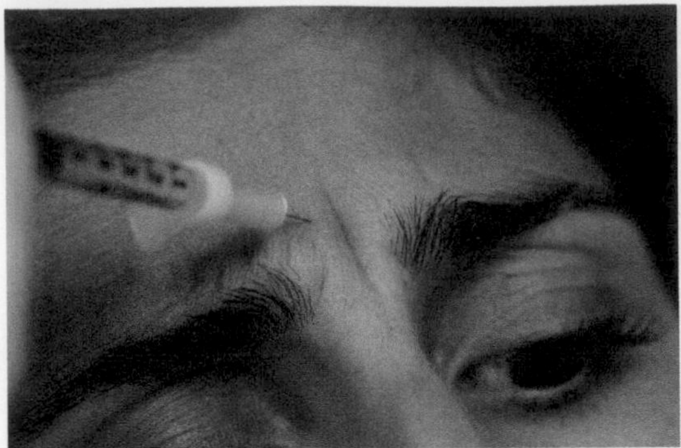

Fig. 4. In this patient, a single midline rhytid is seen on animation. Bilateral injection into the bulk of the procerus on either side is used for treatment in such cases.

uniformly spread across the glabellar region are adequate. Those with deep frown lines or thick muscle may need significantly more to achieve results that they will be satisfied with. Treatment of the frown lines is the only on-label cosmetic indication for Dysport and Xeomin, and along with crow's feet, 1 of 2 for Botox.[11–13]

The patient can assist the practitioner in locating the ideal injection sites by frowning intentionally. Before injecting BTA, it is judicious to aspirate the syringe given the proximity of the supratrochlear and supraorbital vessels in the glabellar region.[14] In addition, it is prudent to maintain a distance of 10 to 15 mm from the bony orbital rim to minimize the incidence of lid ptosis and paralysis of the extraocular muscles.

Periorbital and Midfacial Region

Lateral canthal region

A fan-shaped configuration of horizontal wrinkles that unite in the lateral canthal region is created by the lateral aspect of the orbicularis oculi muscle. These rhytids, known as crow's feet, are commonly treated with Botox injections. Treatment in this region is highly technique sensitive and requires the practitioner to be cognizant of the numerous large, superficial blood vessels to prevent marked ecchymosis, which can persist for weeks. Botox injections for the treatment of crow's feet are completed markedly superficial. BTA injected intradermally will diffuse to the target muscle. However, the practitioner must be extremely cautious to not inject BTA too close to the orbit as the consequences can be devastating. As mentioned earlier, a distance of 10 to 15 mm must be maintained from the bony orbital rim to avoid paralysis of the extraocular muscles and eyelid ptosis (**Fig. 5**). If eyelid ptosis does ensue then the patient can be treated with apraclonidine (Iopidine) ophthalmic solution, which is an alpha adrenergic receptor agonist that stimulates the Mueller muscle to elevate the upper eyelid. Unfortunately, the duration of action of this drug is brief.

A semilunar pattern of injections is used in the lateral canthal region to trail the fan-shaped wrinkles. Ten units of Botox spread across 3 to 4 injection sites is common. Patients with markedly elongated rhytids that extend toward the zygomatic area may need a supplementary row of injections concentrically following the initial set of injections, although at a dose of only 1 to 2 units per site. The most inferior injections must be administered judiciously as descending diffusion of BTA to the upper lip elevators can yield an undesired effect in the perioral region.

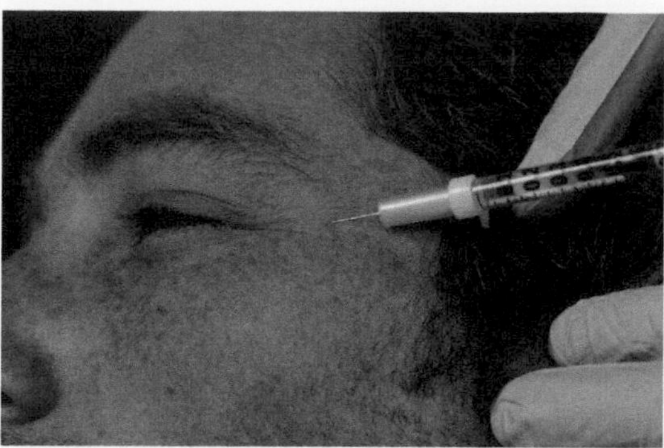

Fig. 5. Treating crow's feet requires very superficial injections that parallel the lateral orbital rim at a distance of 10 to 15 mm.

Lower lid

The bulging of soft tissue in the lower eyelid, known as the jelly roll, is a phenomenon occurring with advancing age that many patients seek treatment for. The cause of this bulge is varied, and it is essential that a correct diagnosis is made so that unwarranted treatment with dire consequences is prevented. Every practitioner performing BTA injections has to possess the ability to differentiate between orbicularis oculi muscle hypertrophy and infraorbital fat pad prolapse.

The anterior border of the orbit consists of the orbital septum, which is a membranous barrier that is practically an extension of the periosteum exterior to the orbital rims. The orbicularis oculi muscle lies superficial to the orbital septum. Weakening of the septum with age permits prolapse of the infraorbital fat pads, which results in a bulge—known as steatoblepharon. The puffy appearance around the eyes (eyelid bags) is secondary to the gravitational and fluid shifting of the fat pads. However, hypertrophic orbicularis oculi muscles can produce a similar bulge, which is especially apparent when a patient smiles or squints. This is predominantly due to the orbital portion of the muscle, which voluntarily and forcefully contracts the palpebral fissure.

A strong indicator of orbicularis hypertrophy is the appearance and disappearance of bulges during animation. Conversely, retropulsion of the globe will allow the practitioner to determine if the bulge is the result of fat prolapse. This is accomplished by gently pressing the globe inward and evaluating the lower lid to see if the fat pads become more prominent. The excess fat and skin in the lower lid can be excised via a blepharoplasty procedure if fat prolapse is responsible for the bulge.

The lower lid bulge due to orbicularis hypertrophy can be treated with BTA injections. Not only will BTA reduce the size of the infraorbital bulge, but it will also give the patient a more awake appearance by allowing the eye to remain open easier. A dose of 1 to 2 units of Botox injected in the pupillary midline approximately 3 mm inferior to the ciliary margin is typically adequate. Care has to be taken when treating this area because excess BTA can inhibit complete eye closure, which will lead to decreased tear production and dry eyes. Treatment in this region should be avoided in patients who have a preexisting compromised capacity to close the lower eyelid, as the risk of keratoconjunctivitis sicca is increased in this patient population.

Nasalis

Horizontal wrinkles that traverse the dorsum of the nose are produced in some people when they frown or squint. Hyperactivity of the nasalis muscle is responsible for these bunny lines. The nasalis originates from the maxilla, extends medially to cover the bridge of the nose, and inserts into the nasal bone. The nares compress when the nasalis contracts and this may produce horizontal rhytids. Two-unit aliquots of Botox equally spaced at 4 injection sites are sufficient to treat this area (**Fig. 6**). In some individuals, the activity of the procerus may accentuate the bunny lines and form furrows across the entire intercanthal length.

Uncommonly, patients will seek treatment for nasal flaring. These patients are uncomfortable with the widening of their nostrils during inspiration. The alar part of the nasalis muscle, the dilator naris, causes the unwanted flare. It originates from the maxilla and the lesser alar cartilage and inserts into the skin at the caudal margin of the nostril. Two to 4 units of Botox injected superficially into each ala significantly reduces the flare.

Perioral Region

Excessive gingival display and nasolabial fold

Excessive maxillary gingival display, or gummy smile, may be treated with BTA if the high smile line results from a hyperfunctional upper lip. There are other causes for a gummy smile so it is important for the practitioner to discern whether a hyperfunctional upper lip is the source or if the condition is due to maxillary vertical excess or hypertrophy of maxillary gingiva. For the latter, definitive treatment is a Le Fort I impaction osteotomy (orthognathic surgery) or gingivoplasty, respectively. If an attempt is made to treat these conditions with BTA, then the result would be an unnatural appearance that most patients find unattractive.

For patients who are candidates, BTA injections to the levator labii superioris alaeque nasi (LLSAN) muscle will decrease elevation of the upper lip, and thus reduce gingival display. The LLSAN is responsible for the final few millimeters of upper lip elevation and also contributes to the deep nasolabial fold that forms in some patients.[15] This muscle originates from the superior aspect of the frontal process of the maxilla, traverses inferiorly in an oblique direction on either side of the nose, and has insertions at the lateral upper lip and the alar cartilage. Two to 5 units of Botox to each LLSAN may be needed for the treatment of excessive maxillary gingival display and deep nasolabial folds. The LLSAN can be palpated just lateral to the piriform aperture where the maxilla meets the inferior aspect of the nasal bone (**Fig. 7**). BTA injections in this region are highly technique sensitive as overtreatment may result in loss of upper lip animation that can manifest as an asymmetric smile.

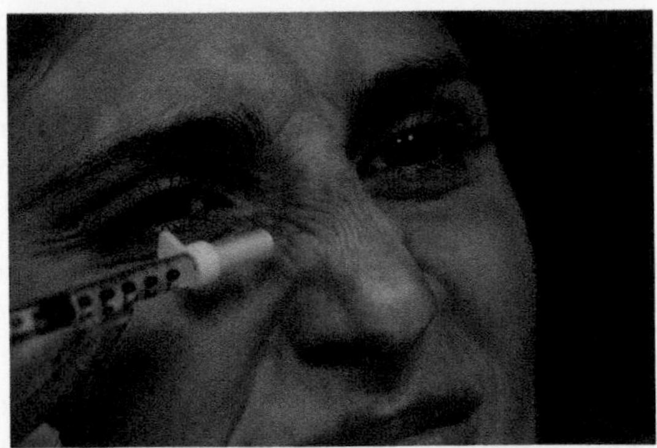

Fig. 6. Hyperactive nasalis treatment at the area of greatest contracture.

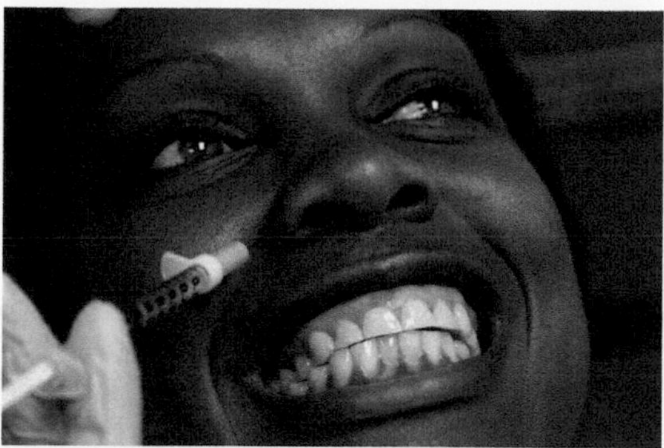

Fig. 7. Excessive gingival display is treated by injection of BTA at the depth of the nasolabial fold just lateral to the alar-facial junction.

Perioral lines

The upper lip vertical rhytids, known as lipstick lines, are produced by the orbicularis oris muscle, and are commonly seen in aging patients—particularly smokers and those with sun damage. Continual puckering of the lips, as when playing an instrument, whistling, or smoking, accelerates the formation of these vertical rhytids by activating the orbicularis oris. This sphincter muscle originates from the oral commissure, where its fibers merge with other perioral elevator muscles to form the modiolus. Animation of the lips, such as protrusion and pursing, is made possible by the various subdermal insertions of the orbicularis oris near the midline. Depending on the patient, 1 to 2 units of Botox at 2 to 4 injection sites in the upper lip are sufficient. Injections in this region are placed superficially, in the dermal layer, due to the fineness of the rhytids.[16] To provide the practitioner with a visualization of the deepest folds the patient is asked to repeatedly purse his or her lips (**Fig. 8**). It is important for patients to understand that total elimination of the lipstick lines is not possible without complete paralysis of the orbicularis oris muscle. Overtreatment may result in problems with speech and oral competence.

Most patients receiving Botox treatment for upper lip rhytids concomitantly receive dermal filler injections. The filler product restores volume and aids in softening the wrinkles, and BTA is used to attenuate the force of the orbicularis oris and weaken it. In addition, Botox prolongs the effect of the filler material by relaxing the underlying musculature.

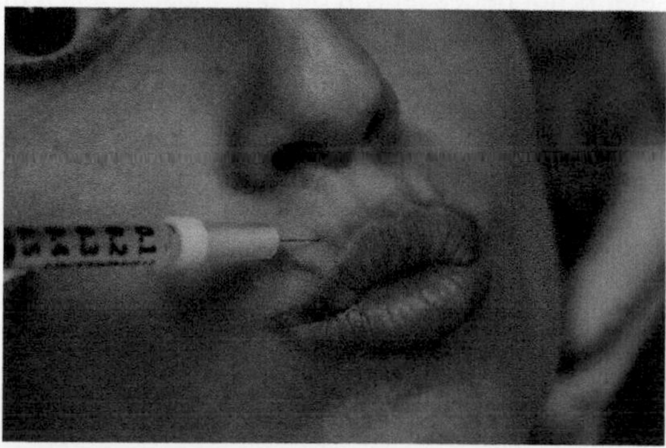

Fig. 8. Asking the patient to pucker his or her lips highlights the deepest folds of lipstick lines.

Oral commissure

The creases below the oral commissures, known as the marionette lines, are the result of the depressor anguli oris muscle. This triangularly shaped muscle originates from the inferior border of the mandible with its broad end and inserts at the oral commissure or angle of the mouth. Its function is to draw the corners of the mouth inferiorly and laterally. Paralysis of the depressor anguli oris permits the perioral elevator muscles to act unopposed. Although the difference after treatment is subtle, patients still notice the change and are satisfied with the results.

Two to 5 units of Botox injected bilaterally will subtly soften the marionette lines by allowing greater elevation of the oral commissures. To isolate the depressor anguli oris, the practitioner asks the patient to display the mandibular teeth by winding the lower lip down. Care must be taken to inject BTA into the belly of the muscle—not into its superior portion. BTA injections placed too far superiorly can cause paralysis of the depressor labii inferioris muscle which may result in drooling and lower lip incompetence. In addition, the injection sites cannot be placed too far inferiorly as paralysis of the marginal mandibular branch of the facial nerve will cause an asymmetric smile. Therefore, it is important to place the needle at least 1 cm away from the inferior border of the mandible when targeting the belly of the depressor anguli oris.

Mentalis

Chin dimpling occurs in some patients when they raise their lower lip during speech or mastication. This appearance, known as peau d'orange or popply chin because it resembles an orange peel, is due to the mentalis muscle. This paired muscle originates from the incisor fossa of the mandible and runs inferomedially to insert into the dermis of the chin. The mentalis is often referred to as the pouting muscle because it protrudes the lower lip.

Patients who find their chin dimpling unattractive can seek BTA treatment. A total of 2 to 5 units of Botox injected around the chin in the regions with the most prominent dimpling are adequate. It is imperative for the practitioner to place the injections superficial and away from the origin of the mentalis as overtreatment may result in speech problems. Specifically, articulation of the consonants B, M, and P will be adversely affected because they require lower lip elevation. In addition, injections placed too far laterally may paralyze the depressor labii inferioris and lead to lower lip incompetence.

Masseter

Although the masseter is not necessarily a perioral muscle, it is a muscle of mastication that is essential to oral function. It is a notably thicker muscle in comparison with the muscles of facial expression and consists of superficial and deep heads that merge at their insertion. The larger superficial head originates from the anterior two-thirds of the zygomatic arch, courses inferoposteriorly, and inserts onto the lateral mandibular ramus and angle. The smaller deep head originates from the posterior third of the zygomatic arch and courses vertically inferior to insert onto the lateral ramus—marginally higher than the superficial head. Jointly, the 2 heads of the masseter function to elevate and protrude the mandible and assist with lateral excursive movements; important anatomy located superficial to the masseter include branches of the facial nerve, the parotid gland and duct, and transverse facial artery.

There are 2 indications for treating the masseter with BTA: cosmetic and pain reduction. Some patients are displeased with the appearance of their hypertrophic masseters. BTA can be used to slim the posterior lower face by gradually causing atrophy of the masseters.[17] In addition, patients who have myofascial pain or temporomandibular dysfunction secondary to parafunctional habits, such as bruxism or clenching are also candidates for BTA treatment to reduce the contraction force of the masseters. Treatment of the masseter with BTA is distinct because the objective is to attenuate the bulk of the muscle as opposed to softening rhytids.

The most prominent areas of masseter hypertrophy are identified by having the patient clench his or her teeth—marking these areas with a surgical pen can be helpful (**Fig. 9**). Five to 10 units of Botox per injection site is a good starting point, with multiple injection sites per masseter being common. However, some patients may need as much as 100 units for bilateral treatment. Follow-up assessment after several weeks will allow the practitioner to determine if supplemental injections are required.

DERMAL FILLERS

In addition to BTA, dermal fillers are another product available in the armamentarium of general dentists for nonsurgical, minimally invasive cosmetic facial treatment. With aging, there is a gradual loss of facial volume due to loss of dermal collagen, lipoatrophy, gravity, and environmental factors—among other reasons. A youthful appearance through volume restoration can be achieved with the use of injectable fillers.

The ideal filler agent must possess certain attributes; it should be biocompatible, noncarcinogenic, nonallergenic, create predictable and long-lasting results, be easy to use, and nonmigratory. Various types of filler products have been available over the past several decades, but hyaluronic acid (HA) and synthetic fillers have fairly recently revolutionized the dermal filler market. Furthermore, fillers may be used in conjunction with BTA to fulfill the patient's desire of turning back the clock. Fillers can be categorized based on several characteristics, such as: filler component (natural, synthetic, or autologous); mechanism of action; and duration of treatment effects.

Dermal fillers are most commonly injected using the linear threading and serial puncture techniques. Via linear threading, the filler is injected evenly along a direct trajectory while withdrawing the needle. When the serial puncture technique is performed, small droplets of filler material are injected in multiple locations.[18]

Hyaluronic Acid (Natural Filler)

HA is a naturally occurring polymer of glycosaminoglycan and is a fundamental constituent of the extracellular matrix of all animal tissues. HA has a very high affinity for water; it can bind a thousand times its weight in water—this forms the foundation of its

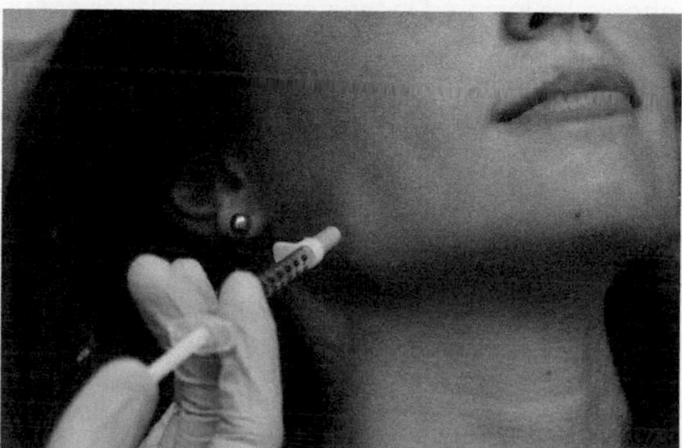

Fig. 9. The masseter is treated in the areas of greatest hypertrophy. Injections for this muscle are typically deeper than used in other areas of the face.

function in soft tissue augmentation. HA does not exhibit specificity for any species or tissue type; therefore, it does not require allergy skin testing since it will not elicit an immunologic response.

Natural HA is enzymatically degraded by hyaluronidase and free radicals, and metabolized by the liver into water and carbon dioxide. Commercial HA is crosslinked with ether bonds to stabilize the filler. The crosslinking process prolongs the duration of HA by making it more resistant to degradation. HA for soft tissue augmentation is produced via a bacterial fermentation process using *Streptococcus equi*. In addition, HA fillers can be manufactured as monophasic or biphasic products. Monophasic fillers are cohesive gels and biphasic fillers are composed of HA particles.[19]

The most commonly used HA fillers are the Restylane and Juvederm series of products—both approved by the FDA for cosmetic soft tissue augmentation. Restylane was approved in 2003 and Juvederm was approved in 2006. Restylane is a biphasic filler and contains 100,000 particles per mL. Juvederm is a monophasic filler that has a higher HA concentration and greater degree of crosslinking compared with Restylane—making it particularly viscous. The higher viscosity may potentially increase the duration of the product, although both types of HA fillers typically have a longevity of 6 to 12 months.[20]

HA fillers provide exceptional results when injected intradermally. The facial regions most commonly treated with HA include the nasolabial folds, the perioral region, lips, marionette lines, cheeks, tear troughs, and jawline. The upper facial regions, such as the forehead and glabellar are best treated with neurotoxin, although the experienced practitioner may concomitantly use Botox and fillers in these regions for exceptional outcomes. The most common side effects with HA fillers are ecchymosis, edema, induration, and pain—all of which are fairly short-lived.

Nonresorbable Synthetic Fillers

Silicone

Medical-grade liquid silicone is a polymer of dimethylsiloxane. Silikon 1000, an injectable silicone, was approved by the FDA in 1997 for the treatment of retinal detachment. The FDA determined that off-label use for soft tissue augmentation was legal as long as the practitioner did not advertise it as such. Liquid silicone is recognized as a foreign body when injected into tissue and gets encapsulated by collagen. This occurs over several weeks and causes gradual growth as secondary collagen is added to the fibrous capsule. Therefore, it is crucial that the practitioner inject silicone in 0.01 mL microdroplets and undercorrect as multiple treatment sessions will be required.[4] Silicone should be injected in the deep dermal layer or subcutaneous tissue and sessions should be spaced at intervals of 4 to 6 weeks. Treatment regions for the experienced practitioner include any part of the face that is usually treated with fillers; although it is most commonly used in the perioral area, such as the lips and nasolabial folds.

Liquid silicone is a permanent filler and irreversible; therefore, it is not recommended for use by the novice practitioner. It can be stored at room temperature and does not promote growth of bacteria. Care must be taken to keep silicone injections conservative because large volume aliquots will migrate through tissue planes, form nodules and granulomas, and destroy tissue.

Polymethylmethacrylate

Bellafill is a suspension of 20% polymethylmethacrylate (PMMA) microspheres and 80% bovine collagen solution. The PMMA microspheres are 30 to 42 μm in diameter. The smooth surface of the microspheres decreases the risk of a foreign body tion and their small size prevents phagocytosis and enzymatic degradation. Therefore, the microspheres stay intact on injection to provide a permanent scaffold onto which new soft tissue may form once the collagen from the injection is degraded. The results are seen immediately. PMMA should be injected at the junction between the deep dermal layer and the subcutaneous tissue. Most practitioners use Bellafill for deep rhytids in the perioral region, such as nasolabial folds, perioral lines, and marionette lines.

Because of the bovine collagen carrier, patients have to undergo an allergy skin test before treatment. PMMA is contraindicated in patients prone to keloid formation.[18] To prevent the filler from being visible or palpable, PMMA injections should be avoided in thin skin areas. Side effects include granuloma formation, an irregular distribution, and chronic pruritus.

Resorbable Synthetic Fillers

Polylactic acid

Sculptra is an injectable filler composed of poly-L-lactic acid particles. It is a synthetic lactic acid polymer that is biodegradable, biocompatible, and immunologically inert. It is the same material as Vicryl suture, does not require skin testing, and can be stored at room temperature. Sculptra was approved by the FDA in 2004 for the treatment of facial lipoatrophy in HIV patients. Polylactic acid is commercially available as a powder and has to be reconstituted with sterile water before use.

The effect of building volume with Sculptra is gradual. When polylactic acid is injected, the particles are recognized as a foreign body and are engulfed by macrophages. Via phagocytosis, the particles are degraded into microspheres which promote an inflammatory reaction that stimulates collagen to enclose the microspheres.[21] This granulomatous response progressively builds fibrous soft tissue, which results in the formation of volume.

Injections should always be placed subdermal. It is important for the practitioner to remember that the primary indication for use of polylactic acid is to restore volume, as opposed to softening fine rhytids. Treatment regions include the cheeks, temples, and nasolabial folds. The patient is instructed to continue to massage the treatment area at home. It may take 3 to 6 months for volume to be reestablished and patients may need to return for repeat injections at an interval of 4 to 6 weeks to achieve the desired effect. Although the foundation that is gained with polylactic acid is not permanent, the effect does last for 18 to 24 months. Side effects include edema, ecchymosis, and the delayed appearance of palpable granulomas that may require surgical excision.

Calcium hydroxyapatite

Radiesse is an injectable filler composed of calcium hydroxyapatite (CaHA) microspheres suspended in a gel carrier composed of carboxymethylcellulose. It is approved by the FDA for cosmetic soft tissue augmentation. Similar to polylactic acid, it is biodegradable, biocompatible, and immunologically inert. Radiesse is not expected to provoke a chronic inflammatory reaction since CaHa is a normal component of bone. CaHA allows for volume restoration by providing a scaffold that stimulates collagen formation. Resorption of the carboxymethylcellulose gel promotes fibrous soft tissue ingrowth.[22]

CaHA should be injected in the deep dermal layer or subcutaneous plane depending on the area of treatment. Most practitioners use Radiesse for deep glabellar furrows, the cheek and malar region, nasolabial folds, and lips. The effects of CaHA have a duration of 12 to 18 months. The CaHa particles are enzymatically degraded over a period of 9 to 12 months. A relatively common side effect is nodule formation in the lips secondary to poor injection technique. These nodules can be treated with corticosteroid injections. Persistent nodules may require surgical excision.

Autologous Fat

Neuber first reported on autologous fat grafts to reconstruct facial defects in 1893. Autologous fat is a popular procedure to this day as there is no additional cost for materials and there is no risk of an allergic reaction or rejection. Historically, overcorrection of the defect by 30% to 50% was prudent due to expected resorption. However, suspending the autologous fat in platelet-rich plasma, along with other advances in fat transfer, have shown promise in increasing the longevity of fat grafts. Harvested fat requires a blood supply to survive. The growth factors found in platelet-rich plasma are believed to induce angiogenesis. Despite the advent of contemporary techniques, most practitioners agree that there will be some postoperative fat resorption. Thus, patients have to be made aware that multiple sessions may be required.

Numerous harvesting sites exist, such as the umbilical region of the abdomen, medial and lateral thighs, and hips/flanks. To prevent an asymmetric harvest and uneven tissue contour, it is recommended to mark the harvest sites with a surgical pen and to obtain fat bilaterally. Tumescent anesthesia is used to infiltrate the harvest sites. Fat harvesting cannulas are used to aspirate about 4 times the anticipated volume of fat required for grafting via standard liposuction technique. To avoid damaging the adipocytes, it is essential to use a low negative pressure during liposuction. The aspirated fat has to be separated from blood, fatty acids, and local anesthetic via centrifugation. The cleansed fat is then mixed with platelet-rich plasma. A large-bore needle (16 or 18 gauge) is used to transfer the fat to the anesthetized recipient sites once multiplanar dissection with a blunt tip cannula is completed.[4]

To ensure fat graft survival, the practitioner has to inject lobules of fat that are about 1 mm in diameter because larger fat droplets have an increased risk of central necrosis. In addition, the fat has to be transferred in a layered technique so that there is an even distribution. Fat is injected into the subcutaneous tissue and no more than 0.1 mL of fat should be injected at a time. Autologous fat may be transferred to essentially any region of the face with volume loss, but most practitioners prefer to use it for the cheeks, tear troughs, and temples. Fibrosis may occur if fat is injected into the dermal layer. It is imperative to avoid intravascular injection because that would cause a fat embolism that could potentially lead to a stroke or blindness.

SUMMARY

Dentists who are highly trained to treat the maxillofacial region have an opportunity to use Botox and dermal fillers in their practice to serve the needs and desires of their patients. These nonsurgical, minimally invasive procedures require the practitioner to have a thorough comprehension of how to correctly use these products to achieve esthetic results.

ACKNOWLEDGMENTS

Special thanks to Jared Miller DDS, Joshua Weiler DDS, Lynda Asadourian DDS, and Saidah Jack-Glidden.

DISCLOSURE STATEMENT

The authors have nothing to disclose.

REFERENCES

1. Barash JR, Arnon SS. A novel strain of *Clostridium botulinum* that produces type B and type H botulinum toxins. J Infect Dis 2014;209(2):183–91.
2. Horowitz BZ. Botulinum toxin. Crit Care Clin 2005;21(4):825–39.
3. Nestor MS, Ablon GR. Duration of action of abobotulinumtoxinA and onabotulinumtoxinA: a randomized, double-blind study using a contralateral frontalis model. J Clin Aesthet Dermatol 2011;4(9):43–9.
4. Niamtu J. Cosmetic facial surgery. 2nd edition. Edinburgh (Scotland): Elsevier; 2018.
5. Nigam PK, Nigam A. Botulinum toxin. Indian J Dermatol 2010;55(1):8–14.
6. Schantz EJ, Johnson EA. Properties and use of botulinum toxin and other microbial neurotoxins in medicine. Microbiol Rev 1992;56(1):80–99.
7. BOTOX Cosmetic (onabotulinumtoxinA) for injection, for intramuscular use [Package insert]. Irvine (CA): Allergan, Inc; 2018.
8. Sadick NS, Herman AR. Comparison of botulinum toxins A and B in the aesthetic treatment of facial rhytides. Dermatol Surg 2003;29:340–7.
9. Niamtu J. Complications in fillers and botox. Oral Maxillofac Surg Clin North Am 2009;21:13–21.
10. Rodriguez ED, Losee JE, Neligan PC. Plastic surgery, volume three: craniofacial, head and neck surgery. 3rd edition. London: Elsevier; 2013.
11. BOTOX® Cosmetic (onabotulinumtoxinA) official site. Welcome! Irvine (CA): Allergan, Inc; 2019. Available at: http://www.botoxcosmetic.com/. Accessed July 1, 2019.
12. Dysport® for temporary improvement of moderate to severe frown lines. Fort Worth (TX): Galderma Laboratories, L.P.; 2018. Available at: http://www.dysportusa.com/. Accessed July 1, 2019.
13. XEOMIN® (incobotulinumtoxinA) for injection, for intramuscular use. Raleigh (NC): Merz North America, Inc; 2019. Available at: http://www.xeominaesthetic.com/. Accessed July 1, 2019.
14. Guttenberg SA. Cosmesis of the mouth, face and jaws. Chichester (UK): Wiley-Blackwell; 2012.
15. Norton NS. Netter's head and neck anatomy for dentistry. 2nd edition. Philadelphia: Elsevier; 2012.
16. Haggerty CJ, Laughlin RM. Atlas of operative oral and maxillofacial surgery. Ames (IA): John Wiley & Sons; 2015.
17. Park NY, Ahn KY, Jung DS. Botulinum toxin type A treatment for contouring of the lower face. Dermatol Surg 2003;29(5):477–83.
18. Papel ID, Frodel JL, Holt GR. Facial plastic and reconstructive surgery. 3rd edition. New York: Thieme; 2009.
19. Gold MH. Use of hyaluronic acid fillers for the treatment of the aging face. Clin Interv Aging 2007;2(3):369–76.
20. Brandt FS, Cazzaniga A. Hyaluronic acid gel fillers in the management of facial aging. Clin Interv Aging 2008;3(1):153–9.
21. Burgess CM. Principles of soft tissue augmentation for the aging face. Clin Interv Aging 2006;1(4):349–55.
22. Jacovella P. Use of calcium hydroxyapatite (Radiesse®) for facial augmentation. Clin Interv Aging 2008;3(1):161–74.

Diagnosis and Treatment Approaches to a "Gummy Smile"

Harry Dym, DDS*, Robert Pierre II, DMD

KEYWORDS

- Gummy smile • Altered passive eruption • Lip repositioning
- Excessive gingival display • Vertical maxillary excess

KEY POINTS

- Excessive gingival display is a common esthetic concern for many patients and increases the risk of an unacceptable esthetic dental result.
- Before delivering treatment, it is paramount for the clinician to identify the cause, as they may be multiple, which will dictate the treatment plan.
- Potential causes may include lip length, lip activity, clinical crown length, altered passive eruption, and vertical maxillary excess.
- Surgical options to treat excess gingival display can include: gingivectomies, crown lengthening, lip repositioning, Botox injection, orthodontics, and orthognathic surgery.

INTRODUCTION: NATURE OF THE PROBLEM

Excessive gingival display, also known as a "gummy smile" is a common esthetic concern among dental patients. The excessive gingival display while smiling has been largely viewed as unaesthetic, leading to many patients seeking some form of treatment to address this issue. The etiology that plays into the gummy smile are often multifactorial, which is why an accurate diagnosis is paramount before any surgical treatment. In this article, we discuss the etiology, classification, diagnostic guidelines, and the current treatment options that can be rendered based on the etiology of the gummy smile.

The gummy smile has been largely defined as a nonpathological condition causing esthetic disharmony, in which more than 3 to 4 mm of gingival tissue is exposed when smiling.[1] **Fig. 1** shows a classic presentation of excessive gingival display while smiling. The anatomic landmarks that factor into the gummy smile are the maxilla, lips,

Department of Oral & Maxillofacial Surgery, The Brooklyn Hospital Center, 121 Dekalb Avenue, Brooklyn, NY 11201, USA
* Corresponding author.
E-mail address: hdymmdds@yahoo.com

Dent Clin N Am 64 (2020) 341–349
https://doi.org/10.1016/j.cden.2019.12.003
0011-8532/20/

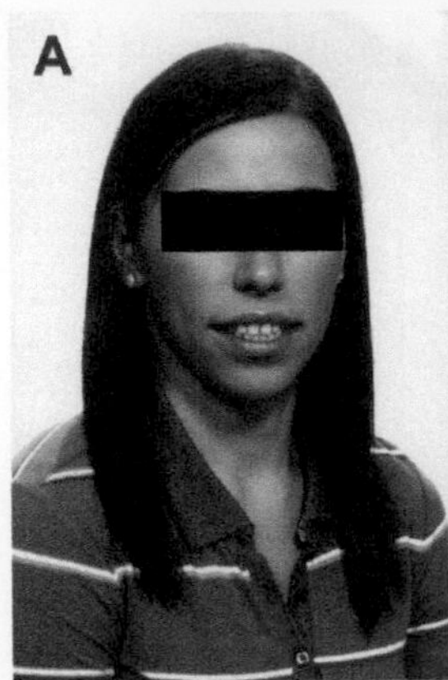

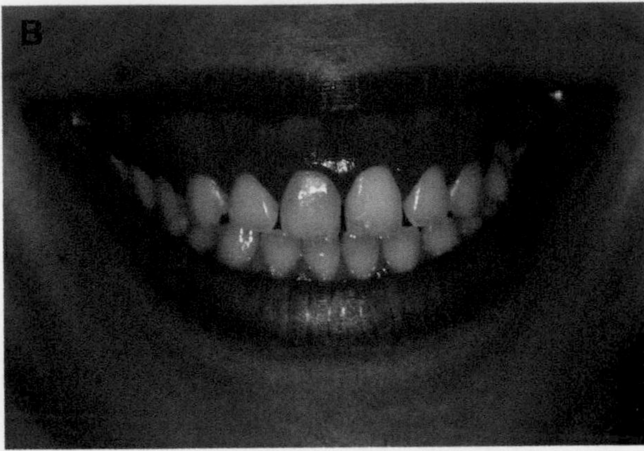

Fig. 1. (*A*) Preoperative full-face view with relaxed lips. (*B*) Preoperative enface view in smile. (*From* Panduric DG, Blaskovic M, Brozovic J, et al. Surgical treatment of excessive gingival display using lip repositioning technique and laser gingivectomy as an alternative to orthognathic surgery. J Oral Maxillofac Surg. 2014;72:404.e2–e3; with permission. (Figure 1 in original).)

gingival architecture, and teeth.[1] All of these anatomic structures must lie in harmony with one another to achieve an esthetic smile. When diagnosing and treating patients with a gummy smile, the clinician must accurately understand and identify the etiology. In addition, multiple etiologies can simultaneously be responsible for the excess gingival display (**Box 1**) and each cause must be accurately identified.[1] Knowing the etiology, whether single or multiple, will dictate which treatment modality will be most appropriate for the patient.

DIAGNOSIS OF EXCESSIVE GINGIVAL DISPLAY

When a patient presents with a chief complaint of their gummy smile, several steps must be taken to arrive at an accurate diagnosis. Furthermore, to correctly identify the etiologic, anatomic, and pathologic causes of a gummy smile, a well-defined diagnostic process should be used as shown in **Box 2**.[1]

Box 1
Potential causes of excessive gingival display

1. Short lip length
2. Hypermobile/hyperactive lip activity
3. Short clinical crown
4. Dentoalveolar extrusion
5. Altered passive eruption
6. Vertical maxillary excess
7. Gingival hyperplasia

Data from Pavone AF, Ghassemian M, Verardi S. Gummy smile and short tooth syndrome-Part 1: Etiopathogenesis, classification, and diagnostic guidelines. Compend Contin Educ Dent. 2016;37(2):102–7; and Bynum J. Treatment of a "gummy smile": understanding etiology is key to success. Compend Contin Educ Dent. 2016;37(2):114–22.

Box 2
Diagnostic assessment of the gummy smile

1. Patient medical history
2. Facial analysis
3. Lip analysis: static versus dynamic
4. Rest position analysis
5. Dental analysis: crown length and incisal margin
6. Periodontal examination

Data from Pavone AF, Ghassemian M, Verardi S. Gummy smile and short tooth syndrome-Part 1: Etiopathogenesis, classification, and diagnostic guidelines. Compend Contin Educ Dent. 2016;37(2):102–7.

Medical History

Obtaining a thorough medical history is always of great importance when arriving at a diagnosis. Key elements include the patient's age and overall health.[1] The patient's age can indicate the eruptive stage of the dentition, and the overall health can indicate to the clinician any contributing factors to the patient's condition.[1]

Facial Analysis

A thorough evaluation of the facial profile of the patient can provide useful information to help identify the cause of the gummy smile. The facial thirds can be evaluated in the frontal and lateral views to determine any deficiencies or excess in the midface.[1] An increase in the ratio of the middle third of the face may indicate vertical maxillary excess (VME).[1] Many authors will agree that VME is the most common extraoral cause of the gummy smile.[1] Cephalometric analysis can be used to help identify VME.[1] Patients with VME usually end up having a skeletal class II relationship. Most patients with moderate to severe VME will require some form of orthognathic surgery as the form of treatment.

Lip Analysis

An analysis of the upper lip to assess for excessive gingival display should be done in both static and dynamic positions.[1] Upper lip length and lip mobility should be assessed to identify the contributing factor to the gummy smile. The upper lip length is measured from subnasale to upper lip stomion with an average of 20 to 22 mm. Measurements less than this can be classified as a short lip and patients may present with lip incompetence and a gummy smile. In the dynamic analysis, hypermobility of the levator labii superioris muscles results in a higher position of the lip and increase exposure of the teeth and gingiva while smiling.[1] Therefore, when it comes to the lips, the cause of the gummy smile can either be from the lip length, the hypermobility of the lip or both.

Dentalveolar Analysis

During the dental analysis, the clinician should analyze the 3D position of the incisors in the rest position.[1] The interlabial gap can be assessed and measure with normal gap distance ranging from 0 to 4 mm.[1] When there is a large interlabial distance exposing an excessive amount of incisal margins, VME, overeruption, or short lip should be suspected.[1] The horizontal and vertical dimensions of the clinical crown should be measure and analyzed. A short clinical crown could be due to wear of the incisal edge or altered eruption.[1] By analyzing the incisal edge and the patient's age the clinician can determine if length discrepancy is located at the incisal margin or at the gingival margin.[1]

Periodontal Analysis

The initial evaluation during the periodontal examination aims to diagnose the pathologic and nonpathological changes in the architecture of the periodontium.[1] Probing depths, clinical attachment levels, and gingival recession should all be assessed and measured. If the patient presents with a clinical short tooth, the etiology must be identified as to whether it is due to inflammation, gingival hyperplasia, or altered eruption.[1]

Altered Passive Eruption

Altered passive eruption is defined as a condition in which the relationship between teeth, alveolar bone, and the soft tissues create an excessive gingival display.[2] Normal tooth eruption occurs in an active and passive phase. The active phase involves the movement of the tooth out of the alveolar bone into occlusal position.[2] The passive phase is the exposure of the crown as a result of apical migration of the gingival tissues.[2] The apical migration occurs in 4 stages as listed in **Box 3**. Altered passive eruption is the failure of the gingival/dental complex to migrate apically past stage 2, with the most obvious sign being a short looking tooth.[2] When making the diagnosis of altered passive eruption, the lips need to be assessed in repose and while smiling.[2] Ruling out a hypermobile lip is necessary before making the diagnosis of altered eruption. A normal translational movement of the lip from rest is about 6 to 8 mm and up to 10 mm in a hypermobile lip situation.[2] If the patient is deemed to have a hypermobile lip then the clinician should consider lip repositioning surgery or botulinum toxin A injections. Dental-alveolar extrusion is commonly treated with orthodontic intrusion.[2] Treatment options are discussed later in this article. A key element to arriving at a diagnosis is noting the location of the cementoenamel junction (CEJ) in the gingival sulcus. The CEJ normally resides just apical to the free gingival margin of the crown. Conversely, the CEJ can reside up to 10 mm apical to the free gingival margin in altered passive eruption.[2] If the CEJ can be detected in the gingival sulcus, and all other etiologies have been ruled out, a diagnosis of altered passive eruption can be made.

SURGICAL TREATMENT OPTIONS

It cannot be overstated that, before any surgical treatment, the etiology must be identified to guide the appropriate treatment. After an etiology has been determined, the clinician should develop the appropriate treatment options to present to the patient,

Box 3
Normal tooth eruption

Stage 1: Teeth in plane of occlusion, JE on the enamel

Stage II: Epithelial attachment rests partly on enamel and cementum apical to CEJ

Stage III: JE lies completely on cementum with base of sulcus at CEJ

Stage IV: All of stage III with a portion of the root clinically exposed

Abbreviations: CEJ, cementoenamel junction; JE, junctional epithelium.

Data from Chan DK. Predictable treatment for "gummy smiles" due to altered passive eruption. Inside Dentistry. 2015;11(7).

including all risks, benefits, and alternatives.[3] The clinician must listen to the patient's overall goal and must curtail the treatment to the patient's specific needs. Not every patient will want to undergo orthognathic surgery to address their VME, so the clinician must present alterative treatment options to achieve the patient's overall goal with realistic expectations. Different surgical methods are discussed in this section based on the etiology of the excessive gingival display.

LIP REPOSITIONING

The hallmark of an "ideal smile" entails the exposure of the entire length of the maxillary teeth with approximately 1 to 3 mm of gingival exposure. Lip repositioning surgery can be used to address excessive gingival display when the etiology is mild VME or a hypermobile lip.[4] Lip repositioning narrows the vestibule limiting muscle pull, which restricts gingival display while smiling.[4] The procedure can also be used in conjunction with crown lengthening or a gingivectomy.

Lip repositioning has been documented as being performed by various methods. The intended goal is to remove a strip of mucosa and shortening the vestibule, thereby restricting the muscle pull of the elevator muscles during smiling.[5] This can be done traditionally using a scalpel, electrocautery, or even a laser surgical approach.

Rubinstein and Kostianovsky first presented the procedure of surgical lip repositioning in 1973 in the plastic surgery literature.[6] The procedure has been subject to many modifications, including preservation of the maxillary labial frenum.[6] **Box 4** outlines the traditional surgical approach taken to perform lip-repositioning surgery. The amount of mucosa to remove is based on the "twice the amount of gingival display rule."[6] It is common practice to prescribe oral antibiotics (amoxicillin 500 mg 3 times a day), nonsteroidal anti-inflammatory drugs (ibuprofen 600 mg 4 times a day), and 0.12% chlorohexidine rinse twice a day as postoperative prescriptions.[6] Postoperative instructions as outlined in **Box 5** should be given written and verbally to the patient

Box 4
Surgical steps in lip repositioning

1. 0.12% Chlorhexidine rinse for 1 minute preoperatively
2. Administer local anesthesia in vestibular mucosa and lip between left and right upper first molar (2% lidocaine w/1:100k epinephrine)
3. Mark incision outline with sterile surgical marking pen
4. Partial thickness horizontal incision made 1 mm coronally to mucogingival junction from first molar to first molar
5. Second horizontal incision was made in the labial mucosa 10 to 12 mm apical to first incision
6. Connect the 2 incisions at the mesial line angles of the right and left maxillary first molar in elliptical outline
7. Remove strip of outlined mucosa by a superficial split thickness dissection
8. Control bleeding with electrocoagulation as needed
9. Take care to avoid damaging minor salivary glands in submucosa
10. Use 4 to 0 silk sutures to close incision lines in interrupted fashion

Data from Alammar A, Heshmeh O, Mounajjed R, et al. A comparison between modified and conventional surgical techniques for surgical lip repositioning in the management of the gummy smile. J Esthet Restor Dent. 2018;30:523–31.

Box 5
Postoperative instructions for lip repositioning

1. Apply ice packs over the upper lip for several hours
2. Soft diet for first week
3. Minimize lip movement when smiling or talking during the first 2 weeks postoperatively
4. No brushing around the surgical site for 14 days
5. Manage postoperative pain with analgesics
6. Suture removal at 2 weeks

Data from Alammar A, Heshmeh O, Mounajjed R, et al. A comparison between modified and conventional surgical techniques for surgical lip repositioning in the management of the gummy smile. J Esthet Restor Dent. 2018;30:523–31.

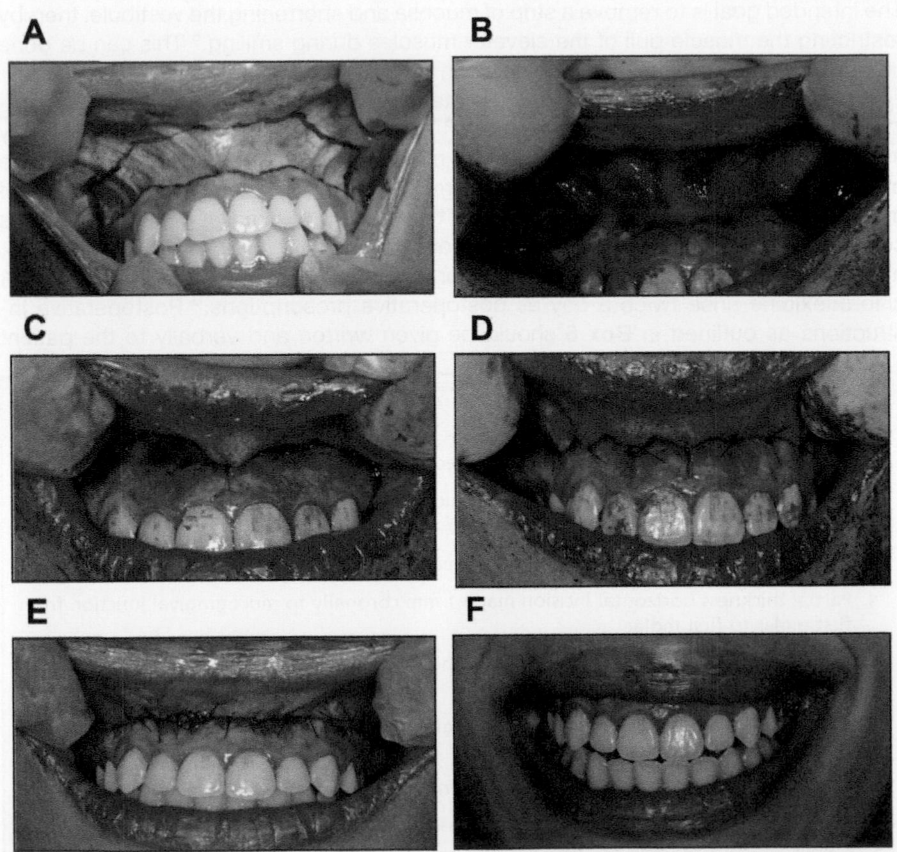

Fig. 2. Surgical steps. (*A*) Incision area outlined according to the "Twice Gingival Display." (*B*) Incision area after superficial incision is finished. (*C*) Midline anchoring suture. (*D*) Remaining anchoring sutures opposite to papillae. (*E*) Both anchoring and stabilizing sutures. (*F*) Immediate postoperative picture. (*From* Foudah M. Lip repositioning: An alternative to invasive surgery a 4 year follow up case report. Saudi Dental Journal. 2019;31:S82; with permission.)

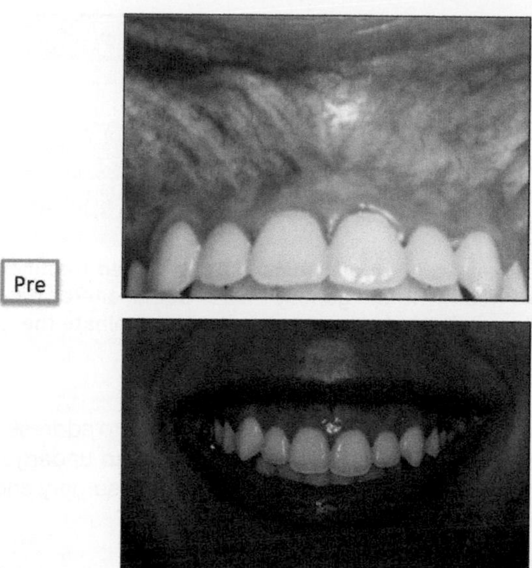

Fig. 3. Preoperative pictures. (*From* Foudah M. Lip repositioning: An alternative to invasive surgery a 4 year follow up case report. Saudi Dental Journal. 2019;31:S82; with permission.)

before discharge.[6] In **Figs. 2–4**, you can see the distinct changes in the amount of gingival display from preoperative to postoperative after having the lip-repositioning surgery performed.[7] Contraindications to lip repositioning include minimal zones of attachment and severe VME.[8] Postoperative complications that should be discussed with the patient include, pain, bruising, swelling, mucocele formation, and possible relapse.[9]

Causes of relapse include the following[7]:

- Not following the "twice the gingival display" rule during the incision
- Cutting in the keratinized attached gingiva
- Performing the procedure with limited amount of keratinized attached gingiva
- Incising deep into the connective tissue and muscle fibers
- Cases with high muscle pull

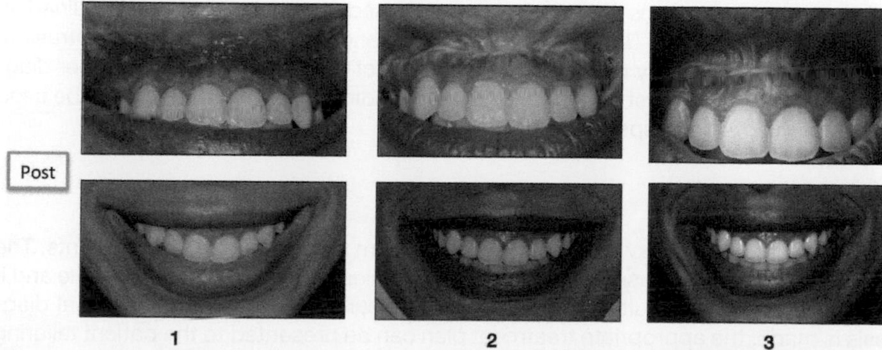

Fig. 4. Postoperative pictures: 1, two-week follow-up; 2, one-year follow-up; 3, four-year follow-up. (*From* Foudah M. Lip repositioning: An alternative to invasive surgery a 4 year follow up case report. Saudi Dental Journal. 2019;31:S83; with permission.)

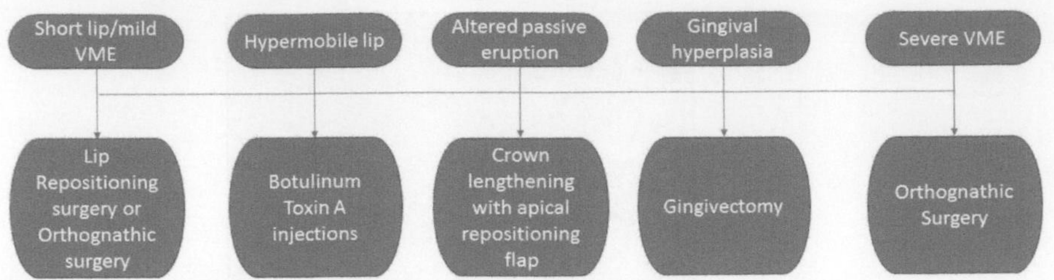

Fig. 5. Diagnosis of excessive gingival display with associated treatment plan. (*Data from* Chan, DK. Predictable treatment for "gummy smiles" due to altered passive eruption. Inside Dentistry. 2015;11(7); and Mahn D. Lip repositioning to eliminate the gummy smile. Inside Dentistry. 2017;13(3).)

Lip-repositioning surgery is a safe predictable method to address excessive gingival display and a viable option for those patients unwilling to undergo orthognathic surgery. However, in the case of severe VME, orthognathic surgery should be performed rather than lip repositioning.

BOTULINUM TOXIN A (BOTOX)

Treatment with botulinum toxin A for facial rejuvenation is currently the most common nonsurgical esthetic procedure in the United States.[10] Botox, derived from *Clostridium botulinum* bacterium, inhibits presynaptic acetylcholine release at the neuromuscular junction thereby inducing muscle paralysis. When the etiology of the gummy smile is found to be a hypermobile/hyperactive upper lip, Botox injection can be a viable treatment option to counteract the hypermobility. Patients undergo injections into the levator labii superioris and the levator labii superioris alaque nasi muscles bilaterally.[10]

The 3 sites of injection on each side are as follows: 2 mm lateral to alar-facial groove, 2 mm lateral to first injection in same horizontal plane, and 2 mm inferior between first 2 sites.[10] Approximately 4 to 6 units of Botox are used on each side. However, increase in the severity of gingival display could warrant a slightly higher dosage of Botox as needed. Treatment of a gummy smile with botulinum toxin A is an effective minimally invasive procedure that can significantly improve smile esthetics for the patient.[10]

The most important phase of treating the gummy smile is identifying the etiology. Different treatment plans can be rendered based on the etiology as outlined in **Fig. 5**. Lip repositioning, Botox injections, crown lengthening, dentoalveolar intrusion, and orthognathic surgery can all be used to correct the gummy smile. A proper diagnosis should be made first and then the corresponding surgical approach can be used based on the patient's specific needs.

SUMMARY

Excessive gingival display is a true esthetic concern that concerns many patients. The gummy smile can be caused by a variety of etiologies as discussed in this article and it is up to the clinician to ultimately arrive at an accurate diagnosis. Once a final diagnosis is made, the appropriate treatment plan can be presented to the patient tailoring it specifically to the patients' needs and concerns. As more research continues, we will likely see new treatment ideas and modifications to existing surgical approaches to the gummy smile.

DISCLOSURE

The authors have nothing to disclose.

REFERENCES

1. Pavone AF, Ghassemian M, Verardi S. Gummy smile and short tooth syndrome—Part 1: etiopathogenesis, classification, and diagnostic guidelines. Compend Contin Educ Dent 2016;37(2):102–7.
2. Chan DK. Predictable treatment for "Gummy Smiles" due to altered passive eruption. Inside Dent 2015;11(7).
3. Bynum J. Treatment of a "Gummy Smile": understanding etiology is key to success. Compend Contin Educ Dent 2016;37(2):114–22.
4. Mahn D. Lip repositioning to eliminate the gummy smile. Inside Dent. 2017.13 (3).
5. Farista S, Yeltiwar R, Kalakonda B, et al. Laser-assisted lip repositioning surgery: novel approach to treat gummy smile. J Indian Soc Periodontol 2017;21(2):165–8.
6. Alammar A, Heshmeh O, Mounajjed R, et al. A comparison between modified and conventional surgical techniques for surgical lip repositioning in the management of the gummy smile. J Esthet Restor Dent 2018;30:523–31.
7. Foudah M. Lip repositioning: an alternative to invasive surgery a 4 year follow up case report. Saudi Dent J 2019;31:S78–84.
8. Deepthi K, Yadalam U, Ranjan R, et al. Lip repositioning, an alternative treatment of gummy smile—a case report. J Oral Biol Craniofac Res 2018;8:231–3.
9. Panduric DG, Blaskovic M, Brozovic J, et al. Surgical treatment of excessive gingival display using lip repositioning technique and laser gingivectomy as an alternative to orthognathic surgery. J Oral Maxillofac Surg 2014;72:404.e1-11.
10. Suber J, Dinh T, Prince M, et al. Onabotulinumtoxin A for the treatment of a "Gummy Smile". Aesthet Surg J 2014;34(3):432–7.

Role of Piezo Surgery and Lasers in the Oral Surgery Office

Tarun Kirpalani, DMD, Harry Dym, DDS*

KEYWORDS

• Piezo • Laser • LANAP • Oral surgery

KEY POINTS

- Piezo surgery is a useful adjunct in oral surgical procedures because it helps limit any soft tissue damage secondary to bony surgery.
- Piezo surgery may limit the amount of sinus membrane perforations during the performance of lateral sinus bone augmentation procedures.
- Laser surgery has a place in soft tissue and hard tissue cutting procedures, and may also have value in the treatment of nerve injuries and periodontal regenerative procedures.

PIEZO SURGERY/INTRODUCTION

The term piezo is derived from the Greek work *piezein*, which means pressure.[1] It was developed by Italian oral surgeon Tomaso Vercelloti in 1988 to overcome the limits of traditional instrumentation in oral bone surgery by modifying and improving conventional ultrasound technology.[2] The process consists of crystals and ceramics that become deformed when exposed to electric flows resulting in oscillating movements with ultrasound frequency that has the power to precisely cut bone structures without causing injuries to soft tissue.[3] The frequency is usually set between 25 and 30 kHz causing microvibrations of 60 to 210 μm amplitude that provides the handpiece with power exceeding 5 W.[2] The product is targeted mainly at bone removal and soft tissue protection, but some models have a modified setting that can be used for excision of soft tissue lesions. The selective and thermally harmless nature of this instrument results in low bleeding tendency.[4]

During surgical use, the inserts should be moved forward and backward continuously at a high speed with minimum pressure, and the only absolute contraindication in its use is with patients who have a pacemaker. A contact load of 150 g provides the greatest depth of cut because the excessive pressure on the insert leads to a

Department of Oral and Maxillofacial Surgery, The Brooklyn Hospital Center, 121 Dekalb Avenue, Brooklyn, NY 11201, USA
* Corresponding author.
E-mail address: Hdym@tbh.org

Dent Clin N Am 64 (2020) 351–363
https://doi.org/10.1016/j.cden.2019.12.007

reduction in oscillations and hence the cutting ability.[5] Pressure with the piezo acts counterproductively by limiting movement of the instrument tip and generating more heat.[2] Therefore, patience here is a virtue, and applying excess pressure to hasten the cut may prove counterproductive.

A number of piezoelectric devices with similar mechanical parts are available on the market. Typically, devices will come with settings preset for the intended procedures. There are also a range of inserts and tips available on the market that vary in size, shape and material (**Fig. 1**). They can be coated with titanium and diamond of different grades. Some examples include the scalpel, cone compressor, bone harvester, and sharp-tipped saw. This is in contrast with conventional microsaws or drills in which the surgeon must apply a greater degree of pressure.[2]

ADVANTAGES OF THE PIEZO TECHNIQUE RELATIVE TO DRILLS AND SAWS

1. Greater precision and safety in bone surgery.[3]
2. Less adverse damages to soft tissues.
3. Less potential for associated bone necrosis.
4. A link flood system that ensures work and comfort of the surgeon by increasing visibility through the cavitation effect—physical effect—resulting from ultrasound vibration with water that removes debris from the cutting area.
5. Better healing and reduced postoperative swelling of patients.
6. Different angles permit it to be used in areas where it is difficult to see and reach.[1]
7. The absence of macrovibrations make patients feel comfortable during oral surgery procedures under local anesthesia and intravenous sedation.

DISADVANTAGES OF PIEZO SURGERY

1. This procedure should not be used in patients with pacemakers.[1]
2. The financial cost is a consideration.
3. The duration for procedures tends to be longer.
4. There is a learning curve with its use.

Piezo Use in Oral Surgery

1. *Dentolalveolar surgery*: The Piezo device can be used to assist in all types of dentoalveolar surgery, including endodontic and periodontal surgeries.[2,3]It has the theoretic ability to decrease the potential damage to both the lingual nerve and the inferior alveolar nerve during the removal of wisdom teeth, though there are no studies to prove this point. Liu and colleagues[6] performed a systematic review and meta-analysis of randomized controlled trials comparing the piezo versus

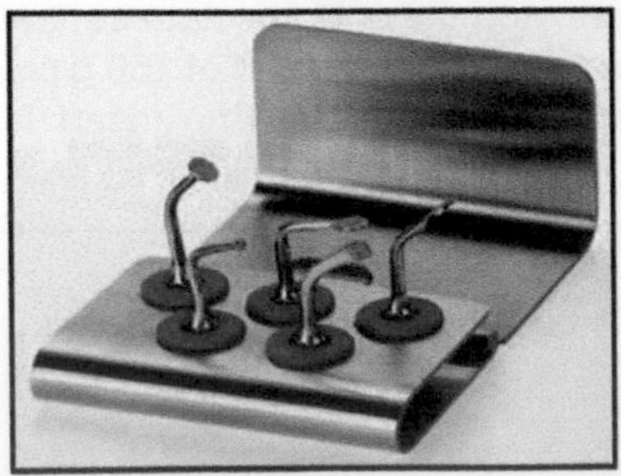
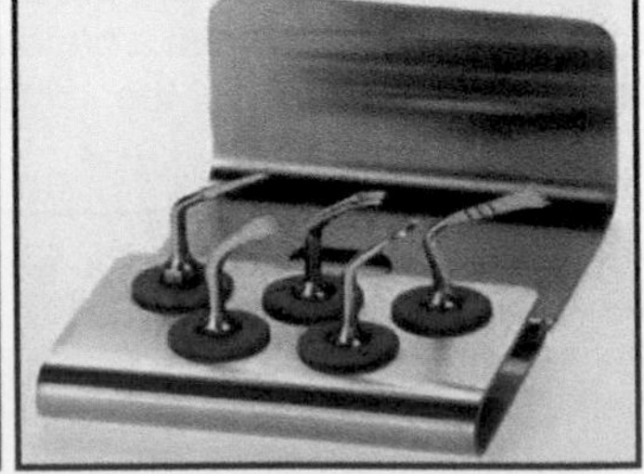

Fig. 1. Different piezo inserts. (*From* Aly LAA. Piezoelectric surgery: Applications in oral & maxillofacial surgery. Future Dental Journal 2018;4:107; with permission.)

conventional rotary instruments for third molar surgery. The study enrolled a total of 402 patients in which the piezo surgery group showed a lower postoperative pain score, less swelling, and greater mouth opening relative to the conventional group. However, more operation time was needed with the piezo and there was no statistically significant difference in postoperative analgesic use by either group. Although studies are limited, it has not been associated with impaired third molar wound healing or increase in dry sockets.[4] Tsai and colleagues[7] evaluated the periodontal condition after third molar removal that showed no statistical difference of average pocket depth or attachment level on the distal side of the second molar when using the piezo versus conventional drills.

2. *Dental implantology:* Implant site preparation could allow for the enlargement of only 1 socket wall by using specially designed inserts (**Fig. 2**).
3. *Ridge splitting techniques:* Classic ridge splitting involved using chisels with rotation and oscillating saws. These techniques were time consuming, technically more difficult, and carried a higher risk of damage to adjacent soft tissues and teeth. The piezo has made this procedure easier and safer to perform with lower risk of thermal necrosis and vertical cusp can be made without damaging adjacent soft tissues and teeth (**Fig. 3**).
4. *Maxillary sinus lifts*: This procedure can be accomplished via a lateral window approach with less risk of perforation of the Schneiderian membrane. Reports show perforation with conventional techniques ranging from 14% to 56%, with the percentage decreasing to as low as 5% with the piezo in some papers in the literature.[8] The bony access window can be created with a diamond-coated square or ball insert, and the sinus membrane can be elevated with rounded and soft tissues inserts (**Fig. 4**).
5. *Inferior alveolar nerve lateralization technique:* These are an alternative to augmentation techniques if implants are planned in edentulous jaws. This decreases the risk of damage to the nerve at the osteotomy lines. Schaeren and colleagues[8] showed that direct exposure of a nerve to piezosurgery does not dissect the nerve, but only induces some structural or functional damage. In most cases, the nerve is able to regenerate with the perineurium intact, in contrast with conventional drills or oscillating saws (**Fig. 5**).
6. *Maxillary and mandibular osteotomies in orthognathic surgery*: This technique is particularly useful when doing a multiple piece maxillary surgery and maintaining vitality of the teeth in the line of osteotomy. Beziat and colleagues in 2007 provided one of the largest studies of the use of the piezo in craniomaxillofacial surgery

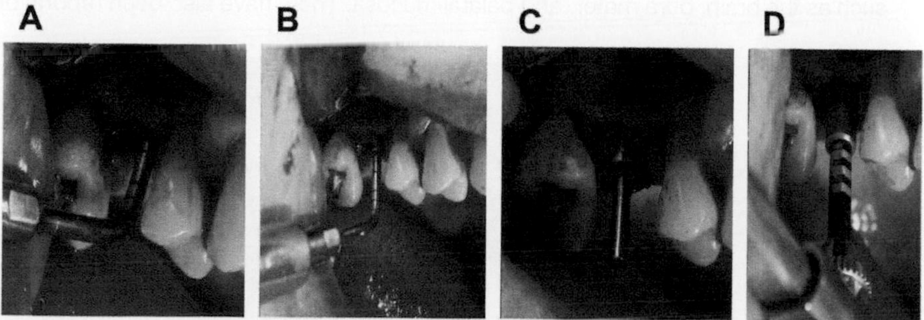

Fig. 2. (*A-D*) shows sequential piezo preparation of an implant site in the right maxilla. (*From* Aly LAA. Piezoelectric surgery: Applications in oral & maxillofacial surgery. Future Dental Journal 2018;4:107; with permission.)

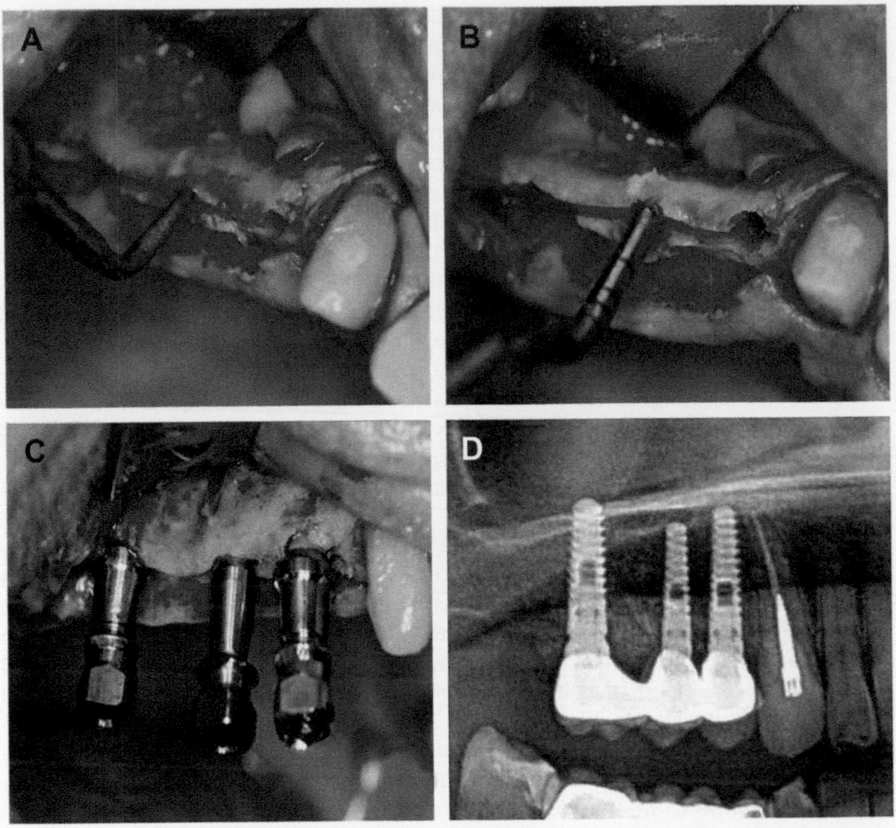

Fig. 3. Alveolar Crest with horizontal bone deficiency can be split and expanded using a piezo insert. (*A*) shows crestal osteotomy made by piezo. (*B*) shows the ridge being expanded. (*C*) shows implants placed with expanded ridge. (*D*) shows a periapical xray of the implants placed. (*From* Aly LAA. Piezoelectric surgery: Applications in oral & maxillofacial surgery. Future Dental Journal 2018;4:105–11; with permission.)

including 144 cases of Lefort 1 and 134 cases of bilateral sagittal split osteotomies, as well as other osteotomies used to treat craniofacial disorders.[1] The conclusion from their article was that the piezo allows for precise cutting and spares soft tissue such as the brain, dura mater, and palatal mucosa. There have also been reports of

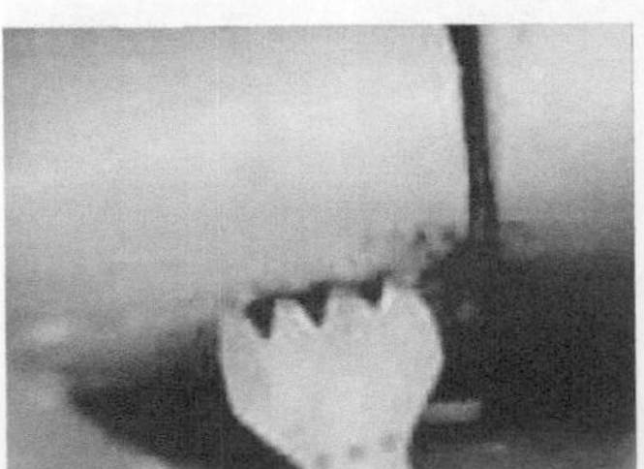

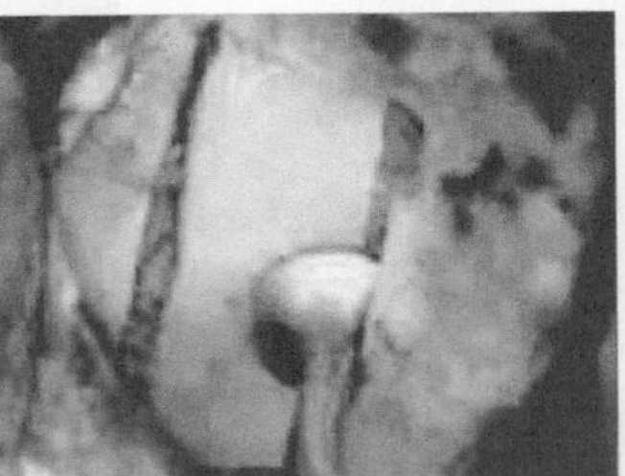

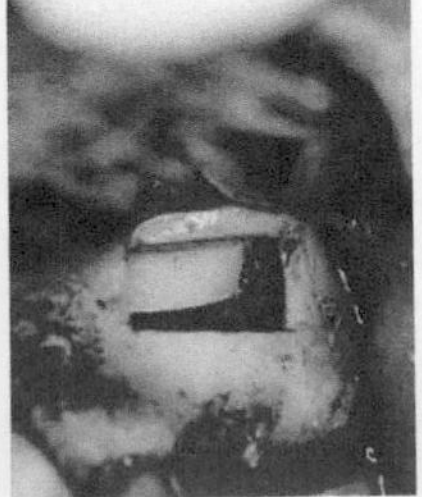

Fig. 4. Maxillary sinus lifting by piezo via lateral window approach. (*From* de Azevedo ET, Costa DL, Przysiezny PE, et al. Using piezoelectric system in oral & maxillofacial surgery. Int J Med Surg Sci. 2015;2(3):553; with permission.)

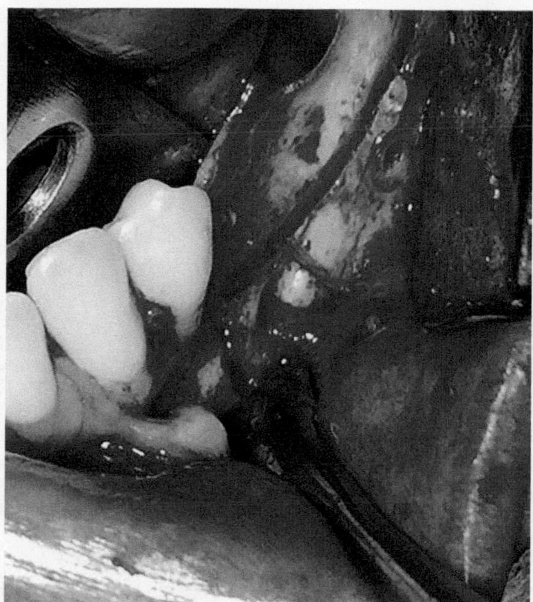

Fig. 5. Inferior alveolar nerve lateralization technique with piezo. (*From* de Azevedo ET, Costa DL, Przysiezny PE, et al. Using piezoelectric system in oral & maxillofacial surgery. Int J Med Surg Sci. 2015;2(3):552; with permission.)

less blood loss from an average of 772 mL in conventional orthognathic surgery versus 537 mL in piezo orthognathic surgery.[8] Landes and colleagues[9] showed that inferior alveolar nerve neurosensation was retained in 98% of their piezo bilateral sagittal split osteotomy cases versus 84% of their conventional bilateral sagittal split osteotomy cases at 3 months postoperative (**Fig. 6**).

7. *Aesthetic facial surgery:* This technique is particularly useful for lateral osteotomies in rhinoplasty procedures with less likelihood of lacerating the nasal tissues and damaging associated vessels. It can also be used in otologic procedures.
8. *Distraction osteogenesis:* The piezo creates precise osteotomies owing to micrometric and linear vibrations. There is also less flap damage, which means better vascularization that leads to more successful bone formation by this process (**Fig. 7**).
9. *Enucleation of maxillofacial cysts/resecting odontogenic tumors:* This procedure allows for careful removal of thin bone overlying the cyst to reduce damage to the epithelial wall. This technique could mean a reduction in the rate of recurrence of the pathology.
10. *Temporomandibular joint surgery:* The piezo device is particularly useful for temporomandibular joint ankylosis cases when performing condylectomies. The LED illumination, continuous irrigation, precise cutting, and preservation of vascular structures, such as the maxillary artery located medially, makes this procedure more effective and safer with a piezo device.
11. *Bone graft harvesting:* The piezo device makes it easier to harvest grafts of optimum dimensions. This technique can involve lateral ramus block grafts or symphysis block grafts. The different angled inserts also help with the osteotomy angulations needed for such harvest (**Fig. 8**). A study by Happe[10] in 2007 studied 40 patients that had mandibular ramus harvests that highlighted

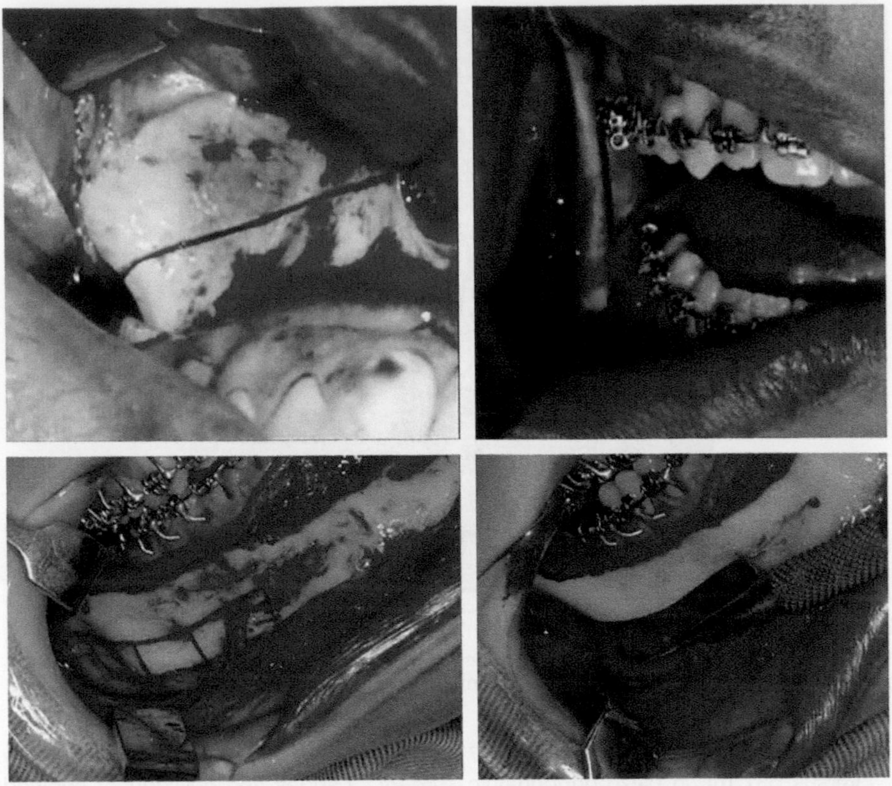

Fig. 6. Lefort 1 osteotomy, sagittal split osteotomy, and subapical total osteotomy by piezo. (*From* de Azevedo ET, Costa DL, Przysiezny PE, et al. Using piezoelectric system in oral & maxillofacial surgery. Int J Med Surg Sci. 2015;2(3):553; with permission.)

the ability of the piezo to provide precise, clean, and smooth cutting with excellent visibility. All grafts integrated without complication, provided enough bone for implant placement with less resorption of the grafts than those harvested by conventional techniques.

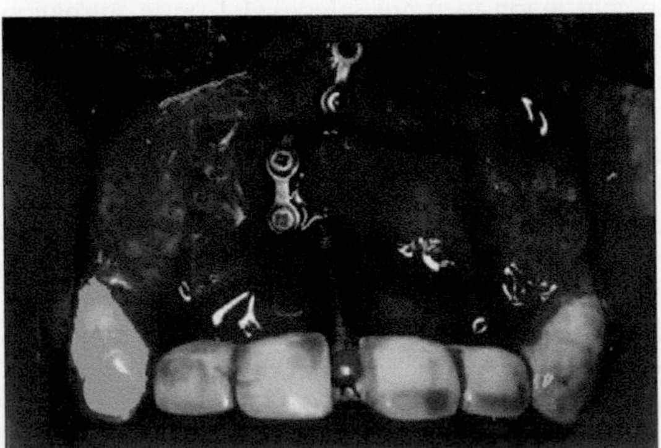

Fig. 7. Osteotomies made for vertical distraction osteogenesis of anterior maxilla. (*From* Aly LAA. Piezoelectric surgery: Applications in oral & maxillofacial surgery. Future Dental Journal 2018;4:110; with permission.)

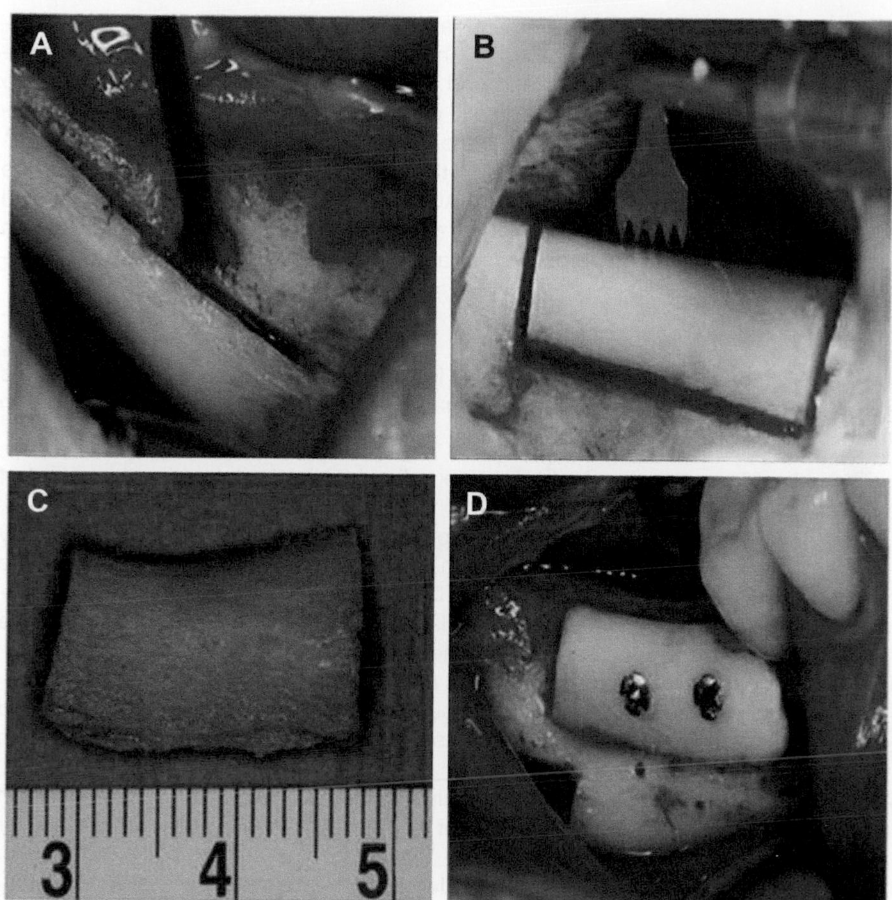

Fig. 8. Lateral ramus harvest with piezo. *(A-B)* show osteotomies made by the piezo. (*C*) shows the lateral ramus graft harvested. (*D*) shows the graft fixated to the recipient site. (*From* Aly LAA. Piezoelectric surgery: Applications in oral & maxillofacial surgery. Future Dental Journal 2018;4:109; with permission.)

THE LASER-ASSISTED NEW ATTACHMENT PROCEDURE

Laser radiation is monochromatic with directionality, coherence, and brightness. There are different types of lasers in dentistry with varying degrees of rays penetrating the tissues based on variable parameters, such as power level, pulse repetition rate, pulse width ,and energy density.[11] Its potential is affected by the absorption coefficient in water. The Nd:YAG (1064 nm) and diode (809–980 nm) are soft tissue lasers with greater depth of penetration than the carbon dioxide (10,600 nm) and Er:YAG (2940 nm) lasers. The radiation can also be in a continuous, pulsed, or running pulse form. Also interesting to note is that laser beam is infrared and invisible, so light is incorporated into the device to act as an aiming beam.[12]

Laser effects on tissues includes coagulation of tissue, hemostasis, disinfection, and detoxification by ablating bacterial endotoxins with colonization inhibition, as well as biomodulation of cells causing better healing of tissues.[13]

The paradigm of periodontal treatment has shifted from resective to more regenerative procedures over the past 2 decades. The laser-assisted new attachment procedure (LANAP) was developed by Gregg and McCarthy, with histologic criteria met to prove the regeneration of the periodontally compromised root using LANAP. Regeneration is defined as formation of new bone, cementum, and periodontal ligament.[14]

One of the first laser therapies used in this manner was introduced in 1990, the Perio-Lase MVP 7, which was an Nd:YAG 106 nm laser in free running pulsed mode. This LANAP protocol evolved in the 1990s and has been advocated in achieving bone regeneration. It received clearance from the US Food and Drug Administration in 2004.[14]

What Is the Protocol?

This LANAP has a specific protocol and is indicated for patients with pocket depths greater than or equal to 4 mm.[14] Its claimed success lies in the systematic way in which it is done:

1. The patient is anesthetized and bone sounding is done to determine the extent of infrabony pockets.
2. An optic tip measuring 0.3 to 0.4 μm is placed parallel to the root surface to carry away the epithelial lining of the pocket in a coronal to apical motion. The first pass of the laser is at 3 W with a free running 100-ms pulse. This selective photothermolysis removes unhealthy, infected, and inflamed epithelium of the pocket sparing the intact connective tissue separation of the layers of tissues at the rete pegs.
3. Ultrasonic scalers are used to clean the root surface.
4. The second pass is at 3 W at a 650-mspulse. This establishes a sticky fibrin blood clot that secures the pocket from detritus matter and perpetuates the healing from the inside out.
5. The gingival tissues are compressed against the root surfaces with no placement of sutures of surgical glue, including splint of any teeth with mobility of grade II or more.
6. Occlusal adjustments are performed to decrease the traumatic forces of occlusion.
7. Postoperative instructions are given for dietary restrictions and proper oral hygiene instruction with an emphasis on periodontal maintenance. Recall is done at 1 week, 1 month, and then every 3 months for maintenance. Probing is ruled out for 6 months to 1 year to permit tissues to heal at the cementum fiber-periodontal ligament interface.

Why Does It Work?

1. Laser energy is only absorbed by the diseased tissues.[14]
2. There is a bactericidal effect on pigmented bacteria.
3. The thermal fibrin clot secures the pocket crevice.
4. Coronal to apical movement of tissues is restricted by the clot acting as a barrier.
5. The epithelium is allowed to heal from the inside out by activation of pluripotent cells from the periodontium.

Purported Advantages of the Laser-Assisted New Attachment Procedure

1. Minimally invasive with better patient compliance.
2. Decreased postoperative pain and morbidity.
3. Less likely to develop hypersensitivity.
4. Less recession.
5. Faster healing.
6. Natural regeneration around teeth and implants.

Discussion of the Literature on the laser-assisted new attachment procedure

The first study that advocated and supported the use of LANAP was done by Yukna and colleagues[15] in 2007. It was a longitudinal, blinded study that histologically showed evidence that sites treated by LANAP displayed regeneration as opposed to no regeneration in control sites. The study showed that when infrabony pockets were treated with LANAP, new connective tissue attachments adjacent to the alveolar bone were seen, but no long junctional epithelium was observed.

In 2014, Nevins and colleagues[16] performed a prospective 9-month human clinical evaluation of LANAP therapy in which 8 patients with advanced periodontitis had 930 sites studied preoperatively and postoperatively. Clinical measurements included clinical attachment loss, probing depths, and recession. The results showed a mean decrease in probing depths by 1.48 mm, mean clinical attachment loss decrease of 0.84 mm, and a mean increase in recession of 0.66 mm. Hence, the clinical results show regeneration of periodontal attachment with the use of LANAP with a decrease in the clinical attachment loss. The authors, however, noted that further investigation with long-term clinical trials are needed to compare the stability of clinical results with conventional therapy. From these data, dentists should decide if advocating this treatment for a relatively small change in clinical attachment loss is worth offering such a treatment.

In contrast, there are some review articles in the literature that could not conclude that LANAP had better results that conventional nonsurgical periodontal treatment. An article by Shah and colleagues[12] in 2015 stated that the current literature is inconclusive owing to limited sample sizes, a lack of adequate controls, a lack of blinded studies, and the fact that most studies did not assess clinical attachment level after treatment, which is the gold standard of assessing periodontal treatment outcomes. This author proposes conventional periodontal therapies with laser therapy as an adjunct.

Cobb[11] in 2010 states in his review article that there are several systemic reviews of the literature that have suggested that there is little evidence to support the purported benefits of lasers in the solo treatment of periodontal disease compared with traditional nonsurgical periodontal therapy. This author also concludes that the body of evidence is inadequate to support evidence-based decision making. Eleven articles were reviewed evaluating LANAP versus conventional nonsurgical periodontal therapy. The data showed an average probing depth reduction of 0.09 mm between lasers and the control, a gain in clinical attachment level of 0.33 mm between lasers and controls, and no differences in reductions in bleeding on probing or subgingival microbial loads. These numbers are not statistically significant and do not support the use of lasers in the treatment of chronic periodontitis over nonsurgical periodontics.

Another review article by Behdin and colleagues[17] in 2015 studied 9 articles comparing LANAP with surgical periodontics. The parameters studied were probing depths, clinical attachment levels, and gingival recession. In flap surgery with or without laser treatment, no statistical difference in the outcomes were found. Similarly, in guided tissue regeneration with enamel matrix derivative, the mean difference in all parameters was negligible with or without laser treatment. Hence, this evidence does not support the use of dental lasers, even as an adjunct to resective or regenerative surgical periodontal therapy.

LOW-LEVEL LASER THERAPY IN THE MANAGEMENT OF TEMPOROMANDIBULAR JOINT DISORDER AND TRIGEMINAL NEUROSENSORY DEFICITS

Low-level laser are also known as soft lasers, low reactive lasers, low-energy laser, and low intensity level laser. The lower level laser therapy (LLLT) using these lasers is referred to as biostimulation or biomodulation by stimulating or suppressing a biological process.[18]

There are many different lasers used in LLLT, and they generally function between 1 and 75 mW. Examples include the helium–neon laser, the gallium–aluminum–arsenide diode laser, the gallium–arsenide diode laser, argon ion laser, the defocused CO_2 laser, and the defocused Nd:YAG laser. They all produce minor changes in surface temperature.

Personal protective equipment, particularly eye protection, should be worn when such therapies are being used. Contraindications for its use include active cancer, pregnancy, hypersensitivity to sunlight, infected wounds, and any treatment over a chest with a pacemaker.

How Does It Work?

There are various biological mechanisms that have postulated how LLLT works.[18]

- Decrease in receptor sensitivity.
- Increase in pain tolerance owing to changes in cell membrane potential.
- Shortening of the inflammation phase.
- Increase in collateral vessels.
- Increase in oxygen consumption by tissues.
- Earlier resolution of interstitial edema.
- Bactericidal effects on microflora.
- Suppressive effects on immune reactions.
- Increased enzyme activation.
- Stimulation of wound healing.
- Reduction in scar formation in nerve crush injuries.

Uses in Oral and Maxillofacial Surgery

In oral and maxillofacial surgery, LLLT has been used to treat oral pathology (such as aphthous stomatitis, aphthous ulcers, herpetic labialis, and gingivostomatitis), soft tissue injuries, mucositis, nerve repair, bone wound healing after odontectomy, pain in patients with medication-related osteonecrosis of the jaw and temporomandibular joint dysfunction. This brief section concentrates on its use in inferior alveolar nerve repair and temporomandibular joint dysfunction.

Nerve conduction effects

Inferior alveolar nerve and lingual nerve injuries can happen after third molar extraction, vestibuloplasties, bilateral sagittal split osteotomies, or trauma. Abnormalities in sensation that persist longer than 6 months leave some degree of long-term disability, with permanent damage to the trigeminal nerve expected if there is no sensory recovery within 1 year.[19]

LLLT has been advocated as a possible treatment for patients with paresthesia in the distribution of the trigeminal nerve. The hypothesis is that, when LLLT is applied to the injured peripheral nerve, it prevents a decrease in action potential, obviates scar formation, increases vascularization, mitigates degeneration of the surrounding muscle, and accelerates regeneration of the injured nerve.[18] At the molecular level, the lasers can stimulate the reinnervation by penetrating up the nerve axon or the adjacent Schwann cells, thus affecting the metabolism of the damaged neural tissues to produce proteins associated with nerve growth or causing the release of tropic factors causing ingrowth of adjacent uninjured nerves.[19] There have been various studies that have supported its use in this manner.

A recent paper by Pol and colleagues[19] in 2016 evaluated the efficacy of superpulsed LLLT on neurosensory recovery of the inferior alveolar nerve after oral surgical procedures (extractions, implants, cystectomies, orthognathic surgeries, and anesthesia). They studied 57 patients with paresthesias of the inferior alveolar nerve; group 1 had the paresthesias for less than 6 months and group 2 with paresthesias more than 6 months. Each patient underwent to 10 laser treatments with 1 per week with a gallium arsenide diode laser. The wavelength of the infrared radiation was 904 to 910 nm superpulsed at 200 ns of pulse duration applied 1 cm from the involved area 5 minutes intraorally and 5 minutes extraorally. The extent of neurosensory recovery was determined using the following parameters: soft touch, 2-point discrimination, pin prick, thermal test, as well as the visual analog scale. The control was the other nonaffected side of the patient. The results demonstrated that between 54.2% and 83.3% of patients had a significant neurosensory recovery as evident in the objective and subjective test, with such results supporting the potential of LLLT to aid in neurosensory recovery in both groups. After LLLT, the value of the visual analog scale decreased and showed a statistically significant difference. The author supports the use of LLLT owing to its noninvasive nature, good tolerance by patients, and lack of adverse effects. However, they agree that more studies are needed with larger sample sizes.

Another article by Santos and colleagues[20] in 2018 studied the effectiveness of LLLT on sensorineural recovery after sagittal split osteotomies. It was a randomized, double-blinded, split mouth design on patients who underwent bilateral sagittal split osteotomy and received LLLT on one side and a placebo on the other as the control. This study was also split into 2 groups as the previous one was; group 1 was within 30 days of the procedure with group 2 was treated 6 months after the procedure. Patients received LLLT on one side and placebo treatment on the other. All 20 patients who received LLLT in groups 1 and 2 showed marked improvement in sensorineural recovery over the course of the sessions, with group 1 showing better results. The authors concluded that LLLT was effective in the recovery from sensorineural disorders after orthognathic surgery during the short postoperative period, particularly in the fifth session. The earlier the treatment the better the results. It was also noted that the prognosis varies considerable with the degree of injury.

Miloro and Criddle[21] in 2018 published an article in the *Journal of Oral and Maxillofacial Surgery* that was a prospective, double-blinded, randomized, controlled clinical trial of patients that had inferior alveolar nerve and lingual nerve deficits. The study aimed to determine if postoperative neurosensory improvement happened over a 3-month period differed between the control group and an LLLT group. Thirty-five patients were studied with nerve injuries from third molar surgery, implant placement, or local anesthesia administration. Results were obtained from a subjective visual analog scale and objective clinical neurosensory testing. Improvement was observed in 40.7% of patients with LLLT compared with 38.5% improvement in controls with both inferior alveolar nerve and lingual nerve. No differences were noted between the study group based on time of injury to treatment. However, no statistical difference in improvement was found between the LLLT and placebo groups, so it failed to support the use of LLLT in such injuries. It is important to note that this study did not take into account the severity of the nerve injury, which could have affected the significance of the results.

Temporomandibular joint disorders

LLLT has been suggested for the management for temporomandibular joint dysfunction through its analgesic, anti-inflammatory and biostimulating effects. The mechanism of the analgesic effect, however, is not well-understood. The working hypothesis is that there are increased pain thresholds through the alteration of neural stimulation with beta endorphins and the inhibition of medullary reflexes. It is also postulated that LLLT can affect the synthesis of prostaglandin, causing arachidonic acid to enter endothelial tissues and smooth muscles allowing them to generate vasodilation and anti-inflammation.[22]

Kulekcioglu and colleagues in 2003 investigated the effectiveness of LLLT with temporomandibular joint dysfunction in patients with both a myogenic and arthrogenic components.[18] They observed significant reduction in pain, the number of tender points, increased mouth opening and lateral jaw movements in both treatment groups versus the placebo.[18]

A review article in 2014 by Chang and colleagues[22] provided a systematic review in which 7 reports were studied. The conclusion of this article was that the use of LLLT with wavelengths of 780 nm and 830 nm on the masticatory muscle or joint capsule for temporomandibular joint pain had a "moderate analgesic effect," but that the optimal parameters have not yet been determined.

Some authors have proposed laser therapy be used in combination with conventional therapies. Others doubt the validity of such claims, stating that the evidence is not convincing. A study by Emshoff and colleagues[23] in 2008 studied the effectiveness of LLLT in the management of temporomandibular joint pain during function in a random, double-blinded study. They studied 52 patients with unilateral temporomandibular joint pain that had failed conservative therapy, including warm compresses, splints, and a soft diet. These patients received 3 treatments per week of 2 minutes each at the closed and open mouth positions for 8 weeks, with one side receiving active helium–neon LLLT versus the other side receiving a sham LLLT. The probe was placed directly on the skin at the center of the upper joint space. Temporomandibular joint pain during function was evaluated at baseline, then at 2, 4, and 8 weeks after the first laser therapy. The results showed no difference in temporomandibular joint pain with function from the LLLT versus the control group in this study. This was attested to the placebo effect. The author states that a more tailored application of LLLT should be developed to take into account the multifactorial aspect of temporomandibular joint dysfunction.

It is clear that further studies are needed to support the use of LLLT in treating temporomandibular joint dysfunction. The studies need to be more specific about the type of temporomandibular joint dysfunction being treated, that is, myofacial pain versus capsulitis versus synovitis versus degenerative changes with Wilkes staging, and so on. In addition, the parameters of care for the use of such low-level laser therapy also needs to be more clearly defined.

DISCLOSURE STATEMENT

The authors have nothing to disclose regarding any financial or any sort of relationship with any commercial company or materials mentioned in this article.

REFERENCES

1. Aly LAA. Piezoelectric Surgery: Applications in oral & Maxillofacial Surgery. Future Dental Journal 2018;4:105–11.
2. Pavlikova G, Foltán R, Horká M, et al. Piezosurgery in oral and maxillofacial surgery. Int J Oral Maxillofac Surg 2011;40:451–7.
3. De Azevedo ET, Costa DL, Pryzysiezny PE, et al. Using Piezoelectric Sysmte in Oral and Maxillofacial Surgery. Int J Med Surg Sci 2015;2(3):551–5.
4. Stübinger S, Kuttenberger J, Filippi A, et al. Intraoral piezosurgery: preliminary results of a new technique. J Oral Maxillofac Surg 2005;63:1283–7.

5. Claire S, Lea SC, Walmsley AD. Characterisation of bone following ultrasonic cutting. Clin Oral Investig 2013;17(3):905–12.
6. Liu J, Hua C, Pan J, et al. Piezosurgery vs conventional rotary instrument in the third molar surgery: a systematic review and meta-analysis of randomized controlled trials. J Dent Sci 2018;13:342–9.
7. Tsai SJ, Chen YL, Chang HH, et al. Effect of piezoelectric instruments on healing propensity of alveolar sockets following mandibular third molar extraction. J Dent Sci 2012;7:296–300.
8. Schaeren S, Jaquiéry C, Heberer M, et al. Assessment of nerve damage using a novel ultrasonic device for bone cutting. J Oral Maxillofac Surg 2008;66:593–6.
9. Landes CA, Stübinger S, Ballon A, et al. Piezoosteotomy in orthognathic surgery versus conventional saw and chisel osteotomy. Oral Maxillofac Surg 2008;12: 138–47.
10. Happe A. Use of piezoelectric surgical device to harvest bone grafts from the mandibular ramus, report of 40 cases. Int J Periodontics Restorative Dent 2007;27:241–9.
11. Cobb CM. Lasers and the treatment of chronic periodontitis. Dental Clinics America 2010;54:35–53.
12. Shah AM, Khan K, Admen F, et al. A review of the use of laser in periodontal therapy. International Dental Journal of Student's Research 2015;3(2):79–82.
13. Cobb CM. Lasers in periodontics: a review of the literature. J Periodontol 2006; 77(4):545–64.
14. Jha A, Gupta V, Adinarayan R. LANAP, periodontics and beyond: a review. J Lasers Med Sci 2018;9(2):76–81.
15. Yukna RA, Carr RL, Evans GH. Histological evaluation of an Nd:YAG laser assisted new attachment procedure in humans. Int J Periodontics Restorative Dent 2007;27(6):577–87.
16. Nevins M, Kim SW, Camelo M, et al. A prospective 9 month human clinical evaluation of LANAP therapy. Int J Periodontics Restorative Dent 2014;34(1):21–7.
17. Behdin S, Monje A, Lin GH, et al. Effectiveness of laser application for periodontal surgical therapy: systematic review and meta-analysis. J Periodontol 2015; 86(12):1352–61.
18. Kahraman S. Low level laser therapy in oral and maxillofacial surgery. Oral Maxillofac Surg Clin North Am 2004;16:277–88.
19. Pol R, Gallesio G, Riso M, et al. Effects of superpulsed, low level laser therapy on neurosensory recovery of the inferior alveolar nerve. J Craniofac Surg 2016;27: 1215–9.
20. Santos FT, Sciescia R, Santos PL, et al. Is low level laser therapy effective on sensorineural recovery after bilateral sagittal split osteotomy? Randomized trial. J Oral Maxillofac Surg 2019;77:164–73.
21. Miloro M, Criddle TR. Does low level laser therapy affect recovery of lingual and inferior alveolar nerve injuries? J Oral Maxillofac Surg 2018;76:2669–75.
22. Chang WD, Lee CL, Lin HY, et al. A meta analysis of clinical effects of low level laser therapy on temporomandibular joint pain. J Phys Ther Sci 2014;26: 1297–300.
23. Emshoff R, Bösch R, Pümpel E, et al. Low level laser therapy for treatment of temporomandibular joint pain: a double-blinded and placebo-controlled trial. Oral Surg Oral Med Oral Pathol Oral Radiol Endod 2008;105:452–6.

Intraoral Scanner, Three-Dimensional Imaging, and Three-Dimensional Printing in the Dental Office

Levon Nikoyan, DDS[a,b,*], Rinil Patel, DDS[a]

KEYWORDS

• 3D scanners • 3D CBCT • 3D printers • Dental implants

KEY POINTS

- The use of three-dimensional imaging in dental office.
- Implementation of digital workflow into dental practice.
- Methods of using computer-assisted design and manufacturing in the dental practice.

INTRODUCTION AND BACKGROUND

The history and mechanism of image acquisition of cone-beam machines have been discussed in many publications.[1] Small footprint and high clinical value return set 3-dimensional (3D) cone-beam computed tomography (CBCT) apart from other technologies in the clinical setting. The use of cone-beam technology brings an unprecedented diagnostic ability to the dental setting. CBCT is at the core of the digital workflow in the dental office, and the information obtained from these machines combined with digital intraoral scanners (IOSs) and 3D printers facilitates a precise and predictable treatment.

CLINICALLY RELEVANT TECHNICAL DATA

CBCT is an invasive diagnostic modality. The terminology describing the radiation emitted during radiographic exposure and how it is measured has been recently modified.[2] Effective radiation is the most important term in everyday clinical practice. It is a

[a] Department of Dentistry and Oral and Maxillofacial Surgery, Woodhull Hospital, 760 Broadway, Brooklyn, NY 11206, USA; [b] Private Practice, Forward Oral Surgery, 248-62 Jericho Tpke, Floral Park, NY 11001, USA
* Corresponding author. Forward Oral Surgery, 248-62 Jericho Tpke, Floral Park, NY 11001.
E-mail address: levondds@gmail.com

Dent Clin N Am 64 (2020) 365–378
https://doi.org/10.1016/j.cden.2019.12.004
0011-8532/20/

measure of the radiation that is determined based on the affected type of tissue. Because organs have variable sensitivity to radiation, a so-called tissue weighting factor exists as a multiplication factor. Gonads, for example, are twice as sensitive to radiation when compared with a structure located in the head and neck region. Therefore, for the amount of exposure, the effective radiation is higher for gonads than for dentoalveolar structures. The *effective radiation* is measured in milli-Sieverts. A single periapical radiograph has an effective dose of 0.005 mSv, and an average panoramic radiograph has an effective dose of 0.02 mSv. The effective radiation dose from a cone-beam scanner is highly variable with values as low as 0.02 mSv and as high as 1.2 mSv.[3]

The other clinically essential details are the multiple projections within a given computed tomography (CT), their names, and their best uses. Just like bitewings are excellent in detecting interproximal caries, for example, some of the views within a CT are more suitable than others for a particular treatment. **Fig. 1** summarizes these views and essential uses. The terminology is consistent with medical CT scans and provides an essential method of communication between practitioners.

USE OF THREE-DIMENSIONAL IMAGING IN THE DENTAL OFFICE

General Dentistry

The use of 3D imaging in a dental office for the detection of caries remains quite limited. Two-dimensional intraoral radiographs still provide the most information for a given dose of radiation. 3D CBCT imaging, regardless of quality, results in significant artifacts (especially as the number of metal restorations nearby increases), and detection of caries, fractures, and decay is notoriously difficult with a high rate of false positives.[4] Suspected fractures when detected on 3D CBCT are generally significant enough to be visualized on plain films, whereas the smaller fractures are challenging to spot on 3D CBCT. Although the cross-section may allow better visualization of vertical and oblique fractures, the use of 3D CBCT for the detection of fractures remains to be improved. Recently, software advances have improved artifact reduction and provide better caries detection and a decrease in false positives.[5]

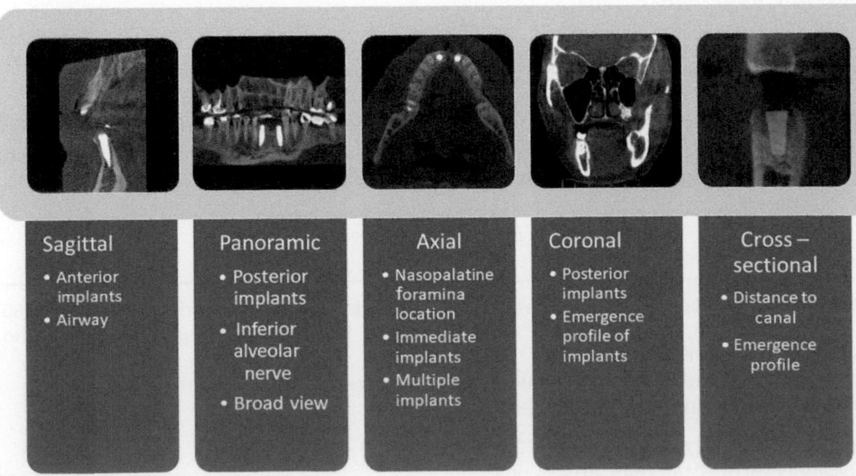

Sagittal
• Anterior implants
• Airway
Panoramic
• Posterior implants
• Inferior alveolar nerve
• Broad view
Axial
• Nasopalatine foramina location
• Immediate implants
• Multiple implants
Coronal
• Posterior implants
• Emergence profile of implants
Cross – sectional
• Distance to canal
• Emergence profile

Fig. 1. Different views from 3D CBCT.

Endodontics

The use of cone-beam imaging is quite widespread in endodontics. In particular, the small field-of-view imaging has gained increasing popularity in practice.[6] This type of imaging has a distinct advantage in dental anatomy representation, decreases radiographic artifacts, and is better able to evaluate healing after endodontic treatment. 3D imaging in endodontics also provides better reduction in the incidence of missed canals and avoidance of complications involving maxillofacial structures. It is also likely that the use of cone beam increases diagnoses of lesions suspected to be pathologic but is in fact superimposition of normal anatomy (maxillary sinus, nasopalatine duct, salivary gland depression). The most significant challenges in the use of CBCT in endodontics is the initial expense of ownership, lack of standardized protocol adopted by practitioners, and liability associated with the sheer volume of diagnostic information. The cost of ownership can be overcome by the availability of equipment financing options offered by many dental suppliers. The American Association of Endodontics has published excellent position papers on the appropriate use of CBCT in the initial diagnosis as well as endodontic treatment.[7] However, in-office rigid radiographic treatment protocols are needed to provide treatment that is consistent with the ALARA principle (as low as reasonably achievable) and maximizes patient care. In what clinical situations and for what teeth requiring endodontic treatment will the cone beam be taken? Is cone beam to be used during the root canal treatment, such as verification of canals or only diagnosis? How would that happen logistically and still keep the field sterile? Is the cone beam to be used for posttreatment evaluation, and if so, what is the plan if adverse treatment is detected radiographically?

When interpreting 3D imaging, the clinician is exposed to considerable diagnostic liability. To successfully interpret cone-beam radiographs, the dentist needs a thorough understanding of head-neck anatomy and a solid background in 3D radiology. Although many dental schools have acquired cone-beam machines, the incorporation of this advanced imaging modality into the curriculum is slow and is taught without integration with patient care.[8] This liability can be further minimized by obtaining a radiology interpretation of the cone beam and by reducing the field of view to include only the area of importance.

Oral Surgery

The use of 3D CBCT for dental and oral maxillofacial surgery is quite common. Most common indications are visualization of root structures of teeth and their proximity to anatomical structures (such as maxillary sinuses and the inferior alveolar canal). When considering dental surgery and the use of 3D CBCT, there are certain assumptions that are made by general dentists, surgeons, and patients that have not been validated by clinical research. First and foremost, obtaining the 3D CBCT itself does not affect the overall risk of complications associated with the inferior alveolar nerve.[9] Second, even with the use of cone-beam technology, there is almost no change in technique for the extraction of wisdom teeth.[10,11] In most instances, the same surgical principles are used whether the mandibular canal is on the buccal or the lingual. Some practitioners find CBCT useful in deciding between coronectomy and extraction.[12] 3D CBCT remains a technologically advanced tool and should not be used solely to determine the management of third molars. The treatment is determined based on a multitude of factors, such as the presence of disease, pain, and pericoronitis.[13] In the most severe impaction cases whereby the patient would not accept the small risk of a neurosensory deficit, there is no need to obtain a cone beam, and the 2-dimensional panoramic radiographic image is sufficient because the treatment approach is not changed.

The Use of Three-Dimensional Imaging in a Dental Office to Detect Pathologic Condition

CBCT can also aid in the management of oral and maxillofacial pathologic condition. CBCT has poor soft tissue differentiation, and its use in the management of malignancies remains limited. Dentoalveolar pathologic condition, however, is an excellent indication for 3D CBCT. **Fig. 2** shows a section of the cone beam for a patient with odontogenic keratocyst immediately after decompression.

Arguably the first method of formulating the pathologic differential diagnosis should be a 2-dimensional film, and if it does not allow enough visualization, then a 3D CBCT should be obtained. The cone beam provides better localization and better quality of the image so that the differential diagnosis can be more realistic. **Fig. 3** demonstrated a panoramic image of the pathologic lesion found on orthodontic examination and failure of adult teeth eruption. The same patient after 3D CBCT (**Figs. 4** and **5**) was obtained; note both of the premolars and the location of the actual lesion are now visible. This type of image significantly improves the ease of surgical access.

USE OF THREE-DIMENSIONAL CONE-BEAM COMPUTED TOMOGRAPHY FOR DENTAL IMPLANTS

The mainstream use of cone-beam imaging remains for dental implants. There are specific advantages that 3D imaging provides when considering placing dental implants. For this section, the authors separate implant treatment into planning, the actual procedure for dental implants, and the detection of potential complications associated with dental implants.

The planning for dental implants is significantly more predictable with the use of cone beam. The use of CBCT provides a more efficient workflow in dental practice. For example, a patient who needs dental implants obtains a 3D CBCT in the dental office. The dentist uses a variety of available software to review the 3D radiograph, plans

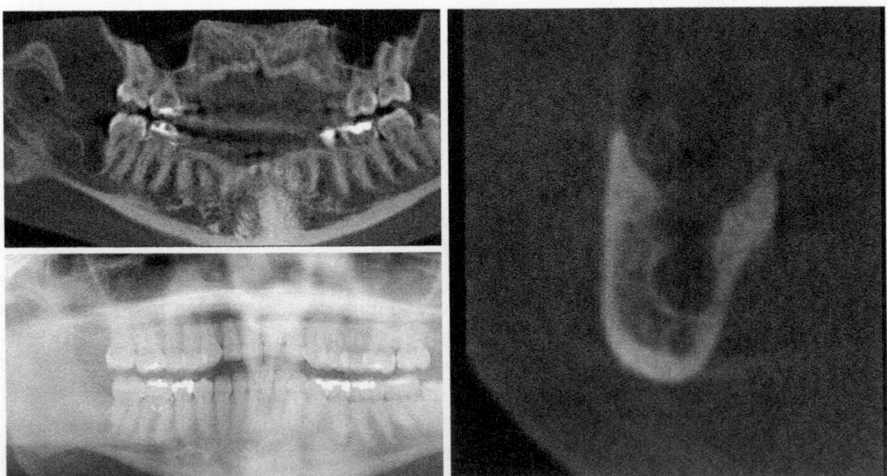

Fig. 2. Pan lower left. CT upper left and cross-section right.

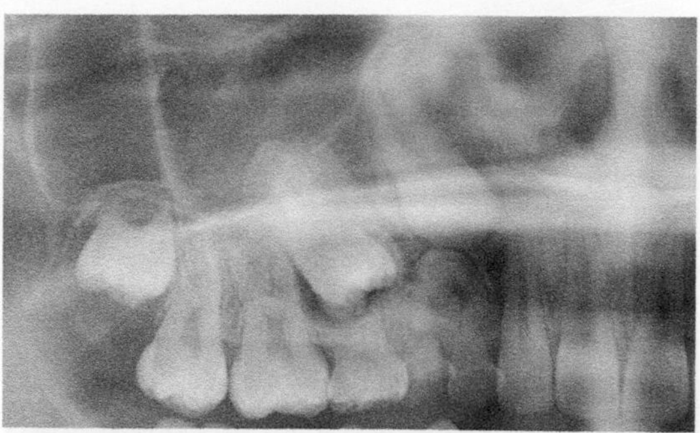

Fig. 3. Plain film. Is there a premolar missing?

the dental implant placement while virtually determining the size, length, and width of the dental implant, then assures that this actual implant is available in stock and schedules the appointment for the surgery. This workflow eliminates the need for having a significant number of different implant sizes in stock, reduces the overall expense, and provides a better and more efficient workflow.

The cone-beam imaging provides predictable planning for dental implant surgery. Because no magnification is present, the exact width and length of the implant can be determined. The implant can be planned virtually on a variety of available software, and many possible complications can be predicted ahead of time. Many of the modern computer programs also provide a method to place a virtual crown, further improving the position of the implant. Because implant surgery is a restoratively driven procedure, the virtual crown presents an opportunity to visualize the simulated final result and interact with implant components to anticipate the need for custom components and restorative complications (**Fig. 6**).

Finally, **Fig. 7** summarizes important anatomic considerations that every implant surgeon must have in mind when preparing for the procedure.

In the most severe cases whereby buccolingual and vertical control is needed to avoid vital anatomic structures, cone beam combined with guided surgery is an excellent strategy to provide consistently safe and reproducible results. The use of guides for implant surgery has exploded, although, initially, when surgical guides came into existence, they were nothing more than suck-down stents with an access hole through the middle of the tooth. These guides were the methods of communication between the restorative dentist and the surgeon. From the surgical point of view, these guides were of minimal use, and they were quite often used for the first few minutes of the surgery to mark the osteotomy and were rapidly discarded afterward.

Furthermore, these guides did not account for local anatomy or bone resorption and provided no vertical control for the fixture. Occasionally, the general dentist placed radiopaque material within the proposed path of the osteotomy. When combined with cone beam, these guides would confirm the position of alveolar bone along the osteotomy path. The most significant limitation of these guides is the lack of flexibility. Mainly, the guide has limited value if the alveolar bone is not within the marked path, because modifications to the surgical protocol are not possible.

Currently, the most popular types of guides combine dentition scans (obtained conventionally or by scanning the dentition with an IOS) with the 3D imaging. These guides usually have an opening to accept manufacturer-specific metal cylinders to control precise width. It is also possible to obtain the pilot-only guide to accommodate the pilot drill only. Regardless of which of these options was chosen, these guides provide information gathered from a patient-specific 3D radiograph. Currently, many

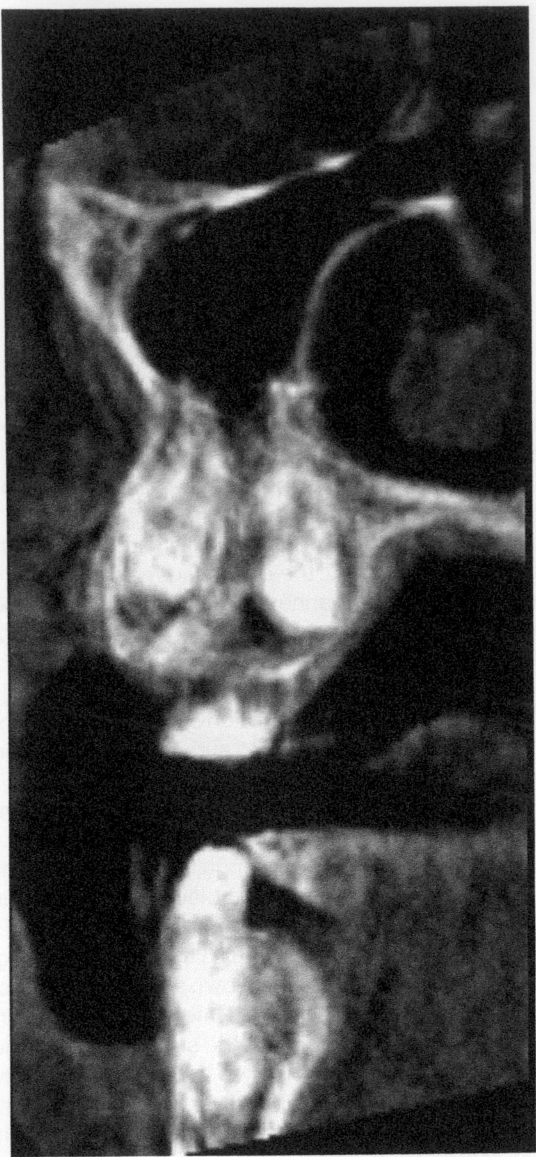

Fig. 4. Cross-section view.

dental implant companies have guided surgical kits that allow different sizes of cylinders to be inserted into the surgical guide with a specific goal of controlling the width and direction from the very first drill until the insertion of the implant. Furthermore, when a guided surgical kit is used, generally speaking, the vertical position of the implant would be controlled as well as the guided surgical kit, allowing the control of the depth when the actual implant is inserted. Therefore, it is possible now to control not only the angulation of the implant but also the vertical depth, which is critical not only for successful implant-retained prosthesis but also if any temporization is intended.

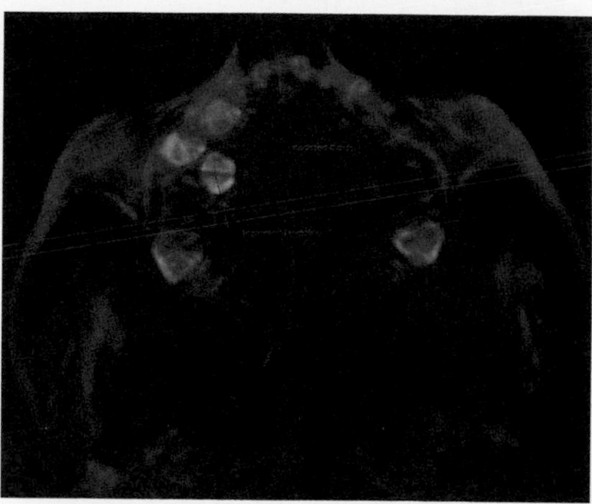

Fig. 5. Axial view.

Cases requiring multiple dental implants with extractions and immediate temporization are the most complex implant procedures. The success of the immediate temporary is directly dependent on precise dental implant placement in the vertical and horizontal plane and the quality of the initial impression. Although it is possible to freehand these surgeries and then use trial and error to find appropriate multiunit abutments, the predictability of such an approach is quite limited. **Fig. 8** illustrates a case whereby dental implants were placed without regard for the final restoration, without preoperative 3D CBCT, and without accessing the initial maxillomandibular relationship. **Fig. 9** shows multiple views of a well-planned case executed with immediate temporization.

To successfully deliver a multi-implant retained provisional with cross-arch stability (such as hybrid restoration), a CT-based guided approach is needed. The entire case

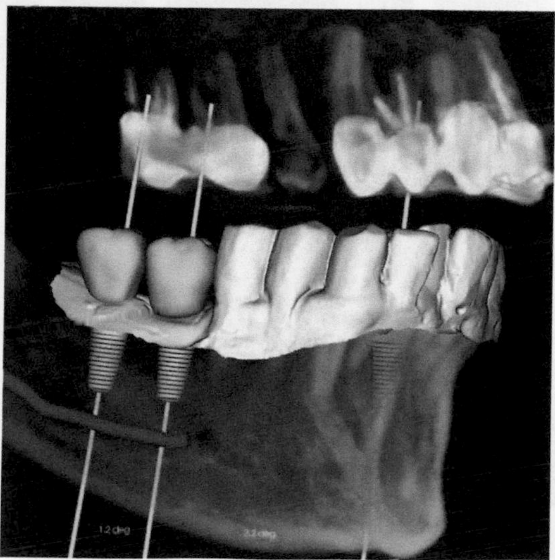

Fig. 6. Dental implants, virtual crowns, and superimposed model.

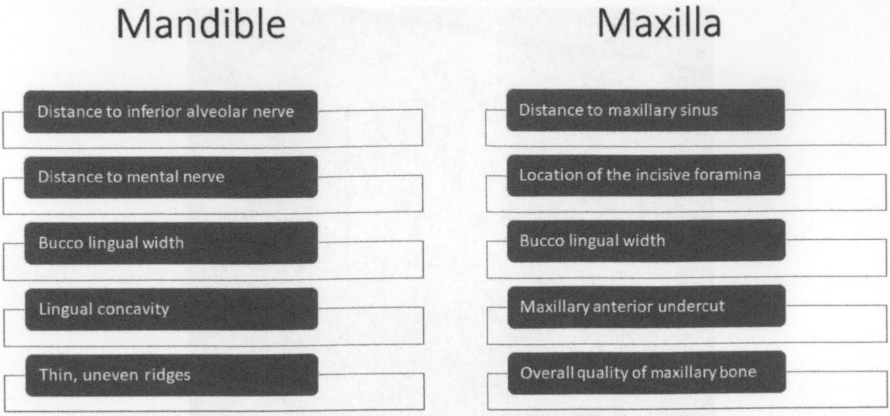

Mandible

- Distance to inferior alveolar nerve
- Distance to mental nerve
- Bucco lingual width
- Lingual concavity
- Thin, uneven ridges

Maxilla

- Distance to maxillary sinus
- Location of the incisive foramina
- Bucco lingual width
- Maxillary anterior undercut
- Overall quality of maxillary bone

Fig. 7. Important anatomic considerations for implant surgery.

(just like a single unit implant) is planned with the final restoration in mind. **Fig. 10** summarizes the required steps in chronologic order.

Although the use of surgical guides provides consistent and safe surgery, it also increases the cost and delays the overall treatment time. With the conventional method of planning, it takes approximately 3 weeks to have the manufactured guide in the office ready for surgery. Although implant surgery is not an urgent procedure, there is a significant waiting time needed for osteointegration, and required extra time for guide

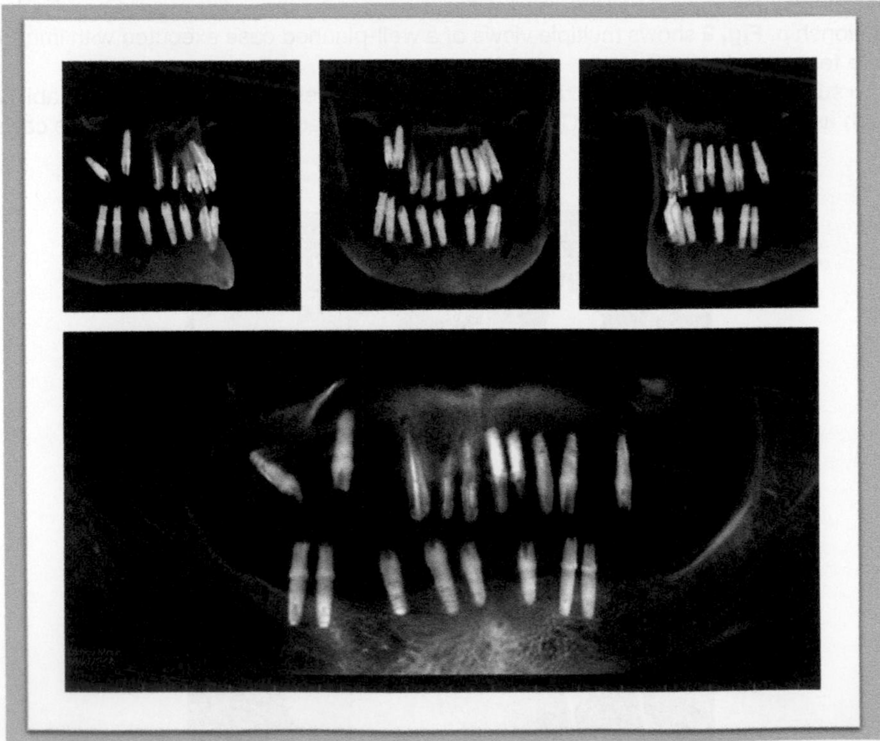

Fig. 8. Poorly planned case. CT taken 5 years after initial treatment.

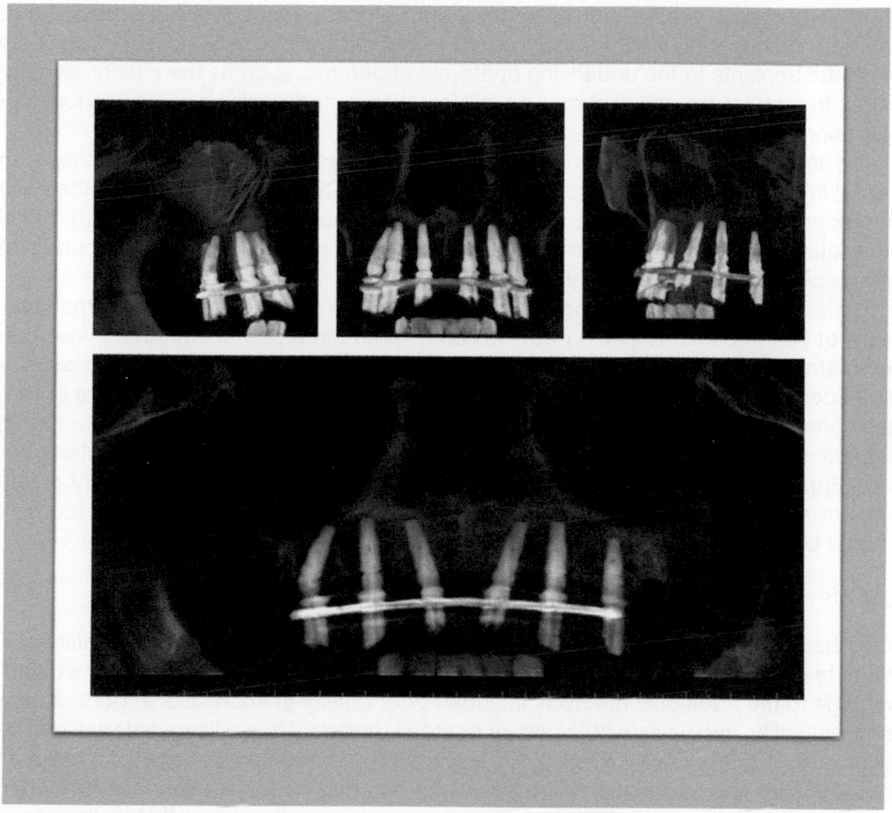

Fig. 9. Case planned with 3D CBCT, guided immediately temporized.

manufacturing adds to the overall patient anxiety and anticipation. There is also an inherent error that occasionally influences the precision of surgical guides. The 3D printed surgical guide is only as good as the quality of the obtained cone beam and registry of the patient's dentition. It is, therefore, important that the practitioner understands how to identify potential problems with the guide (such as the guide not fitting, a discrepancy in the implant platform position from clinically acceptable position) and has a viable plan of action if that guide does represent patient's actual, current situation. A patient's 3D CBCT should always be available for review, and a viable backup plan should exist.

The use of 3D CBCT imaging is also applicable in postoperative visualization of implant placement and early detection of potential problems with dental implants. The use of 3D CBCT immediately postoperatively provides a unique display of the

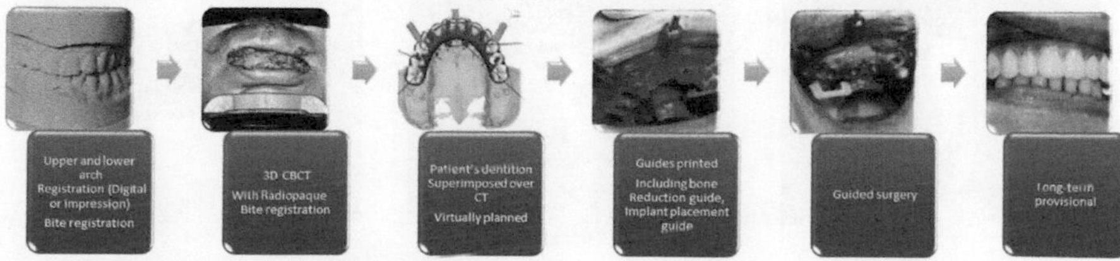

Fig. 10. Workflow for complex implant cases.

angle, emergence profile, as well as the depth of the implant. Another advantage of having a postoperative dental scan would include visualization of possible proximity of dental implants to the underlying anatomic structures, such as the inferior alveolar nerve. Immediate treatment should be implemented if compression of the inferior alveolar nerve is detected.[14]

The use of cone-beam imaging for the detection of early and late complications with dental implants has been discussed extensively. 3D CBCT could be used in the early postoperative healing period to visualize better complications associated with dental integration. Soft tissue ingrowth and development of periapical pathologic condition are visible on cone-beam imaging (**Fig. 11**).

Furthermore, cone-beam imaging could be used in early diagnosis and management of peri-implantitis. When detected early, premature peri-implant bone loss can be treated more effectively. The cross-sectional images of peri-implant bone loss provide specific areas of bone loss, the number of threads of the implant that are potentially affected, as well as help to develop a better management plan. In late dental implant complications, it is critical to identify if the failure is surgical or prosthetic in nature (**Fig. 12**). Although there are many different types of surgical management of late implant-related complications, removal of the implant, bone graft, and replacement should be considered as well.[15]

USE OF INTRAORAL SCANNERS IN THE DENTAL OFFICE

IOSs have become an alternative way of capturing dental impressions. Traditionally, alginate impressions were taken and poured into plaster or stone models. The disadvantage to the traditional methods included poor quality of impressions, poor dimensional stability, and voids within plaster or stone models. These disadvantages can be eliminated with the use of IOSs. IOSs incorporate a handheld camera to capture an image in standard tessellation language (STL), a computer to download the formatted image, and software to analyze and allow the user to view the image.[16] With the use of IOSs, dentists can better evaluate anatomic structures, formulate treatment plans, and communicate with other clinicians and technicians.

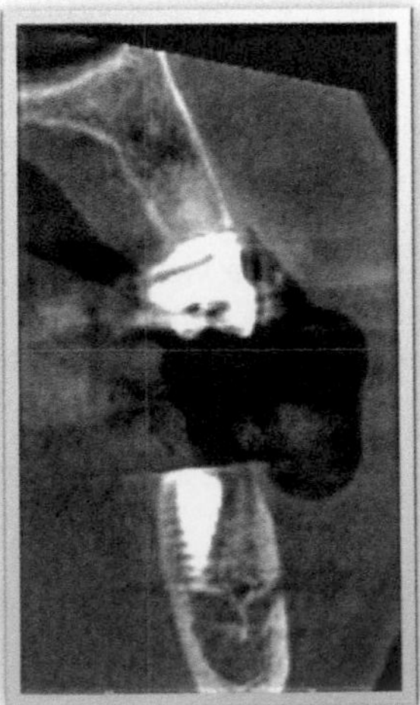
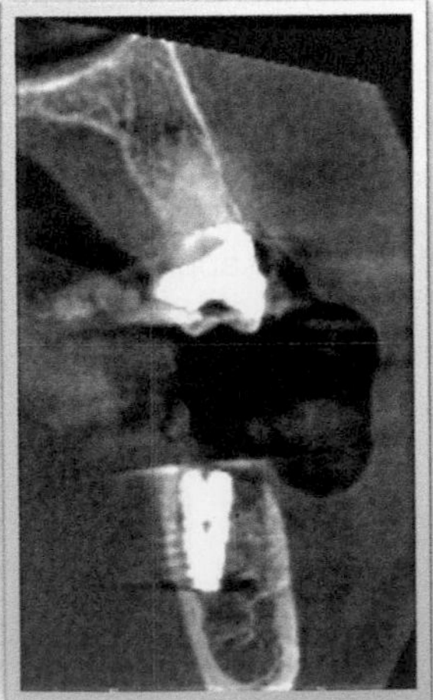
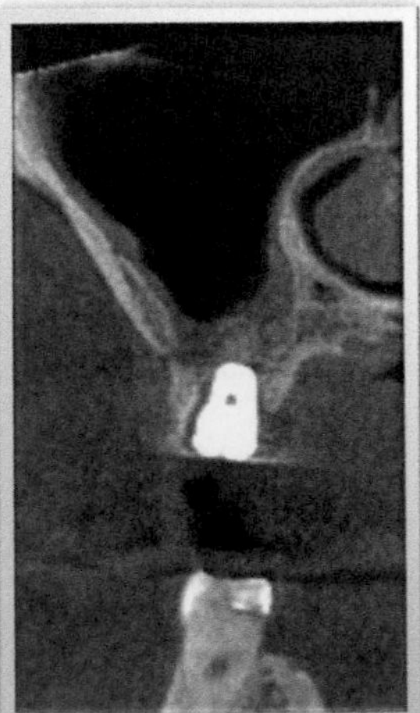

Fig. 11. Cross-sectional images of early failure. Note radiolucency around the implants.

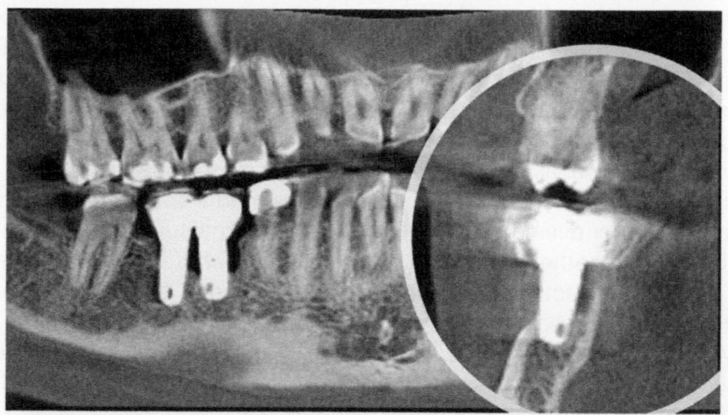

Fig. 12. Late implant failure. Note loss of bone on the buccal and lingual.

The first step in taking an impression with an IOS depends on the type of camera. When capturing dental tissues, the reflective or polished surfaces may prevent the software from triangulating specific points of interest (POI) to one another. To overcome this, the user must either change the orientation of the camera, use a camera with a polarizing filter, or powder-coat the dental tissue.[16,17] Once the oral cavity is ready to be captured, IOSs work by projecting a light source onto an object, which is then analyzed and converted by software to create POI. The POIs are then triangulated with each other to create a 3D model.[16,17] These POIs are transferred to the computer and converted into an STL-file type. Although other file formats exist, STL is the most common and widely used. The STL file is then loaded on specialized software to render the original image and to allow changes to be made before the 3D printing process begins.

IOSs have several advantages: they decrease patient discomfort, allow for better communication with the dental technician and patients, simplify clinical procedures, decrease the need for plaster casts, and are time efficient. However, disadvantages include difficulty detecting deep margins on prepared teeth, the learning curve associated with its use, and the initial costs of the technology. However, 1 study comparing the estimated costs of digital impressions and conventional impressions estimated $37.66 and $102.10 per patient, respectively.[17,18]

THREE-DIMENSIONAL PRINTING

The age of digital dentistry is now and not in the future. Modern digital technology affects everyday clinical practice. Even the most conservative and technologically unsavvy dentist is dependent on technology like computer-assisted design and computer-assisted manufacturing (CAD/CAM), stereolithography (SLA), and STL. Even if the dental practice is entirely free of digital scanners and printers, and the only method of impressions is conventional, most of the laboratories convert the "analog" impression into digital on the initial workup.

3D printing technology as a concept of volumetric object generation is not new.[19] CAD/CAM began in dentistry as a closed, all-in-one system, such as CEREC (Dentsply Sirona). Over the past 20 years, there has been a shift to more open and compatible systems that allow communication of multiple separate components. This transition enables a multitude of image acquisition devices (IOSs, CT scans) to be used to generate and transfer the images to printing devices. Most of the modern IOSs can produce and export to SLA format (STL), and most SLA printers can handle dental applications. SLA is not the only 3D printing technology available to generate plastics. Currently, 2 other 3D printing technologies for plastics exist: fused deposition modeling (FDM) and selective laser sintering.[20] FDM is the most widely used technology in consumer-level modeling. SLA is the most commonly used technology to generate clinically relevant models in medicine and dentistry. Most recently, the Formlabs (Formlabs, Somerville, MA, USA) SLA printer has gained popularity in dental practice because of its lower cost of initial investment, smaller size, and ease of use. The manufacturer even has a return on investment calculator.[21] The most important question is not whether to use the technology, but whether to outsource the SLA printing of plastics products or incorporate it into practice. It is not an easy question to answer and cannot be reliably obtained from a simple questioner. The type of dental practice, willingness to engage the "technology," and hidden costs involved are all important considerations. A more practical method of estimation is to simulate a workflow for office and imagine doing it every day (**Fig. 13**).

DIGITAL WORKFLOW FOR DENTAL IMPLANTS

Establishing a completely digital workflow requires the utilization of every component, no outsourcing, and the most significant initial expense and training. A digital IOS is used to capture the patient's dentition. Cone-beam 3D CBCT is obtained, and in the implant planning, software images from the scanner and cone beam are combined. The software is used to "clean up" and remove artifacts and to plan the final implant-retained restoration and the implant placement based on the intended restoration. A surgical guide is designed in the software and sent to the 3D printer in house. If provisional is planned, it is also sent to the printer. The manufactured guide is used to place the implants in the intended position, and the patient enters the healing stage. The generated data are saved and can be used in the future. After the healing period, a new intraoral scan is needed to register the soft tissue changes that occurred during the healing period. The final restoration is designed and printed, or the final design file can be transferred to a dental laboratory for milling. The process outlined above can be an overwhelming one. There are many aspects of the workflow that require special

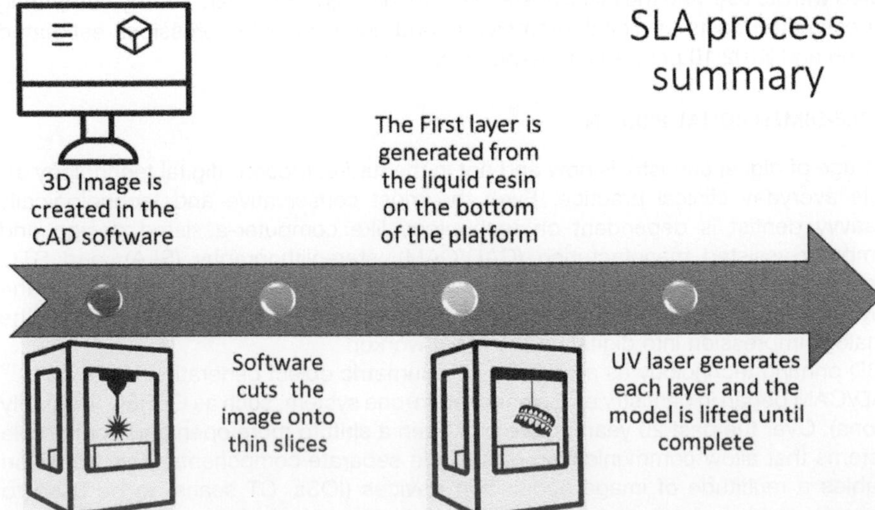

Fig. 13. Three-dimensional printer workflow.

consideration: purchasing all the required components, installation, consumable supplies, and software needed to communicate between scanners, cone beams, and printers. One of the most important additional considerations is the human factor. There is a learning curve involved and time required in scanning, designing, and delivering the fully digital components. Who is responsible for each of these steps, and will this flow take away the dentist's valuable time in actively treating patients?

Method 2 is a hybrid between a fully digital office and an "analog" one. It uses some but not all of the components of the digital workflow. Which equipment one uses would depend on the availability and the comfort level of the practitioner. In a modern implant practice, for example, the practitioner may have an intraoral 3D scanner, CT scan, and all of the software needed to plan and design the components but not the 3D printer. In that case, after gathering all of the information, the 3D scan data (in DICOM) and STL files are sent to the guide production laboratory.

SUMMARY

The use of the 3D CBCT imaging dental office has become unquestionably a common imaging modality. The authors have discussed multiple treatments that would benefit from the use of this technology. Furthermore, they have outlined how cone-beam technology fits into the overall digital workflow. Because digital dentistry is still relatively new, many dentists have not fully incorporated every part of this flow into their practices. Dental implant surgery can be performed without the use of a cone-beam or any of the components of the digital workflow. However, as the expectations of the implant dentistry are further increased, the surgery of placement of implants becomes complicated and increasingly precise. Nowhere is it truer than for full arch restorations. When performed without any of the components of the digital workflow, this approach will lead to more extensive surgical exposure (more pain and swelling), the greater stock of restorative components needed, and significantly more chair-side required to temporize the treatment. The advances in the digital workflow now make it possible to predictably treat these cases in a relatively expeditious fashion and lower stress environment for the dentist.

DISCLOSURE STATEMENT

The authors have nothing to disclose.

REFERENCES

1. Nasseh I, Al-Rawi W. Cone beam computed tomography. Dent Clin North Am 2018;62(3):361–91.
2. Hicks D, Melkers M, Barna J, et al. Comparison of the accuracy of CBCT effective radiation dose information in peer-reviewed journals and dental media. Gen Dent 2019;67(3):38–46.
3. Smith-Bindman R, Lipson J, Marcus R, et al. Radiation dose associated with common computed tomography examinations and the associated lifetime attributable risk of cancer. Arch Intern Med 2009;169(22):2078–86.
4. Wenzel A. Radiographic display of carious lesions and cavitation in approximal surfaces: advantages and drawbacks of conventional and advanced modalities. Acta Odontol Scand 2014;72(4):251–64.
5. Gaalaas L, Tyndall D, Mol A, et al. Ex vivo evaluation of new 2D and 3D dental radiographic technology for detecting caries. Dentomaxillofac Radiol 2016; 45(3):20150281.

6. Scarfe WC, Levin MD, Gane D, et al. Use of cone beam computed tomography in endodontics. Int J Dent 2009;2009:634567.
7. Fayad MI. The impact of cone beam computed tomography in endodontics: new era in diagnosing and treatment planing. In: Endodontics: colleagues in excellence. American Association of Endodontists; 2018.
8. Parashar V, Whaites E, Monsour P, et al. Cone beam computed tomography in dental education: a survey of US, UK, and Australian dental schools. J Dent Educ 2012;76(11):1443–7.
9. Petersen LB, Vaeth M, Wenzel A. Neurosensoric disturbances after surgical removal of the mandibular third molar based on either panoramic imaging or cone beam CT scanning: a randomized controlled trial (RCT). Dentomaxillofac Radiol 2016;45(2):20150224.
10. Manor Y, Abir R, Manor A, et al. Are different imaging methods affecting the treatment decision of extractions of mandibular third molars? Dentomaxillofac Radiol 2017;46(1):20160233.
11. Aravindaksha SP, Balasundaram A, Gauthier B, et al. Does the use of cone beam CT for the removal of wisdom teeth change the surgical approach compared with panoramic radiography? J Oral Maxillofac Surg 2015;73(9):e12.
12. Matzen LH, Christensen J, Hintze H, et al. Influence of cone beam CT on treatment plan before surgical intervention of mandibular third molars and impact of radiographic factors on deciding on coronectomy vs surgical removal. Dentomaxillofac Radiol 2013;42(1):98870341.
13. Management of third molar teeth. American Association of Oral and Maxillofacial Surgeons; 2016. Available at: http://www.aaoms.org/docs/govt_affairs/advocacy_white_papers/management_third_molar_white_paper.pdf.
14. Steinberg MJ, Kelly PD. Implant-related nerve injuries. Dent Clin North Am 2015;59(2):357–73.
15. Matsumoto W, Morelli VG, de Almeida RP, et al. Removal of implant and new rehabilitation for better esthetics. Case Rep Dent 2018;2018:9379608.
16. Richert R, Goujat A, Venet L, et al. Intraoral scanner technologies: a review to make a successful impression. J Healthc Eng 2017;2017:8427595.
17. Mangano F, Gandolfi A, Luongo G, et al. Intraoral scanners in dentistry: a review of the current literature. BMC Oral Health 2017;17(1):149.
18. Resnick CM, Doyle M, Calabrese CE, et al. Is it cost effective to add an intraoral scanner to an oral and maxillofacial surgery practice? J Oral Maxillofac Surg 2019;77(8):1687–94.
19. Duret F, Preston JD. CAD/CAM imaging in dentistry. Curr Opin Dent 1991;1(2):150–4.
20. Cho W, Job AV, Chen J, et al. A review of current clinical applications of three-dimensional printing in spine surgery. Asian Spine J 2018;12(1):171–7.
21. Formlabs I. ROI 2019. Available at: https://formlabs.com/roi/. Accessed July 01, 2019.

Neuropathic Pain and Burning Mouth Syndrome

An Overview and Current Update

Harry Dym, DDS[a,*], Spencer Lin, DMD[b], Jaykrishna Thakkar, DDS[a]

KEYWORDS

- Burning mouth syndrome • Glossodynia • Trigeminal neuropathic conditions

KEY POINTS

- Burning mouth syndrome/glossodynia and trigeminal neuropathic conditions can have serious negative impact on a patient's overall quality of life.
- These conditions are often hard to diagnose and even harder to fully treat and manage, but it is important for dentists/oral and maxillofacial surgeons to be aware of these conditions and modalities of their treatment.
- Often the only method for arriving at the proper diagnosis is for patients to undergo traditional approaches for treatment of presenting signs and symptoms, and it is the unexpected failure of interventional therapies that leads ultimately to a proper diagnosis.

The overwhelming reason that causes most patients to visit the dentist or oral and maxillofacial surgeon is the onset (either acute or chronic) of some form of orofacial pain. Clinicians who wish to develop a successful practice must be knowledgeable in performing a thorough systematic head/neck and oral examination as well as in interpreting appropriate imaging studies so as to be able to arrive at the correct diagnosis in order to properly alleviate the patient's pain.

The predominant cause of most patients' orofacial pain upon visiting a dental/oral surgery provider will be of dental or periodontal origin. Patients presenting with pain secondary to a temporomandibular joint disorder (TMD) is another frequent reason for patients seeking respite from their facial pain. TMD involves the masticatory system, the temporomandibular joint (TMJ), or more commonly a combination of the two. The National Institutes of Health reported in 2014 that the prevalence of TMD with signs and symptoms range from 5% to 12%, based on studies from around the globe.[1]

Other possible causes of oral/facial pain are sinus conditions, salivary infections, headaches, migraines, vascular disorders, and neuropathic pain syndromes. Patients

[a] Dentistry and Oral & Maxillofacial Surgery, The Brooklyn Hospital Center, 121 DeKalb Avenue, Brooklyn, NY 11201, USA; [b] Division of Oral and Maxillofacial Surgery, Woodhull Medical Center, 710 Flushing Avenue, Brooklyn, New York 11206, USA

* Corresponding author. The Brooklyn Hospital Center, Outpatient Care Building, 1st Floor 121 DeKalb Avenue, Brooklyn, NY 11201.

E-mail address: hdym@tbh.org

Dent Clin N Am 64 (2020) 379–399

https://doi.org/10.1016/j.cden.2019.12.009

dental.theclinics.com

0011-8532/20/

with chronic facial pain are often also plagued with comorbidities, such as depression, anxiety, along with other chronic pain disorders.

This article focuses on 2 distinct subjects: burning mouth syndrome (BMS)/glossodynia and trigeminal neuropathic conditions. Both of these entities can have serious negative impact on a patient's overall quality of life. These conditions are often hard to diagnose and even harder to fully treat and manage, but it is important for dentists/oral and maxillofacial surgeons to be aware of these conditions and modalities of their treatment. It is not unusual for patients who suffer from trigeminal neuropathic pain to have undergone almost full-mouth root canal therapy only to have all their teeth extracted in a desperate attempt to alleviate their chronic orofacial (neuropathic) pain. Often the only method for arriving at the proper diagnosis is for patients to undergo traditional approaches for treatment of presenting signs and symptoms, and it is the unexpected failure of interventional therapies that ultimately leads to a proper diagnosis.

NEUROPATHIC PAIN

Neuropathic pain is currently defined by the International Association for the Study of Pain as pain caused by a lesion or disease of the somatosensory nervous system.[2–4] The neuropathic pain may present as a dysesthesia or pain from normally nonpainful stimuli. It may be continuous or episodic in nature. By neuropathy, the authors mean a continuous pain signal generated within the nervous system without adequate stimulation of the peripheral sensory neurons. This article reviews various chronic neuropathic pain conditions.

Central Pain Syndrome

Central sensitized pain is defined as increased or amplification of pain within the central nervous system (CNS) that causes pain hypersensitivity and that causes an increased painful response to painful stimuli and nonpainful stimuli, referred to as hyperalgesia and Allodyna. This disease process starts and is perpetuated by the CNS. This disorder may be caused by inflammation, structural mechanisms, and central causes.[5,6]

Patients are diagnosed with centralized pain by the duration and distribution of the pain. If the patient has developed pain for the last 3 months that is consecutive and widespread. These symptoms should also be in addition to sleep disturbance, fatigue, and changes in mood. This disease process can only be diagnosed after a peripheral cause of pain has been ruled out as a diagnosis.[7]

After performing a thorough examination and recording the duration, severity, and location of pain, the provider must perform a thorough musculoskeletal examination and laboratory testing, which includes a complete blood count, erythrocyte sedimentation rate, or a C-reactive protein level. These diagnostic laboratory tests provide a measure of the acute phase response.

According to the European Federation of Neurological Sciences guidelines from 2010, the pharmacologic treatment of centralized neuropathic pain includes tricyclic antidepressants (TCAs) as the first line of treatment, gabapentin, and lamotrigine. Other pharmacologic treatments that have been used include phenytoin, carbamazepine, and clonazepam. Transcutaneous electrical nerve stimulation has been shown to provide alleviation.[8] Surgical intervention is only appropriate after noninvasive methods have failed.

NEUROPATHIC PAIN MECHANISMS

Deafferentation Pain

Through various methods, such as inflammation, injury, and trauma, afferent fibers can become sensitized. Usually this pain is self-limiting and resolves after inflammation and swelling have resolved. In cases where pain is caused by disease or permanent loss of afferent fibers (deafferentation), this pain will progress as central in nature. "This pain modality usually occurs when intact nerve roots, tracts, and nerves are partially or entirely disrupted. This usually occurs after trauma or peripheral nerve injury. This phenomenon can also be present after formation of lesions along central tracts or damage to posterior rootlets."[9]

To the dentist or oral surgeon, it is possible to have patients experience deafferentation pain after an extraction or endodontic procedure. Both of these procedures cause the removal of nerve tissue from/with the tooth. Most patients complain of dull and aching pain, sharp needlelike pain, or burning sensation. The painful sensation is caused by "hypersensitivity of the central neurons, damaged cells, decrease in inhibition, and increase in facilitation at the lesion site."[9] Patients report alleviation of this pain with the help of local anesthetics. Deafferent pain is resistant to morphine treatment but affected by barbiturates.

Patients who have undergone radical neck dissections and have had branches of the trigeminal nerve sacrificed may present with deafferentation pain.

Sympathetic Mediated Pain

Triggered by the autonomic nervous system, "[s]ympathetic mediated pain results from a nociceptive process rather than a noxious stimuli." Signaling begins in the afferent pathway by catecholamines. A-1 adrenoreceptors are increased in the skin of chronic pain conditions, thus increasing sympathetic mediation. Sympathetic neurotransmitters do not activate sensory nerves; however, when the sensory nerves are sensitized because of injury or chronic pain situations, the nerve upregulates the receptors to respond to sympathetic signals. This sympathetic pain presents as flushing, abnormal skin temperature in the painful area, and sweating.[10,11]

Traumatic injury can lead to a chronic pain condition called complex regional pain syndrome (CRPS), which is characterized by continuous pain and hyperalgesia. The efferent pathway continues sympathetic activation, thus continuing the release of catecholamines and facilitating pain.[9] CRPS is thought to be caused by damage to the peripheral and central nervous systems. A surgical procedure (even minor procedures) can in certain individuals act to heighten this condition. This condition following oral procedures has been called "painful traumatic trigeminal neuropathy."

Glossopharyngeal Neuralgia

Glossopharyngeal neuralgia is a far rarer neuropathic condition that involves the distribution of the glossopharyngeal nerve. Like Trigeminal Neuralgia, it is sudden, severe, and most commonly unilateral. Patients feel a stabbing pain along the glossopharyngeal nerve, such as the ear, base of tongue, tonsillar fossa, and beneath the angle of the mandible. The pain can be triggered by yawning, swallowing, chewing, and talking.

PSYCHIATRIC CONTRIBUTION TO PAIN

Chronic pain syndromes usually accompany or are linked to psychogenic factors, such as depression, anxiety, bipolar disorder, and stress, making it very difficult to assess and diagnose pain disorders. Patients with a mental health diagnosis were twice as likely to be prescribed opioids compared with those without a diagnosis according to a prospective study by Closs.[9] It is essential that these factors are recognized during the initial visit. Referring a patient for psychological therapy will assist in the treatment process.

"The nociceptive pathways are modulated by psychological processes which may amplify pain symptoms."[12] These patients must be treated with a multidisciplinary approach. These patients may have long-standing emotional, mental, and work-life stress contributing to their pain. A long discussion in an attempt to understand the patient's pain and then possibly a referral to a mental health organization may assist in managing physical manifestation to a patient's chronic pain status. Serotonin-norepinephrine reuptake inhibitors (SNRIs) and TCA have a strong contribution in the pharmacotherapy involved in treating patients with chronic facial pain, as detailed further in this article.

Migraines

Migraine is an episodic disorder characterized by a severe headache that is associated with nausea, light, and sound sensitivity. This disorder is divided into 2 subtypes: migraine without aura (70% of cases) and with aura (30% of cases). Patients describe aura as an initial sign or symptom, such as flashing lights or blind spots in the vision. Once diagnosis is made by a neurologist or orofacial pain specialist, there is much that a dentist or oral surgeon can do to provide and manage a patient's chronic migraines.[9]

Patients typically present with complaints of severe, unilateral, throbbing headaches that can last from 4 hours to 3 days. Pharmacotherapy includes nonsteroidal anti-inflammatory drugs (NSAIDs) or triptans for acute therapy (described in detail in later discussion under the treatment section). Other commonly used medications include aspirin, ibuprofen, naproxen, ergotamine, sumatriptan, and zolmitriptan.

The practicing oral surgeon and dentist can now provide alternate preventative therapy: botulinum toxin type A. Botox is commonly used for cosmetic procedures to abolish wrinkles and fine lines of the skin and also in the treatment of myofascial pain disorders (described further in later discussion). Evidence suggests that botulinum toxin may inhibit the release of neuropeptides involved in pain perception and inflammation and has become a viable and effective option in the treatment of migraines.[13]

PATHOPHYSIOLOGY

To understand chronic pain diseases, it is important to understand the underlying pathophysiology. Even though it is still not clearly elucidated, there are 2 hypotheses that are present to describe the disease process. The "lesion" described in the definition above for neuropathic pain can be an irritative lesion that affects the somatosensory pathway; this can increase activity in the nociceptive pathway. The second hypothesis indicates that neurons in proximity of the lesion can become hyperactive and hypersensitive through denervation.[7]

The pain conduction pathway is generally described as involving three orders of neurons that transmit the actual pain signal following activation of the nerve fiber. The first order neurons have special receptors called nociceptors-Three type of nociceptors exist mechanical, thermal and polymodal. Signals from these pain receptors are transmitted from the site of injury to the dorsal bone of the spinal cord predominantly by A- delta and C fibers (first order neurons) and once the CNS is activated this signal and information is transmitted by second order neurons to the thalamus and eventually by third order neurons to the higher cortical areas.

CLINICAL PRESENTATION OF NEUROPATHIC PAIN

Patients will typically present with varying pain in severity, intensity, description, and area/location. Patients can report muscle pain that can be cramping, constricting, or crushing. Dysesthesias are common with a burning feeling that can be constant or intermittent. Pain can also be described as shooting, lancinating, or hyperpathic.

The patient will also describe triggers to their pain, such as cold, hot, movement, light touch, and emotional distress.

Neurologic pain can be (1) episodic or (2) continuous. Examples of episodic pain are trigeminal neuralgia and glossopharyngeal neuralgia. Examples of continuous neuropathic pain include herpetic neuralgia, postherpetic neuralgia, traumatic, neuralgia, and Eagle syndrome.

Trigeminal neuralgia is characterized by sharp, unilateral, stabbing pain that extends in one or more branches of the trigeminal nerve. This pain is most often triggered by various stimuli, such as light touch and vibrations. This disease process usually affects 1 side and usually the maxillary and mandibular division of the trigeminal nerve (shown in **Fig. 1**). Trigeminal neuralgia can present because of posterior fossa compressive lesions, intracranial tumors, or demyelinating plaques of multiple sclerosis.[14,15] Continuous afferent input of nerve impulses may produce central sensitization.

Neuroimaging will help distinguish classic TN to secondary TN. MRI is the preferred imaging technique with or without contrast because of the higher resolution.

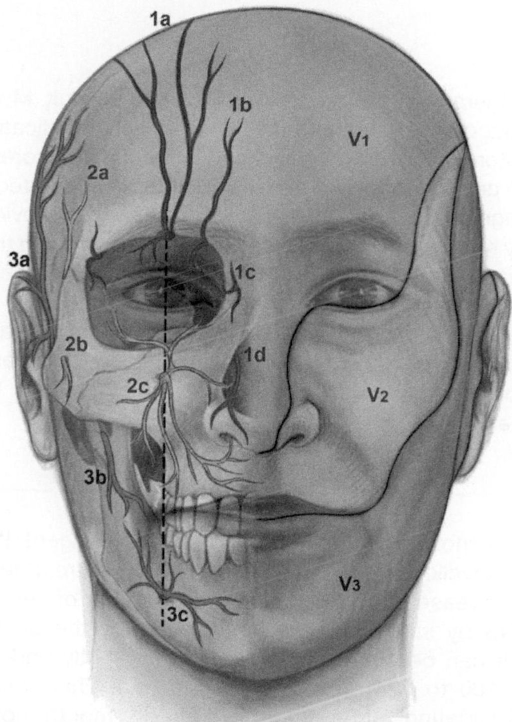

Fig. 1. Cutaneous innervation of the face: ophthalmic nerve (V1), (1a) supraorbital nerve, (1b) supratrochlear nerve, (1c) infratrochlear nerve, (1d) external nasal nerve; maxillary nerve (V2), (2a) zygomaticotemporal nerve, (2b) zygomaticofacial nerve, (2c) infraorbital nerve; mandibular nerve (V3), (3a) auriculotemporal nerve, (3b) buccal nerve, (3c) mental nerve. (*From* Marur T, Tuna Y, Demirci S. Facial anatomy. Clin Dermatol. 2014;32(1):21; with permission.)

According to the International Classification of Headache Disorders, Third Edition, diagnostic criteria include the following: (1) recurrent paroxysms of unilateral pain along the distribution of the trigeminal nerve; (2) pain that lasts from a faction of a second to 2 minutes, severe in intensity, and electric in characteristic; (3) pain precipitated by innocuous stimuli; and (4) pain not accounted for by another diagnosis. The differential diagnosis includes compression of the trigeminal nerve, demyelination from multiple sclerosis.

Anesthesia Dolorosa

Anesthesia dolorosa is also known as painful trigeminal neuropathy following an incidence of trauma, which produces unilateral facial pain and may be accompanied by trigeminal nerve dysfunction. Pain is superimposed in the area of that face that lacks or has impaired sensation. Diagnosis is achieved according to the International Classification of Headache Disorders, Third Edition: facial pain in the distribution of one or both trigeminal nerves, history of identifiable trauma to nerve with hyperalgesia, hypoesthesia, allodynia, and pain developed within 6 months of traumatic event.

Painful trigeminal neuralgia is most common in women (74:1; women:men) and is diagnosed in 5 out of 100,000 people.[16]

TREATMENT

Finding appropriate therapy for neuropathic pain can be difficult. Most treatment therapies include pharmacotherapy that reduces CNS activity, medications that enhance the reuptake of serotonin and noradrenaline and influence adrenoreceptors and electrical stimulation of central/peripheral nerves. Using an integrated multimodal biopsychological management plan is the most efficient way to provide treatment. The provider must timely recognize the pain syndrome by performing a thorough examination. Recognizing that a patient's pain is not only a psychogenic illness allows patients from believing that the pain is only in their head.

Based on a systematic review of randomized clinical trials in various neuropathic pain conditions by the European Federation of Neurological Societies, there are strong recommendations on approaching treatment of neuropathic pain.[1] These recommendations are described in later discussion.

Antidepressants

Amitriptyline

Amitriptyline is a TCA most commonly used as a first-line agent. It is also known as the most effective tricyclic for central poststroke pain in treatment of neuropathic pain. It causes an increase in the synaptic concentration of serotonin and norepinephrine in the CNS by inhibition of their reuptake by the presynaptic neuronal membrane pump. It can be started at 10 to 25 mg nightly and titrated up until a maximum dose of 100 to 124 mg nightly is attained. This antidepressant along with other TCAs is sedating. Side effects include dry mouth, constipation, tachycardia, palpitations, orthostatic hypotension, weight gain, blurred vision, and urinary retention.

SNRIs are commonly used to treat depression by blocking presynaptic serotonin and norepinephrine transport proteins in the presynapsis. The specific class of drugs also have evidence of analgesic qualities similar to TCAs. The evidence for selective serotonin reuptake inhibitors (SSRIs) is not as potent as shown from a systematic review by Saarto and Wiffen.[17]

Carbamazepine (Tegretol)

Carbamazepine (Tegretol) is an anticonvulsant drug most commonly used for bipolar disorder, focal onset of seizures, and trigeminal neuralgia/glossopharyngeal neuralgia. Tegretol has anticonvulsant, anticholinergic, antineuralgic, antidiuretic, and antidepressant properties. It may depress activity in the nucleus ventral of the thalamus and decrease synaptic transmission by limiting influx of sodium ions across the cell membrane or other unknown mechanisms. It is used to treat neuropathic pain as a component of multimodal pain control. It may be initially started at 100 to 200 mg/d and gradually increased over several weeks in increments of 200 mg/d as needed to a maximum dose of 1200 mg/d. Although the side effects are rare, they are serious, such as agranulocytosis, aplastic anemia, and Stevens-Johnson syndrome.

Gabapentin

Gabapentin is similar in structure to γ-aminobutyric acid (GABA) but does not bind to GABAa or GABAb receptors. It binds to high-affinity gabapentin binding sites in the brain that possess the alpha-2-delta-1 subunit, which modulates the release of excitatory neurotransmitters. Gabapentin is a type of anticonvulsant that is commonly used for the treatment of postherpetic neuralgia and neuropathic pain when the adverse effects of TCAs are to be avoided. Gabapentin is also known to relieve allodynia, burning, and shooting pain. Gabapentin is contraindicated in patients who have hypersensitivity to Gabapentin. It can be started at 300 mg daily and increased as needed for pain relief. Most patients feel adequate relief at a dose of 900 to 2400 mg. The most common side effects include somnolence, diarrhea, mood swings, ataxia, fatigue, nausea, and dizziness.[2]

Pregabalin (Lyrica)

Pregabalin binds to the alpha-2-delta subunit of the calcium channel In the CNS at nerve terminals, thus inhibiting excitatory neurotransmitter release. It exerts an antinociceptive and anticonvulsant effect. It is a common medication used for fibromyalgia, neuropathic pain associated with peripheral neuropathy, and spinal cord injury. Pregabalin is contraindicated in patients with hypersensitivity to pregabalin. It can be started at 25 mg once daily to 50 mg 3 times per day. Higher doses can be given to the patient, but the total dose of 600 mg daily should not be exceeded. When the drug is discontinued, it should be tapered over a week or else withdrawal symptoms may present. Some common side effects include dizziness, somnolence, dry mouth, peripheral edema, and weight gain. Pregabalin can also cause sedation and confusion.

Capsaicin

Capsaicin can be administered as a topical cream commonly used for neuropathic pain and muscle/joint pain and provides temporary relief of minor aches and pains of muscles and joints and mild relief in patients with diabetic neuropathy or postherpetic neuralgia. It acts as an agonist to the Vanilloid Receptor Subtype I (TRPVI). and activates ligand-gated cation channels on nociceptive nerve fibers. Binding to the TRPVI Receptor causes desensitization of sensory axons and inhibition of transmission initiation. If the topical cream causes irritation or erythema, it should be discontinued. The patient should apply the cream to the affected area 3 to 4 times daily.

Providing supplementation with analgesics is a very effective dual or triple therapy when treating chronic pain syndromes. After reviewing a patient's medical history, a provider is advised to supplement main-line treatment methods with nonopioid analgesics, opioid analgesics, antidepressants, topical medications, and therapy.

Nonopioid Analgesics

Paraacetylaminophenol/acetaminophen

Paraacetylaminophenol/acetaminophen is an over-the-counter analgesic and antipyretic that is commonly paired with an opioid to provide increased support or lower the dose of opioid needed. A dose of 325 mg to 600 mg every 6 hours is usually prescribed alongside other treatments. An overdose of acetaminophen can cause severe hepatotoxicity. The Food and Drug Administration (FDA) reports the maximum dose of acetaminophen at 4 g/d. It is contraindicated in patients with liver disease.

NSAIDs-naproxen is a type of NSAID that acts reversibly to inhibit the cyclooxygenase-1 (COX-1) and -2 enzyme, causing a decrease in the formation of prostaglandin. It has antipyretic, analgesic, and anti-inflammatory properties. It is one of the most commonly used analgesic medications throughout medicine. It is contraindicated in patients with a history of asthma, urticaria, or anaphylactic reactions. In treating patients with facial pain, start by dosing 500 mg every 12 hours for 2 weeks. The patient should be reevaluated in 2 weeks for improvement. Long-standing use of NSAIDs may cause gastrointestinal disturbances and is also not advised for patients with gastrointestinal conditions. Other NSAIDs include celecoxib (COX-2 inhibitors) and ibuprofen.

MUSCULOSKELETAL PAIN

Facial pain is not limited to neuropathic pain. Patients may confuse neuronal pain with musculoskeletal pain. It is up to the dentist/oral surgeon to perform a thorough examination to distinguish the differences in these conditions and treat appropriately. Most patients who present with complaints of facial pain actually have pain caused by conditions that fall under the TMD classification, and dentists/oral surgeons should be sensitized to this fact.

Most patients who complain of TMJ/TMD pain have a myofascial component. These patients have pain associated with the masticatory muscles, which can become highly inflamed, swollen, or tender because of several causes (**Fig. 2**). An average mouth opening is 40 mm. There may be a limitation on opening because of functional inhibition to opening or because of guarding. Pain on palpation of the temporalis and masseter muscles bilaterally along with pterygoid muscles intraorally will elicit a pain response if inflamed. Check intraorally for wear facets on the dentition and to better assess whether the patient is a bruxer, which may contribute to myofascial pain. This cluster of pain conditions has a 2:1 predilection toward women. In totality, 5% of the population is affected with temporomandibular disorders.[18]

Some patients suffer from painful conditions directly related and limited to the Temporomandibular Joint, such as articular disc derangements with or without reduction, synovitis/capsulitis, or osteoarthritis. These disorders may present as pain to the affected or bilateral sides with pain on opening/closing along with possible popping, clicking, and crepitus. They are diagnosed after evaluation of the disc position and integrity. The anterior displacement of the articular disc and its movement create the click and pop sound that patients complain of when opening and closing the jaw.

The TMJ is considered a diarthrodial joint, a synovial joint, and a compound joint. The articular disc is composed of a dense fibrous connective tissue; it is not vascularized and not innervated.[18]

A conservative approach should be initiated, only progressing as necessary. Multiple treatment modalities with increasing invasiveness include TMJ arthrocentesis, arthroscopy, disc replacement, and full TMJ replacements.

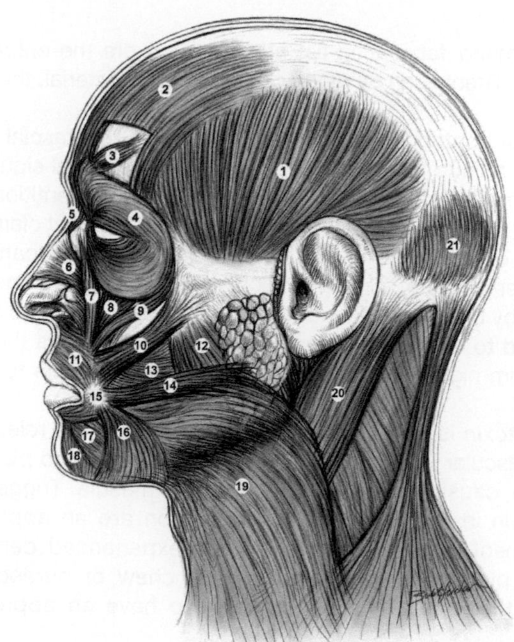

Fig. 2. Mimetic muscles and masticatory muscles: (1) temporalis, (2) frontalis, (3) corrugator supercilii, (4) orbicularis oculi, (5) procerus, (6) nasalis, (7) levator labii superioris alaeque nasi, (8) levator labii superioris, (9) zygomaticus minor, (10) zygomaticus major, (11) orbicularis oris, (12) masseter, (13) buccinator, (14) risorius, (15) modiolus, (16) depressor anguli oris, (17) depressor labii inferioris, (18) mentalis, (19) platysma, (20) sternocleidomastoid, (21) occipitalis. (*From* Marur T, Tuna Y, Demirci S. Facial anatomy. Clin Dermatol. 2014;32(1):15; with permission.)

TREATMENT

It is advised to initially treat patients with primary myofascial pain with conservative treatment and progress in aggressiveness as treatment modalities fail. Pharmacotherapy can be initiated immediately along with other supportive treatments.

Cyclobenzaprine (Flexeril)

Cyclobenzaprine (Flexeril) is a skeletal muscle relaxant that blocks nerve impulses commonly used for TMD and muscle spasms. It is a centrally acting skeletal muscle relaxant related to TCAs and influences both alpha and gamma motor neurons. Its use is contraindicated in patients with hypersensitivity to flexural or during or within 14 days of monoamine oxidase inhibitors as well as in patients with hyperthyroidism, heart failure, arrhythmias, heart block, or conduction disturbances. Dosing begins with 10 mg once daily administered 1 to 2 hours before bedtime. Other methods include taking it twice a day in 5-mg doses every 12 hours. It is important to reevaluate the patient in 2 weeks for improvement.

Naproxen

Naproxen is an NSAID that was described previously.

Bite-splint therapy

The authors recommend fabricating flat stent that covers the entire arch (either the maxilla or mandible). Stents can be made of hard or soft material, the authors prefer to use polished acrylic.

Bruxism is a major contributing factor to the patient's myofascial pain. The experienced dentist and oral surgeon should be aware of the clinical signs that the patient may be a bruxer. The patient will exhibit wear facets on the dentition, and the patient or their partner may volunteer the information that they are night clenchers or bruxers. This habit can also cause inflammation of the muscles of mastication. It is essential that the practitioner palpate all the muscles of mastication and distinguish the response provided by the patient. The authors prefer to make a hard customary acrylic stent either adapted to the upper or lower dentition that covers the entire arch. The stent should be worn nightly and daily as well if patient admits to clenching during the day.

Botulinum neurotoxin is a neuromodulator that inhibits the release of acetylcholine at the neuromuscular junction, depolarizing the motor end plate, which inhibits muscle contraction, causing flaccid paralysis of the muscle. Trigger point injections with botulinum toxin in the muscles of mastication are an approved therapy by the FDA for treatment of myofascial pain. The experienced dentist/oral surgeon would be wise to place their patient on a soft chew or pureed diet, which will assist in allowing the muscles of mastication to have an appropriate period of healing.

BURNING MOUTH SYNDROME

BMS is defined by the International Association for the Study of Pain as burning pain in the tongue or other oral mucous membrane associated with normal signs and laboratory findings lasting at least 4 to 6 months.[19] The International Headache Society in the International Classification of Headache Disorders describes it as an intraoral burning sensation for which no medical or dental cause can be found.[20] Historically, this condition has been referred to by numerous names based on the location or quality of pain and includes scalded mouth syndrome, sore tongue, stomatodynia, burning lips syndrome, burning mouth condition, glossodynia, glossalgia, stomatopyrosis, oral dysesthesia, glossopyrosis, and sore mouth.[1,21,22] However, if burning mouth is a symptom of other local, systemic, or psychogenic diseases, then this is referred to as oral burning disorder; otherwise, the term BMS is used, making it a diagnosis of exclusion.[1] In the cases of ineffective outcomes of treatments, patients with BMS often repeat consultations, which aggravates their anxiety about physical health and, on the other hand, the duration of BMS assumes a chronic tendency.[23]

EPIDEMIOLOGY

There is a higher incidence of BMS in women than men. The ratio between women and men varies from 3:1 to 16:1. Postmenopausal women aged 50 to 89 years had the highest disease incidence, with the maximal rate in women aged 70 to 79 years. After the age of 50 years, BMS incidence in men and women significantly increased across age groups.[24] BMS usually first presents 3 years before to 12 years following menopause and rarely before the age of 30. No studies have reported the prevalence of burning mouth by social, educational, or occupational groups.[25]

CLINICAL FINDINGS

The tongue is most commonly affected, principally the anterior two-thirds and tip on the dorsum and at the anterolateral margins.[26] The anterior hard palate, mucosal aspect of the lip, and mandibular alveolar regions can also be affected, whereas sites such as the buccal mucosa and floor of the mouth are rarely involved.[26] BMS is almost always bilateral and symmetric and does not follow the anatomic distribution of a peripheral sensory nerve.[27]

BMS patients will also often report subjective conditions, such as xerostomia and dysgeusia, as well as sialorrhoea, globus hystericus, halitosis, or dysphagia.[19] Most patients suffering from BMS experience their symptoms without any known triggering factor. A small portion of patients can link the onset of their illness to previous events, such as previous dental procedures, medication use, or infections, implying that neuroplastic/neurologic changes may be responsible for their symptoms. Others report the onset of symptoms following a traumatic life event.

Some signs that are thought to originate from psychological disturbances/anxiety might include the following: (1) frothy saliva indicating a parotid hypofunction and dominance of mucoid submandibular saliva over the serous parotid saliva (anxiety is the most common cause of both acute and chronic xerostomia); (2) dryness of the inner aspect of the lower lip from minor labial gland hypofunction; (3) scalloping of the lateral lingual margins secondary to habitual pressure against the adjacent teeth; (4) buccal mucosal irregularity often with leukoedema, translucent keratosis, and linea alba, also due to pressure against the adjacent teeth; (5) low-grade erythema of the anterior dorsum of the tongue as a result of traumatic abrasion of the filiform papillae against the adjacent teeth and palate and exposure of the sensitive fungiform papillae; (6) low-grade erythema and often slight sensitivity of the coincident anterior hard palate; and (7) low-grade linear erythema of the inner aspect of the lip coincident with the edges of the incisor teeth, mainly on the lower lip.[19] Clinicians have found that patients are highly likely to accept that anxiety or an associated condition is related to their dysaesthesia if they can agree that the visible presentation of clusters taken from this list have no real cause other than anxiety or other psychological/psychiatric bases.[19]

Subjective or objective halitosis is known to be present in some patients with BMS. One such cause is the anaerobic production of volatile sulfur compounds by bacteria in the mouth, and in stress, there is an increased concentration of sulfur compounds in saliva.[28] Within the BMS patient group, the objective assessment of halitosis is an important parameter in the workup. The Evaluation of Halitosis includes both clinical assessment during examination and response of family members and friends to the condition. No reaction from family almost always indicates a subjective awareness without clinical correlation, and 1 consideration is a psychogenic component in origin.[19]

Dysgeusia and changes in the tongue have been documented for many people suffering from BMS. It has been demonstrated that after exposure to a mild stressor, college students' sensitivity to saccharin's bitterness is increased.[29] The dorsum of the tongue changes with age in many patients, with a loss of density and shortening and flattening of the filiform papillae.[19] In areas subjected to habitual and repetitive trauma by rubbing against adjacent tissues, usually the palate or anterior mandibular teeth, the atrophy is bilateral and restricted to the anterior dorsum or the lateral and anterolateral margins of the tongue. Often these habits can be related to stress/anxiety, which can be manifested in tongue thrusting and bruxism, therefore demonstrating that changes in the tongue can result from aging in addition to psychological origins.

CAUSE

Hormonal

Among menopausal or postmenopausal women with BMS, follicle-stimulating hormone was higher, whereas estradiol was significantly lower.[23] There was no difference between the BMS group and the control group for blood analyses regarding white blood cell count, red blood cell count, hemoglobin, and platelet count. One study showed that most patients with BMS who responded to hormone replacement therapy had an increased expression of nuclear estrogen receptor.[30,31]

Smoking

A significant relationship exists between smoking and patients suffering from BMS. Some hypothesize that harmful substances, such as benzopyrene and polycyclic aromatic hydrocarbons, may be the culprit.[23] In addition, cigarette smoking has a positive correlation with taste disturbance.[8]

Medication

Many medications can alter salivary flow by both sympathomimetic and parasympathomimetic actions or by acting directly on salivary cellular processes, so it is often challenging to distinguish between physiologic and psychological causative factors associated with hyposalivation and subjective oral dryness.[19]

Somatization

Some studies suggest that patients with BMS significantly demonstrated symptoms of somatization. Most patients were easily irritated and readily lost their tempers, and many showed hypochondriasis or asthenia and exhibited dismal emotion and being unwilling to exercise, whereas some reported having numb limbs or drumming in the ears.[23]

Adverse Life Events

Patients with BMS were shown to have significant differences in early adverse life events, including interpersonal tension.[23]

Xerostomia

Low unstimulated salivary flow without subjective dryness is associated with age and medication (antihypertensives and analgesics), whereas purely subjective oral dryness is associated with depression, perceived stress, state and trait anxiety, female gender, and antihypertensives.[32] It is important to understand that xerostomia can be multifactorial, comprising both physiologic and psychological reasons, and thus, understanding this concept is important in managing patient's expectations regarding treatment.

Nutritional Deficiencies

Nutritional deficiencies involving vitamins and minerals, especially those associated with anemia (iron and vitamin B12 deficiency), zinc, and vitamin B complexes, have been known to have links with BMS.[33]

CLASSIFICATION

Type 1 BMS is characterized as a burning sensation that is not present upon waking, but which develops in the late morning and progresses during the waking hours, with the greatest intensity of discomfort in the evening. This sensation is present every day.

In type 2 BMS, patients awake with a burning sensation that is constant throughout the day, which often prevents patients from falling asleep. This discomfort is present all day, every day.

Patients with type 3 BMS report intermittent symptoms and symptom-free periods, with variable presence between days and may experience the symptoms at unusual oral sites, such as the floor of the mouth and buccal mucosa.[34]

In patients with primary BMS, the nomenclature of primary BMS is made when no clinical or laboratory test abnormalities are present.

In secondary BMS cases in which there is an identifiable underlying cause for BMS, it is classified as secondary BMS. Some of the reported causes include salivary hypofunction, menopause, oral candidiasis, nutritional deficiencies, endocrinopathies, bruxism, medication adverse effects, dental trauma, mucosal irritation from dentures, and allergic contact stomatitis.[35,36]

PATHOPHYSIOLOGY

Neuropathic

Dysgeusia and phantom taste are often reported in patients with BMS. In the peripheral nervous system, the dysfunction of the trigeminal nerve and chorda tympani nerve induces an alteration of the sensitivity threshold and reflection in the trigeminal nerve area. Maladaptive neural alteration reduces the threshold of pain transmission and transmits an ascending nociceptive signal that is not transmitted under healthy conditions.

In the CNS, alterations of gray matter volume in the pain-related area and brain activity for the nociceptive stimulus have been reported.[37] In BMS brain, alteration of gray matter volume and activity is not prominent in the somatosensory area, but is recognized in the prefrontal cortex, anterior cingulate gyrus, and hippocampus, which belong to the limbic system.[37] Thus, is it proposed that central sensitization is one of the many entities that play a role in BMS.

Patients will very often associate the onset of burning symptoms with a particular life event ranging from dental procedures, respiratory illness, a course of medication, or stressful events. It is suggested that certain dental treatments may cause injury to orofacial tissues and nerves, leading to undesirable neuroplastic changes, which lead in turn to BMS symptoms. Central sensitization producing long-lasting neuroplastic changes in central nociceptive neurons, including increased excitability and occasional spontaneous tonic activity, has also been suggested as a mechanism, as has damage to the taste system, causing oral phantom pain.

Endocrine

Reduced synthesis of ovarian steroids after menopause induces deficiency or dysfunction in adrenal steroids, which abolishes the neuroprotective effects of steroids on neural tissues.[5] It has been shown that epithelial cells scraped from the tongues of patients with BMS demonstrated increased artemin, a glial cell-derived neurotrophic factor (GDNF).[38] Notably, animal studies demonstrated that ovariectomy leads to upregulation of these GDNFs.[39] It is implied that gonadal hormones are necessary for maintaining tongue epithelium thickness and that artemin plays a significant role in keratinization. In addition, artemin overexpression is linked to atrophy of the lingual nerve along with other thinner fibers, such as unmyelinated fibers, which have been seen in findings of BMS patients. Furthermore, animal studies have shown increased levels of artemin in tongue epithelium can induce pain-related behavior resembling heat pain.[40]

One possible hypothesis is the increase in mucosal blood flow of the hard palate, on the tip of the tongue, on the midline of the oral vestibule, and on the lip. Compared with the controls, patients suffering from BMS had increased mucosal blood flow of the oral cavity when stimulated. There were no differences between groups regarding blood flow of peripheral sites, suggesting BMS symptoms may be related to disturbed vasoreactivity.[41]

Another hypothesis proposes a comprehensive mechanism for BMS, taste disturbances, or xerostomia based on a regional neuropathy. The mechanism suggested is via either a regional small-fiber idiopathic neuropathy affecting salivary secretion and oral sensation or a primary idiopathic neuropathy causing sensory neural dysfunction at the receptor level by changing the oral cavity environment. Sensory changes in the tongue and changed salivary composition with normal salivary flow rates have been demonstrated in patients with BMS, xerostomia, and dysgeusia.[42]

Numerous recent studies claim that circadian clock dysfunction can play a key role in the pathogenesis of BMS because pain perception, depression and anxiety, and sleep disorders are linked with circadian disturbances.[43] Because dopamine is an important regulator of circadian rhythms in the CNS and the hypothalamic-pituitary-adrenal (HPA) axis is affected by circadian rhythms, both the HPA axis and dopamine levels may be altered in BMS,[44] suggesting that future treatment may include alterations of the sleep cycle.

Psychological

Several studies suggest the important role of psychological factors, such as anxiety and depressive disorders, in unexplained somatic symptoms, and the prevalence of nonspecific somatoform symptoms is higher in psychologically disturbed patients than in the general population.[45] BMS patients have poorer self-reported overall health and complain of more illnesses, gastrointestinal problems, chronic fatigue, disturbed sleep patterns, headaches, and pain in other locations,[46] and are anxious, introverted, and self-reliant, have low self-esteem, are fearful, prone to worry, feel nervous and tense, in addition to a tendency to show frustration and bitterness.[47] Patients with BMS have significantly higher levels of neuroticism in all its facets: anxiety, anger, hostility, depression, self-consciousness, impulsiveness, and vulnerability.[47] All facets of neuroticism that are significant in BMS are significantly related to the negative affect and lower life satisfaction and complaints of pervasive psychological distress.[47] There also seems to be a direct relationship between a worsening of physical symptoms, increased functional impairments, and a lowering of the quality of life with progression to depression and anxiety in a cause-and-effect relationship.[46]

As with all chronic pain sufferers, it is challenging to distinguish whether depression and anxiety are causes or effects of the symptoms of oral dysaesthesias, such as BMS. Depression and psychological disturbance are common in chronic pain populations and may be secondary to chronic pain rather than the cause of BMS. Mood and sleep disturbances and a decreased desire to socialize may also be secondary, but nonetheless contributing factors, rather than the primary precipitating factors of BMS.[19] Some investigators propose that sleep disturbances and chronic fatigue can be a manifestation of the psychological aspect, anxiety, whereas gastrointestinal symptoms represent the physical counterpart. To further support a somatoform pain disorder model of BMS, anxiolytic drugs, such as SSRI and amisulpride, can cause an improvement in BMS symptoms.[48] The implication is that BMS may indicate distress that causes vulnerable individuals to experience emotional distress as pain.[19]

The exact psychological relation to BMS has been questionable, but numerous studies have shown psychological abnormalities with the condition. Therefore, the initial prescription of a low-dose anxiolytic will usually provide some level of dampening of symptom intensity and so confirm the diagnosis of BMS.[19]

Treatment

The mechanisms of BMS are poorly understood, and there are no standard treatment protocols. However, it may be agreed upon that both physiologic and psychological aspects of the disease must be addressed for successful management of these patients. For the patient to achieve early acceptance of the diagnosis and understanding of the disease process, this can have paramount benefits for the commencement of formal treatment.[19] If not, the common scenario of patients continuing to search for a "real diagnosis" may ensue, as often seen with people with dysaesthesias who often deny to accept the psychological aspect of their disease.

Topical Medication

Clonazepam

A benzodiazepine that acts as an agonist of the GABA receptor was found to be efficacious in reducing symptoms of BMS. Protocols required patients to suck on a 1-mg tablet of clonazepam for 3 minutes, holding the saliva near the pain sites and then spitting out the excess saliva (3 times a day for 14 days).[49] Other protocols included a similar method using 0.5-mg tablets up to 4 times a day. Patients were instructed to suck on a clonazepam tablet for 3 minutes, spit out excess saliva, and hold their saliva near the pain sites. It was found to be effective both short term (<10 weeks) and long term (>10 weeks), showing a 50% reduction in symptoms for most patients; however, people may develop dependence because symptoms can return when medication is not continued. Common side effects include xerostomia, lethargy, and fatigue.[50]

Capsaicin

Prolonged used of this analgesic causes depletion of TRPV1, the afferent receptor responsible for transmitting heat sensation, therefore, desensitizing this pain receptor.[51] However, 0.01% or 0.025% oral capsaicin gel on the dorsal part of tongue 3 times daily for 14 days has been shown to be efficacious.[52] However, patient history of gastric-related disorders must be taken into account because side effects include increased sensation of burning immediately after application.[43]

Low-level laser therapy

Low-level laser therapy (LLLT) is reported to improve peripheral circulation, oxygenate hypoxic cells, and help remove noxious products[53] in addition to blocking c-fiber depolarization, which is an afferent pathway for heat/pain.[20] Most of the current literature on LLTT showed improvements in symptoms compared with placebo, despite the variability in treatment protocol for laser parameters.[20] LLLT delivered at 300-mW continuous wave emission with an average power of 1 W/cm^2 delivered with a 0.6-cm-diameter probe protected with a transparent plastic sleeve, held perpendicularly at the distance of 2 mm. Laser was delivered ~10 seconds per point up to 0.5 cm beyond the symptomatic borders. Patients from this group underwent 2 laser irradiation sessions weekly for 5 weeks and showed a significant reduction in symptoms when compared with patients using topical clonazepam 3 times weekly for 3 weeks.[21]

Spanemberg et al. aimed to clinically assess the effect of difference LLLT protocols in the treatment of BMS patients.[54,55] Spanemberg used a diode laser for 4 groups (wavelength 830 nm, weekly session, 10 sessions); 1 group (IR3W) received infrared laser (wavelength 830 nm, 1 session/wk, 9 sessions); 1 group received red laser (685 nm, 35 mW, 2 J, 72 J/cm, 3 sessions/wk, 9 sessions), and control group (placebo) and found that significant reductions in symptoms were found in all treatment groups compared with placebo.

Lactoperoxidase (Biotine mouthwash) and topical lidocaine have not been shown to be effective because of their short duration of action.[56]

Systemic Medication

Clonazepam

Clonazepam treatment varied from 0.25 to 2 mg daily with overall increasing dosage being positively correlated to efficacy; however, some instances presented in which patients stopped treatment using less than 1 mg daily because of negative side effects.[57] Some studies show that it is not effective in improving mood, xerostomia, and taste dysfunction,[58] but works best when normal salivary flow is present and in those beginning with severe initial symptoms or those who do not use psychotropic medications.[24]

Alpha-lipoic acid

Alpha-lipoic acid is a coenzyme shown to have neuroprotective and antioxidant properties and that is thought to exert neuroregenerative actions. Current literature has conflicting evidence for improvement of symptoms and the proposed side effects of gastrointestinal upset and headaches when compared with placebo; therefore, further research is indicated to determine its effectiveness when used in isolation.[43]

Gabapentin

Gabapentin is an anticonvulsant commonly used for neuropathic pain and is a GABA agonist. Although effective when used alone, GABA in combination with alpha-lipoic acid (300 mg Gabapentin + 600 mg alpha-lipoic acid/day for 60 days) shows a 70% success rate in the reduction of burning sensation.[59]

Catuama

Catuama is an herbal product from Brazil composed of 4 extracts of medicinal plants (catuaba, ginger, guarana, and muira puama) that is sought after for supposed improvement of physical and mental fatigue. Its components have demonstrated antinocioceptive, antidepressant, and vasorelaxant effects in addition to affecting dopaminergic and serotonergic pathways in animal studies. A dose of 310 mg Catuama capsules twice a week for 8 weeks resulted in a 51.5% reduction in symptoms.[54]

Hormone replacement therapy

Conjugated estrogens like premarin, 0.625 mg/d for 21 days, and medroxyprogesterone acetate like farlutal, 10 mg/d from day 12 through day 21, for 3 consecutive cycles can relieve oral burning symptoms for perimenopausal and postmenopausal women.[30] However, the diagnosis for BMS was not made during this study. In addition, this was only successful for select patients with estrogen receptors in the oral mucosa.[60] Therefore, the efficacy of hormone replacement therapy for BMS is not confirmed.

Behavioral Therapy

Cognitive behavioral therapy relaxation and cognitive restructuring are 2 specific techniques relevant to the management of BMS. As the name implies, relaxation techniques include progressive muscle relaxation and focused breathing to alleviate discomfort, whereas cognitive restructuring seeks to identify and modify destructive thoughts related to emotional and behavioral problems.[26] In patients with resistant BMS after receiving pharmacologic treatment, those who received additional cognitive therapy for 12 to 15 sessions had decreased symptoms compared with a placebo group after 6 months, further strengthening the argument that part of BMS has a psychological component.[61]

Clinical management is complex, and there is no uniform treatment protocol, but in each case, both the physiologic and the psychological components of the patient's symptoms must be addressed. The acceptance of psychological factors by the patient is often an important element of BMS management, but this in itself can present a clinically challenging situation.[19] Because BMS is regarded as a multifactorial condition, refraining from bad oral habits, removing local irritating factors, stopping smoking, and keeping good mental health status may help in the prevention of BMS.[23]

SUMMARY

The predominant reasons for oral pain, more often than not, are related to diseased teeth and gums. Dentists and oral surgeons should always perform a thorough examination to rule out these common factors as the etiologic causative agents for a patient's facial and oral pain. Only after an exhaustive examination is performed and common causes are ruled out should one entertain a possible neuropathic cause for the patient's pain. Dentists and oral surgeons should be acutely aware that a continuous performance of dental and oral surgical procedures that can treat so far what Is untreatable in pain relief can only lead to the continuation and perhaps exacerbation of the preexisting medical condition. This article provides a review in neuropathic pain so that patients with intractable pain can be properly diagnosed and properly treated without having to undergo futile dental or oral surgical procedures.

Many general dentists are not properly trained in the area of oral facial pain and as a result fail to recognize neuropathic pain when it arises in their patients. It is clear that the patient's medical conditions, mental state, and social background play an important role in the patient developing certain oral facial pain conditions and require dentists to broaden their approach when evaluating the chronic pain patient. It is hoped that this article will have made the vital point that not all oral pain is dental in origin, and the pain can be approached or treated with a single dental procedure. The complaint of the patient must always be evaluated, and if the patient's pain persists despite multiple dental interventions, a revaluation should be undertaken and alternate treatment modalities be instituted.

Finally, many doctors are confronted by patients who complain of a chronic burning sensation of their tongues and oral cavity. This complaint is quite disturbing and alarming to patients, and it is vital that dentists and oral surgeons be knowledgeable in this area.

DISCLOSURE

The authors have nothing to disclose.

REFERENCES

1. Attal N, Cruccu G, Baron R, et al. EFNS guidelines on the pharmacological treatment of neuropathicpain: 2010 revision. European Journal of Neurology 2010;17:1113–23.
2. Backonja M, Glanzman RL. Gabapentin dosing for neuropathic pain: evidence from randomized, placebo-controlled clinical trials. Clin Ther 2003;25(1):81–104.
3. Balasubramanian R, Klasser G. Medical clinics of NAM, vol. 98. Philadelphia: Elsevier; 2014. p. 1385–405.
4. Barker K, Savage N. Burning mouth syndrome: an update on recent findings. Aust Dent J 2005;50:220–3.
5. Woda A, Dao T, Gremeau-Richard C. Steroid dysregulation and stomatodynia (burning mouth syndrome). J Orofac Pain 2009;23(3):202–10.
6. Woolf CJ. Central sensitization: implications for the diagnosis and treatment of pain. Pain 2011;152:S2.
7. Boivie J, Casey KL. Central pain in the face and head. In: Olesen J, editor. The headaches. Philadelphia: Lippincott Williams and Wilkins; 2006. p. 1063.
8. Thorstensson B, Hugoson A. Prevalence of some oral complaints and their relation to oral health variables in an adult Swedish population. Acta Odontol Scand 1996;54:257–62.
9. Taverner T, Closs SJ, Briggs M. The Journey to Chronic Pain: A Grounded Theory of Older Adult's Experiences of Pain Associated with Leg Ulceration. Pain Manag Nurs 2014;15(1):186–98.
10. Clark GT, Dionne RA. Orofacial Pain. Chichester: Wiley Blackwell; 2012.
11. Granot M, Nagler R. Association between regional idiopathic neuropathy and salivary involvement as the possible mechanism for oral sensory complaints. J Pain 2005;6:581–7.
12. Price DD. Psychological and neural mechanisms of the affective dimension of pain. Science 2000;288(5472):1769–72.
13. Capehart KL. Dentists role in migraine treatments with botulinum toxins. Decisions in Dentistry 2019;44.
14. Abetz LM, Savage NW. Burning mouth syndrome and psychological disorders. Aust Dental J 2009;54:84–93.
15. Al-Maweri SA, Javed F, Kalakonda B, et al. Efficacy of low level laser therapy in the treatment of burning mouth syndrome: a systematic review. Photodiagnosis Photodyn Ther 2017;17:188–93.
16. Sarlani E, Balciunas BA, Grace EG. Orofacial pain—part I: assessment and management of musculoskeletal and neuropathic causes. AACN Adv Crit Care 2005;16(3):333–46.
17. Saarto T, Wiffen PJ. Antidepressants for neuropathic pain: a Cochrane review. J Neurol Neurosurg Psychiatry 2010;81(12):1372–3.
18. Miloro M, Larry J. Peterson. Peterson's principles of oral and maxillofacial surgery. Shelton (CT): People's Medical Pub. House-USA; 2012.
19. Merskey H, Bogduk N. Descriptions of chronic pain syndromes and definitions of pain terms. In: Merskey H, Bogduk N, editors. Classification of chronic pain. 2nd edition. Seattle (WA): IASP Press; 1994. p. 74.
20. International Headache Society. The International Classification of Headache Disorders: 2nd edition. Cephalalgia 2004;24(Suppl 1):9–160.

21. Arduino PG, Cafaro A, Garrone M, et al. A randomized pilot study to assess the safety and the value of low-level laser therapy versus clonazepam in patients with burning mouth syndrome. Lasers Med Sci 2016;31:811–6.
22. Argoff CE, Dubin A, Pilitsis J. Pain management secrets E-Book. Elsevier Health Sciences; 2017.
23. Gao J, Chen L, Zhou J, et al. A case-control study on etiological factors involved in patients with burning mouth syndrome. J Oral Pathol Med 2008; 38:24–8.
24. Ko JY, Kim MJ, Lee SG, et al. Outcome predictors affecting the efficacy of clonazepam therapy for the management of burning mouth syndrome (BMS). Arch Gerontol Geriatr 2012;55(3):755–61.
25. Klasser GD, Fischer DJ, Epstein JB. Burning mouth syndrome: recognition, understanding, and management. Oral Maxillofac Surg Clin North Am 2008;20: 255–71, vii.
26. Savage N, Boras V, Barker K. Burning mouth syndrome: clinical presentation, diagnosis and treatment. Australas J Dermatol 2006;47:77–83.
27. Murnion BP. Neuropathic pain: current definition and review of drug treatment. Aust prescriber 2018;41(3):60–3.
28. Queiroz C, Hayacibara M, Tabchoury C, et al. Relationship between stressful situations, salivary flow rate and oral volatile sulphur-containing compounds. Eur J Oral Sci 2002;110:337–40.
29. Dess NK, Edelheit D. The bitter with the sweet: the taste/stress/temperament nexus. Biol Psychol 1998;48:103–19.
30. Forabosco A, Criscuolo M, Coukos G, et al. Efficacy of hormone replacement therapy in postmenopausal women with oral discomfort. Oral Surg Oral Med Oral Pathol 1992;73(5):570–4.
31. Forssell H, Jääskeläinen S, Tenovuo O, et al. Sensory dysfunction in burning mouth syndrome. Pain 2002;99:41–7.
32. Bergdahl M, Bergdahl J. Low unstimulated salivary flow and subjective oral dryness: association with medication, anxiety, depression, and stress. J Dent Res 2000;79:1652–8.
33. Lamey PJ. Burning mouth syndrome. Dermatol Clin 1996;14:339–54 [PubMed] [Google Scholar].
34. Lauria G, Majorana A, Borgna M, et al. Trigeminal small-fibre sensory neuropathy causes burning mouth syndrome. Pain 2005;115:332–7.
35. Kohorst J, Bruce A, Torgerson R, et al. A population-based study of the incidence of burning mouth syndrome. Mayo Clin Proc 2014;89(11):1545–52.
36. Lamey PJ, Hammond A, Allam BF, et al. Vitamin status of patients with burning mouth syndrome and the response to replacement therapy. Br Dent J 1986; 160(3):81–4.
37. Sinding C, Gransjøen AM, Schlumberger G, et al. Grey matter changes of the pain matrix in patients with burning mouth syndrome. Eur J Neurosci 2016;43: 997–1005.
38. Sardella A, Gualerzi A, Lodi G, et al. Morphological evaluation of tongue mucosa in burning mouth syndrome. Arch Oral Biol 2012;57(1):94–101.
39. Hernández-Aragón LG, García-Villamar V, Carrasco-Ruiz ML, et al. Role of estrogens in the size of neuronal somata of paravaginal ganglia in ovariectomized rabbits. Biomed Res Int 2017;2017:2089645.
40. Shinoda M, Takeda M, Honda K, et al. Involvement of peripheral artemin signaling in tongue pain: possible mechanism in burning mouth syndrome. Pain 2015; 156(12):2528–37.

41. Heckmann SM, Heckmann JG, Hilz MJ, et al. Oral mucosal blood flow in patients with burning mouth syndrome. Pain 2001;90(3):281–6.
42. Gremeau-Richard C, Dubray C, Aublet-Cuvelier B, et al. Effect of lingual nerve block on burning mouth syndrome (stomatodynia): a randomized crossover trial. Pain 2010;149:27–32.
43. Ritchie A, Kramer JM. Recent advances in the etiology and treatment of burning mouth syndrome. J Dental Res 2018;97(11):1193–9.
44. Hagelberg N, Forssell H, Rinne JO, et al. Striatal dopamine D1 and D2 receptors in burning mouth syndrome. Pain 2003;101(1–2):149–54.
45. Hexel M, Sonneck G. Somatoform symptoms, anxiety, and depression in the context of traumatic life experiences by comparing participants with and without psychiatric diagnoses. Psychopathology 2002;35:303–13.
46. Lamey P, Freeman R, Eddie S, et al. Vulnerability and presenting symptoms in burning mouth syndrome. Oral Surg Oral Med Oral Pathol Oral Radiol Endod 2005;99(1):48–54.
47. Firas A. Psychological profile in burning mouth syndrome. Oral Surg Oral Med Oral Pathol Oral Radiol Endod 2004;97:339–44.
48. Maina G, Vitalucci A, Gandolfo S, et al. Comparative efficacy of SSRIs and amisulpride in burning mouth syndrome: a single-blind study. J Clin Psychiatry 2002; 63:38–43.
49. Guimara˜es AL, de Sa AR, Victoria JM, et al. Interleukin-1b and serotonin transporter gene polymorphisms in burning mouth syndrome patients. J Pain 2006;7: 654–8.
50. Taub E, Munz M, Tasker RR. Chronic electrical stimulation of the gasserian ganglion for the relief of pain in a series of 34 patients. J Neurosurg 1997;86(2): 197–202.
51. Kisely S, Forbes M, Sawyer E, et al. A systematic review of randomized trials for the treatment of burning mouth syndrome. J Psychosom Res 2016;86:39–46.
52. Jorgensen MR, Pedersen AM. Analgesic effect of topical oral capsaicin gel in burning mouth syndrome. Acta Odontol Scand 2017;75(2):130–6.
53. Pinheiro AJ, Cavalcanti ET, Pinheiro TI, et al. Low-level laser therapy in the management of disorders of the maxillofacial region. J Clin Laser Med Surg 1997;15: 181–3.
54. Spanemberg JC, Cherubini K, de Figueiredo MA, et al. Effect of an herbal compound for treatment of burning mouth syndrome: randomized, controlled, double-blind clinical trial. Oral Surg Oral Med Oral Pathol Oral Radiol 2012; 113:373–7.
55. Spanemberg JC, Lopez J, de Figueiredo MA, et al. Efficacy of low-level laser therapy for the treatment of burning mouth syndrome: a randomized, controlled trial. J Biomed Opt 2015;20:098001.
56. Femiano F. Burning mouth syndrome (BMS): an open trial of comparative efficacy of alpha-lipoic acid (thioctic acid) with other therapies. Minerva Stomatol 2002; 51:405–9.
57. Cui Y, Xu H, Chen FM, et al. Efficacy evaluation of clonazepam for symptom remission in burning mouth syndrome: a meta-analysis. Oral Dis 2016;22:503–11.
58. Heckmann SM, Kirchner E, Grushka M, et al. A double-blind study on clonazepam in patients with burning mouth syndrome. Laryngoscope 2012;122(4): 813–6.
59. López-D'alessandro E, Escovich L. Combination of alpha lipoic acid and gabapentin, its efficacy in the treatment of Burning Mouth Syndrome: A randomized,

double-blind, placebo controlled trial. Med Oral Patol Oral Cir Bucal 2011;16(5):e635–40.
60. Volpe A, Lucenti V, Forabosco A, et al. Oral discomfort and hormone replacement therapy in the post-menopause. Maturitas 1991;13(1):1–5.
61. Bergdahl J, Anneroth G, Perris G. Cognitive therapy in the treatment of patients with resistant burning mouth syndrome: a controlled study. J Oral Pathol Med 1995;24(5):213–5.

Zygomatic Implants

A Solution for the Atrophic Maxilla

Jonathan Rosenstein, DDS, Harry Dym, DDS*

KEYWORDS

• Zygoma • Implant • Atrophic • Maxilla • Oral surgery

KEY POINTS

- Patients with a severely atrophic or resected maxilla can prove challenging to restore to a functional dentition.
- Although more surgically challenging than traditional implants, zygomatic implants may provide a solution to otherwise nonrestorable maxillae.
- Zygomatic implants have been shown to have high success rates.

INTRODUCTION

In recent decades, endosseous dental implants have become an increasingly popular solution to the problem of replacing lost or missing teeth. Because of the near-constant strides in research relating to dental implants, advances in effectiveness, efficiency, and cost have made dental implants a viable option for a large percentage of the population. However, limitations still exist. Sufficient bony height and width are still required for successful placement and retention of functional dental implants. In some patients, this can present a challenging scenario for the oral surgeon and restorative dentist, both in the placement and in the restoration of the dental implants.

Osseointegration of implants in even a healthy and robust maxilla has been shown to have lower success rates when compared with the mandible. This is especially true for implants placed in the posterior maxilla.[1] In patients with a severely atrophic maxilla, successful dental implant placement is especially difficult. Various solutions have been proposed for restoring the maxillary dentition in a patient with an atrophic maxilla. Options such as onlay bone grafting with autogenous iliac crest bone, sinus lift procedures, ridge split procedures, and even LeFort I surgical downfracture with interpositional bone grafting have been utilized. However, the zygomatic implant may present a far simpler approach to restoring the atrophic maxilla.[2]

Department of Oral and Maxillofacial Surgery, The Brooklyn Hospital Center, 121 Dekalb Avenue, Brooklyn, NY 11201, USA
* Corresponding author.
E-mail address: Hdym@tbh.org

Dent Clin N Am 64 (2020) 401–409
https://doi.org/10.1016/j.cden.2019.12.005
0011-8532/20/

OVERVIEW OF MAXILLARY BONE QUALITY

As referenced previously, the quality and quantity of maxillary bone are often less than that of the mandible. This is mainly because of the type of bone present in the posterior maxilla. Lekholm and Zarb (1985) described 4 main bone types in the maxilla and mandible:

1. Type 1: bone comprised mostly (if not all) of homogenous cortical bone
2. Type 2: bone that contains a core of densely packed cancellous bone, surrounded by at least 2 mm of cortical bone
3. Type 3: bone that contains a core of densely packed cancellous bone, but surrounded by only a thin layer of cortical bone.
4. Type 4: bone comprised of mostly nondense cancellous bone, surrounded by only a thin layer of cortical bone

The higher the overall bone density, the greater the success rate of osseointegration. This is likely because of higher levels of bone-to-implant contact and stabilization, which occurs readily in dense cortical bone as compared with the more loosely organized cancellous bone. Generally, healthy maxillae have been shown to have type 3 bone in the anterior and type 4 in the posterior. In resorbed maxillae, the bone density is often even further diminished.[3] This diminishment in the quality and quantity of maxillary bone is only exacerbated the longer a patient remains edentulous. It has been documented that the maxilla resorbs, on average, 2 mm within the first year after tooth extraction, and then at a rate of 0.5 mm/y, compared with 0.2 mm/y in the mandible.[4]

TREATMENT OPTIONS FOR THE ATROPHIC MAXILLA

In order to solve the problem of low quality and quantity of maxillary bone for placing implants, various treatments have been proposed. For many years, the gold standard of treatment was considered to be bone grafting procedures. This included techniques such as crestal onlay grafts, sinus lifts, and, as mentioned previously, Lefort I osteotomy with interpositional bone grafting. It is beyond the scope of this article to go into these techniques in detail, other than to mention that bone grafting procedures are not always a viable or desirable option for many patients. For patients who have undergone maxillary resection and/or radiation therapy for cancer treatment, bone grafting may not be a viable option, because of compromised vasculature. The same can be said for patients with certain metabolic disorders, congenital deformities, or those in an immunocompromised state. Even in a healthy edentulous patient, factors such as graft donor site morbidity, increased healing time, longer surgical time, and increased chance of infection can all be factors that would deter an individual from wanting to undergo extensive grafting procedures. It has also been reported that there is a lower implant survival rate for areas in the maxilla that have been grafted, compared with native bone.[2] Because of this, a nongrafting option to restore the resected or atrophic maxilla could be of great value to surgeons and patients.

ZYGOMATIC IMPLANTS

As early as 1988, the Branemark System described a standard surgical technique for intrasinus placement of zygomatic implants.[5] Many have documented the placement of these implants for use as supports for an obturator or other larger maxillofacial prostheses for patients who have undergone maxillectomies.[6] Since then, Branemark and others have described various surgical techniques and approaches for placement of zygomatic implants that could be used to restore a patient's dentition. To this end, there have been 2 main treatment designs utilized.[7]

First, for patients with sufficient anterior maxillary bone for traditional implant placement, 1 zygomatic implant should be placed on each side of the posterior maxilla. Two or more traditional endosteal implants should be placed in the anterior maxilla. For patients without sufficient anterior maxillary bone, 2 or more zygomatic implants should be placed on each side of the posterior maxilla.

Both of these designs have been shown to have high rates of success when used to support a fixed dental prosthesis or overdenture. The success of zygomatic implants as supports for full arch restorations has been documented by some to be at 100%.[8] Other studies have shown some failures, but most authors agree that zygomatic implants are successful well over 95% of the time.[9]

It should be noted that the success of zygomatic implants is likely not due to the bone quality of the zygoma, itself. On the contrary, the zygoma is comprised mainly of loose cancellous bone that is not favorable for implant success. The stability of zygomatic implants is thought, instead, to stem from the fact that the implant usually passes through 3 to 4 cortical layers of bone, compared with the single cortical layer that most traditional implants would pass through.[10] This will be explained.

INDICATIONS AND CONTRAINDICATIONS

The obvious indications for zygomatic implants, as mentioned previously, include those patients with a severely resorbed posterior maxilla who require an implant-supported prosthesis. These patients may include those with systemic diseases that cause resorption of the maxilla, patients who had undergone maxillary resection or radiation therapy, immunocompromised patients, or those with congenital deformities such as severe cleft palate. More routine indications could include patients for whom bone grafting would not be desirable because of possible donor site morbidity, increased pain, longer surgical time, or even cultural/religious aversion to foreign bone material.

Contraindications and relative contraindications for zygomatic implants would be similar to those for normal dental implant placement, such as tobacco smoking addiction, head and neck radiotherapy, and bisphosphonate therapy. Additionally, some have stated that because zygomatic implants often pass through the maxillary sinus, their placement may increase the risk of chronic maxillary sinusitis if a patient contracts an upper respiratory tract infection that closes off the sinus ostium. For patients prone to these infections, zygomatic implants may be contraindicated.[11]

Although not a contraindication, it is worthwhile to state a possible drawback to zygomatic implants. Because of their angulation, the head of zygomatic implants will often emerge more pallatally than traditional dental implants. This may make the dental prosthesis excessively bulky in this area, which can cause discomfort to selected patient. The extreme angulation of the zygomatic implant necessitates the use of angled abutments, which come in standard 25°, 35°, 45°, and 55° angulations.

TECHNIQUE FOR PLACEMENT OF ZYGOMATIC IMPLANTS

Various surgical approaches for zygomatic implant placement have been described and shown to be successful. The most common and basic approach, known as the intrasinus approach, will first be explained. Other approaches will then be described as variations or modifications on the intrasinus approach.

Surgical Incision and Flap

A crestal incision is made on the palatal aspect of the maxillary crest from the area of the first molar to opposing first molar. A flap is then elevated to expose the lateral surface of the maxilla until the zygomatic process is revealed, similar to the flap used in a LeFort 1 osteotomy. The infraorbital neurovascular bundle should also be visualized. At this point, because of the placement of the incision, both the buccal and palatal aspect of the alveolar crest should be fully exposed

Lateral Window

A window should be made into the lateral aspect of the maxillary sinus, bilaterally, close to the inferior border of the zygomatic crest. This can be performed with a rotary handpiece and round bur, Piezo, or any such instrument that would normally be used for the osteotomy of a lateral window approach for a maxillary sinus lift. The dimensions of the window should be such that it will facilitate easy visualization of the implant drill and zygomatic implant itself (**Fig. 1**). The suggested size is approximately 10 × 5 mm.

Elevation of Schneiderian Membrane

Similar to the technique used for a lateral window sinus lift, the sinus membrane should be carefully elevated off of the inferior, lateral, and superior walls of the sinus. This is to prevent perforation of the membrane by the implant drill or implant itself. Although this is not necessary for the success of the zygomatic implant, it is ideal, as some have theorized it may decrease the chance of an oroantral communication and future sinus disease. Many current authors, however, are not concerned with this as a significant risk.

Implant Osteotomy

Based on the presurgical and prosthodontic planning, the zygomatic implant drill should be used to start the osteotomy on the alveolar crest at the point from which

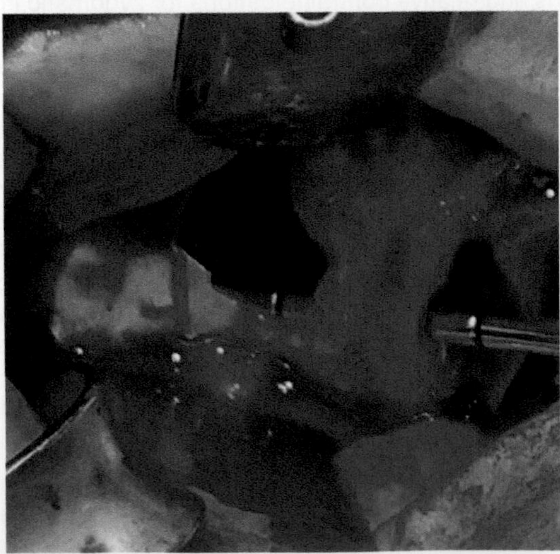

Fig. 1. The dimensions of the window should be such that it will facilitate easy visualization of the implant drill and zygomatic implant.

the head of the implant will emerge. The osteotomy should be continued in a superior-lateral-posterior direction, through the alveolar crest, into the sinus cavity, and eventually end within the superior cortical layer of the zygoma itself. It is important to use a specialized drill guard during osteotomy formation in order to prevent contact between the shaft of the drill and surrounding soft tissue (**Fig. 2**). Just as with traditional endosteal implants, the zygomatic drill burs are used under irrigation and in ascending orders of width until the appropriate size is reached. At this point, a depth indicator is used to confirm appropriate implant length (see **Fig. 1**). These implants are usually between 35 mm and 55 mm in length.

Implant Placement

Once the osteotomies have been completed and the appropriate length and angulation of the implant has been finalized, the zygomatic implant can be placed. It should

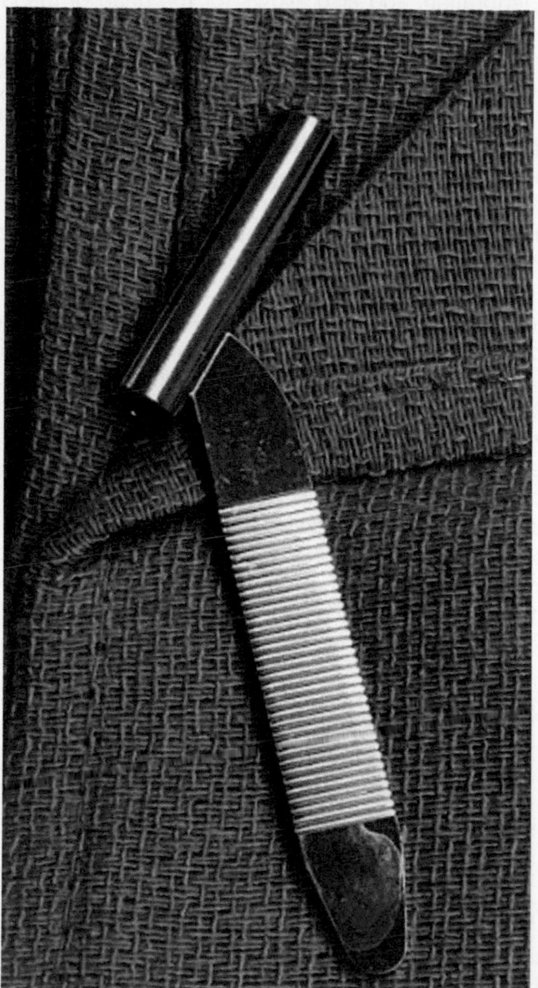

Fig. 2. It is important to use a specialized drill guard during osteotomy formation in order to prevent contact between the shaft of the drill and surrounding soft tissue.

be placed on the rotary handpiece at low speed, being guided along the same route taken with the implant drills. It should be advanced until the apex reaches the superior cortex of the zygoma, and then further rotated until the angled implant head is at the desired position at the maxillary alveolar crest (**Fig. 3**). At this point the cover screw can be placed, and the surgical flap re-approximated and closed with sutures.

Variations on the Intrasinus Approach

A common variation to the intrasinus approach, known as the sinus slot procedure, has been described by Stella and Warner.[12] In this technique, a slot is drilled into the side of the malar bone, extending from 5 mm superior to crest of the alveolar ridge to the superior extent of the contour of the zygomatic buttress. The implant drills, and the path of the implant will follow the line of this slot. This allows the zygomatic implant to pass directly through the lateral wall of the maxillary bone on its way to the zygomatic bone. This bypasses the need for a lateral window, decreases the chances of sinus membrane perforation, and also allows for the head of the implant to emerge at the height of the alveolar crest, rather than the palatal aspect.

Some patients may present with a deep buccal concavity of the lateral surface of the maxilla. Such a concavity may make it impossible to extend the zygomatic implant through the sinus or maxillary bone and into the zygoma, while still having the emergence of the implant head at an appropriate location on the alveolar ridge. In order to accommodate this anatomy, the extrasinus approach was developed. In this technique, the implant will pass from the alveolar ridge, then out through the lateral surface of the maxilla, where it would otherwise have entered the sinus cavity, before re-entering the maxilla at the zygomatic buttress, and then eventually entering the zygoma, itself.[13]

A more recent method, known as the extramaxillary technique, was developed to simplify the surgical technique and to facilitate a more prosthodontically appropriate emergence of the implant head. Similar to the extrasinus approach, the extramaxillary approach does not have the path of implant insertion enter into the sinus. However, in the extramaxillary approach, the implant will only contact the maxilla at the height of alveolar ridge before traveling lateral-superior-posterior and then anchoring the implant apex within the zygoma. In this approach, it is said that the alveolar ridge only accommodates the implant, meaning that it will pass through a channel made just at the lateral surface of the alveolus, in order to allow for ideal prosthodontic placement at the height of the crest, but that no actual anchorage or osseointegration occurs at this location (**Fig. 4**). All of the support for the implant comes from the osseointegration occurring within the zygoma itself.[14]

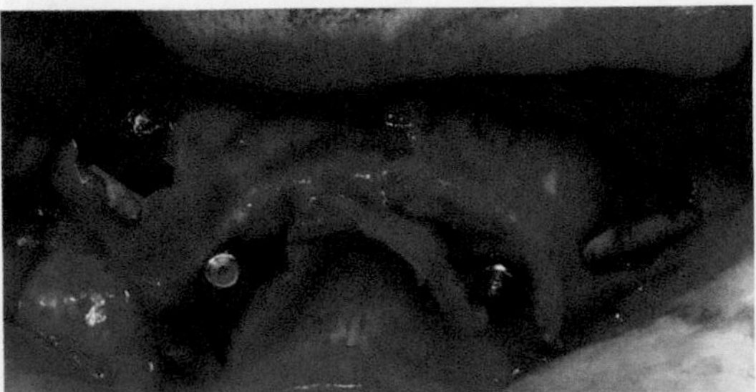

Fig. 3. The zygomatic implant should be advanced until the apex reaches the superior cortex of the zygoma, and then further rotated until the angled implant head is at the desired position at the maxillary alveolar crest.

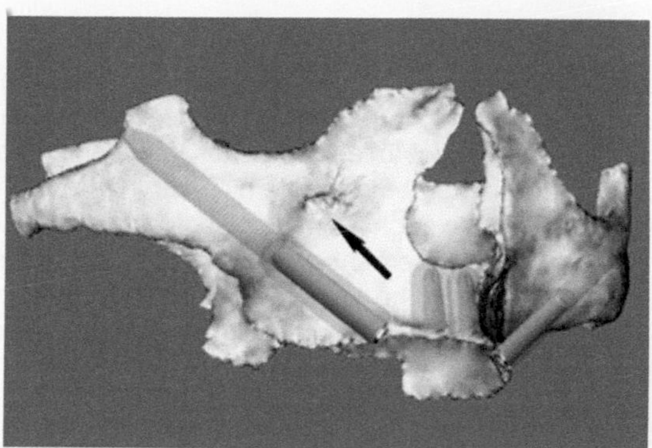

Fig. 4. Implant positions in all-on-4 hybrid situation. One standard maxillary anchored implant and 1 extramaxillary implant were placed bilaterally. Note extramaxillary implant placed posteriorly in inferior edge of zygoma, 3 mm from posterior vertical edge of zygomatic bone. Extramaxillary implant used exclusively zygomatic anchorage. Maxillary crest only accommodates implant, meaning that implant osseointegration only occurs in zygomatic bone. Note infraorbital foramen indicated by arrow. (*From* Maló P, Nobre MDA, Lopes I. A new approach to rehabilitate the severely atrophic maxilla using extramaxillary anchored implants in immediate function: a pilot study. J Prosthet Dent. 2008;100(5):357; with permission.)

Although not a separate technique, it is of note that the advent of computer-guided virtual surgical planning has provided the surgeon with novel ways to improve upon the aforementioned techniques. Using a computed tomography scan of a patient's facial bones, a surgical guide can be fabricated that will be able to accurately predetermine the appropriate length and width of the implant and direct the implant drills and placement of the implant along the preplanned path of insertion. This can obviate the necessity for such a large lateral window in the intrasinus technique, other than for intraoperative verification of implant placement.

COMPLICATIONS

As with any surgical procedure, there are risks and complications involved with the placement of zygomatic implants. Most of the complications associated with zygomatic implants are no different than those associated with standard dental implant placement, such as bleeding, swelling, infection, and failure of osseointegration. Other complications thought to be more strongly associated with zygomatic implants could include sinusitis, oroantral fistula formation, periorbital and conjunctival hematoma or edema, facial pain and edema, and epistaxis.[7] Some of the more serious complications could even include paresthesia of the infraorbital nerve, caused by possible proximity of path of zygomatic implant insertion, orbital floor perforation, and perforation into the infratemporal fossa. In a cadaver study performed by Yuki Uchida and colleagues[15] in 2001, it was shown that deviation from a fairly narrow range could cause severe damage to sensitive anatomic structures. If a line were drawn the point of ideal emergence of the zygomatic head in the alveolar bone to the point at which the temporal and frontal processes of the zygomatic bone meet (ie: jugale), it was shown that directing the implant at an angulation of 43.8° or less above this line could cause perforation of the infratemporal fossa, while directing the implant at an angulation of 50.6° or more above this line could cause perforation of the orbital floor.

SUMMARY

Studies of zygomatic implants placed in patients with severely atrophic or resected maxillae have shown that zygomatic implants constitute a successful and predictable method for supporting fixed or removable prostheses, and can be used to restore the maxillary dentition. These implants demonstrate high survival rates of 98.4% over the course of at least 12 years[9] and lack significant risk factors.[16] Given the relative simplicity of zygomatic implant placement compared with the drawn out process of significant bone grafting to restore the severely atrophic or resected maxilla, zygomatic implants continue to be an ideal, stable, and viable option for many patients who would have difficulty or be unable to undergo more traumatic treatment.

DISCLOSURE

The authors have nothing to disclose.

REFERENCES

1. Meyer U, Vollmer D, Runte C, et al. Bone loading pattern around implants in average and atrophic edentulous maxillae: a finite-element analysis. J Craniomaxillofac Surg 2001;29:100–5.
2. Block MS, Haggerty CJ, Fisher GR. Nongrafting implant options for restoration of the edentulous maxilla. J Oral Maxillofac Surg 2009;67:872–81.
3. Devlin H, Horner K, Ledgerton D. A comparison of maxillary and mandibular bone mineral densities. J Prosthet Dent 1998;79:323–7.
4. Bryant SR, Zarb GA. Outcomes of implant prosthodontic treatment in older adults. J Can Dent Assoc 2002;68:97–102.
5. Branemark PI. Surgery and fixture installation. Zygomaticus fixture clinical procedures. Goteborg (Sweden): Nobel Biocare AB; 1998.
6. Weischer T, Schettler D, Mohr C. Titanium implants in the zygoma as retaining elements after hemimaxillectomy. Int J Oral Maxillofac Implants 1997;12:211–4.
7. Stievenart M, Malevez C. Rehabilitation of totally atrophied by means of four zygomatic implants and fixed prosthesis: A 6-40 month follow-up. Int J Oral Maxillofac Surg 2010;39:358–63.
8. Ahlgren F, Størksen K, Tornes K. A study of 25 zygomatic dental implants with 11 to 49 months' follow-up after loading. Int J Oral Maxillofac Implants 2006;21:421–5.
9. Aparicio C, Ouazzani W, Hatano N. The use of zygomatic implants for prosthetic rehabilitation of the severely resorbed maxilla. Periodontol 2000 2008;47:162–71.
10. Nkenke E, Hahn M, Lell M, et al. Anatomic site evaluation of the zygomatic bone for dental implant placement. Clin Oral Implants Res 2003;14:72–9.
11. Ishak MI, Abdul Kadir MR. Treatment options for severely atrophic maxillae. Biomechanics in dentistry: evaluation of different surgical approaches to treat atrophic maxilla patients. Springer Science and Business Media; 2012.
12. Stella J, Warner M. Sinus slot technique for simplification and improved orientation of zygomaticus dental implants: a technical note. Int J Oral Maxillofac Implants 2000;20:788–92.
13. Aparicio C, Ouazzani W, Garcia R, et al. Prospective clinical study on titanium implants in the zygomatic arch for prosthetic rehabilitation of the atrophic edentulous maxilla with a follow-up of 6 months to 5 years. Clin Implant Dent Relat Res 2006;8:114–22.

14. Maló P, Nobre Mde A, Lopes I. A new approach to rehabilitate the severely atrophic maxilla using extramaxillary anchored implants in immediate function: a pilot study. J Prosthet Dent 2008;100:354–66.
15. Uchida Y, Goto M, Katsuki T, et al. Measurement of the maxilla and zygoma as an aid in installing zygomatic implants. J Oral Maxillofac Surg 2001;59:1193–8.
16. Chana H, Smith G, Bansal H, et al. A retrospective cohort study of the survival rate of 88 Zygomatic implants placed over an 18-year period. Int J Oral Maxillofac Implants 2019;34:461–70.

Treatment of the Dental Patient with Bleeding Dyscrasias

Etiologies and Management Options for Surgical Success in Practice

Leslie R. Halpern, DDS, MD, PHD, FICD[a,*], David R. Adams, DDS[a], Earl Clarkson, DDS[b]

KEYWORDS

• Anticoagulants • Antiplatelet medications • Hemophilia A • Hemophilia B • Hemostatic agents • Thromboprophylaxis • von Willebrand disease

KEY POINTS

- Oral health care providers see patients who are on anticoagulant and antiplatelet therapy for various medical conditions requiring hemostatic control.
- Patients who present with inherited bleeding dyscrasias require perioperative management that involves a knowledge of medicine and surgery in order to avoid an adverse thrombotic event.
- The oral health care provider must be knowledgeable in the treatment of hemostasis both during the intraoperative and postoperative period to avoid undue adverse bleeding.
- Although there is no consensus statement in oral health, the treatment of patients on anticoagulant and/or antiplatelet therapy, as well as inherited disorders, requires an awareness of evidence-based standards that have been applied in other specialties.
- Hemostatic agents are a useful adjunct in the treatment of patients who are at risk for acquired and inherited bleeding disorders.

INTRODUCTION

The oral health care provider sees a significant number of patients in his or her practice who suffer from either acquired or inherited bleeding dyscrasias. Although routine dental procedures are generally low-risk procedures in which there is little chance

[a] Oral and Maxillofacial Surgery, University of Utah School of Dentistry, 530 South Wakara Way, Salt Lake City, UT 84108, USA; [b] Woodhull Medical and Mental Health Center, 760 Broadway, Brooklyn, NY 11206, USA
* Corresponding author.
E-mail address: Leslie.halpern@hsc.utah.edu

Dent Clin N Am 64 (2020) 411–434
https://doi.org/10.1016/j.cden.2019.12.010

of adverse outcomes, patients with inherited or acquired bleeding disorders require careful attention with respect to the assessment of bleeding risk. A significant number of patients receives either oral anticoagulants or antiplatelet therapies as the most effective prophylactic medications to reduce thrombotic sequelae that predispose them to acquired bleeding disorders that can be life-threatening. Other patients who manifest systemic bleeding dyscrasias including inherited coagulation disorders such as hemophilia, von Willebrand disease, Christmas disease (factor IX deficiency), as well as those who suffer from platelet disorders must also be treated within a well-designed set of strategies for best management of hemostasis during surgical intervention and postoperative healing. Appropriate perioperative surgical management by the dental practitioner can help to avoid catastrophic adverse outcomes.

The severity of a bleeding dyscrasia will depend on disease-related factors, whether they be acquired or inherited, as well as patient factors such as type of vascular risk (ie, periodontal disease/inflammation, the number of teeth extracted, bone augmented, and wound surface violated or exposed).[1] Many practitioners agree that there is no standardized approach in the anticoagulant prophylaxis of patients requiring oral and maxillofacial surgical procedures. The purpose of this article is to develop a series of algorithms in the management of acquired and systemic bleeding dyscrasias seen by the oral health care practitioner in his or her practice. These approaches include a discussion of the epidemiology of bleeding disorders in surgical patients, mechanism of hemostasis, and strategies for patient management based on the etiology of the bleeding disorder, whether acquired or inherited.

HEMOSTASIS

The mechanism for normal hemostasis involves 3 events (**Box 1**).[1,2] Each requires a set algorithm within the cascade of clot formation that if interrupted by pharmacologic or genetic insult can result in significant bleeding during surgical intervention. **Fig. 1** provides a flow scheme/cascade depicting locations that can be targets for either genetic or pharmacologic disruption of normal hemostasis. The timing of a bleeding event during surgery will be predicated on whether the dyscrasia is a result of platelet dysfunction, or a breakdown in the pathway of coagulation. Preoperative laboratory tests are often required in order to determine whether bleeding can be a risk in surgical intervention. Several laboratory tests are recommended as evidence of hemostatic efficacy.[3]

Prothrombin Time

Prothrombin time (PT) tests the efficacy of the extrinsic pathway of clotting involving factors, X, VII, V, prothrombin, and fibrinogen. Prothrombin, VII, and factor X are vitamin K dependent and therefore associated with Warfarin therapy (see section on

Box 1
Three phases of hemostasis

1. Vascular phase. The phase of vasoconstriction to slow down the loss of blood
2. Platelet plug. This will initiate an aggregation of platelets and their activation along a scaffolding of subendothelial collagen.
3. Amplification phase. The platelets will release their granules and to trigger coagulation via thromboplastin, enzymes and cross-link to form a fibrin clot.

Adapted from Beirne RO. Anesthetic considerations for patients with bleeding disorders. In: Bosack RC, Lieblich S, editors. Anesthesia complications in the dental office. Ames, Iowa: John Wiley and Sons, Inc.; 2014. p. 103; with permission.

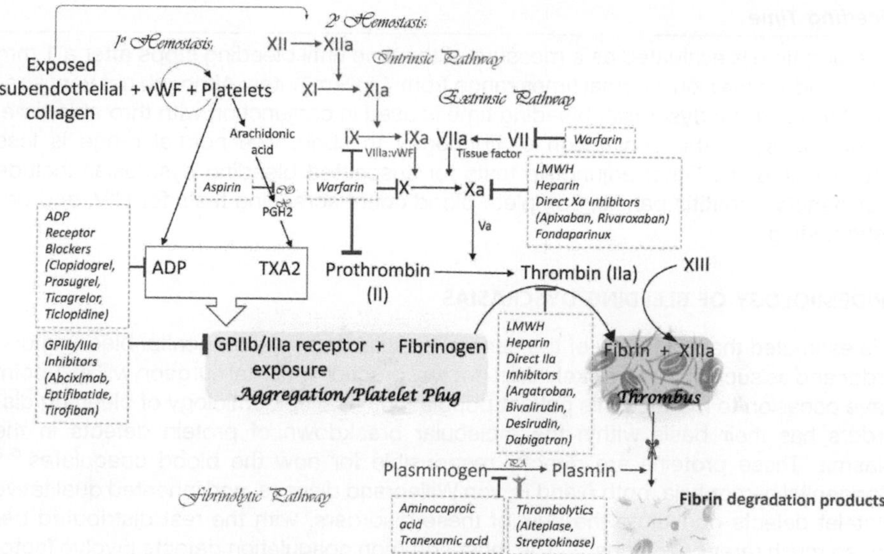

Fig. 1. The effect of anticoagulant/antiplatelet therapy on clot formation. Pathway for coagulation including the location of action by anticoagulants, antiplatelet therapeutics and factor activity of inherited bleeding disorders. (*Adapted from* Beirne RO. Anesthetic considerations for patients with bleeding disorders. In: Bosack RC, Lieblich S, editors. Anesthesia complications in the dental office. Ames, Iowa: John Wiley and Sons, Inc.; 2014. p. 103–11; with permission.)

anticoagulant therapies). The PT is measured using the International Normalized Ratio (INR) that measures the patient's PT in relation to the PT control that is standardized to the World Health Organization value.[4,5] This technique adjusts the actual PT for variations in the reagents used to run the test among hospitals. Under normal conditions the INR is 1.0.

Partial Thromboplastin Time

Partial thromboplastin time (aPTT) tests the adequacy of the intrinsic pathway of clotting involving factors VIII, IX, XI and XII as well as the common pathway (factor V, X, prothrombin, and fibrinogen). Abnormalities of aPTT are often a result of factor deficiencies of the intrinsic and common pathways of clotting. This can be used to identify genetic origins of bleeding problems. The normal value ranges from 22 to 34. aPTT can be used to correlate the effect of anticoagulants and antiplatelets as well as dysfunction of liver physiology.

Qualitative/Quantitative Platelet Dysfunction

The normal range of platelets can vary from 150,000 to 450,000/μL of blood. Absolute counts can identify deficiency (ie, thrombocytopenia but not necessarily function). Platelet function analysis 100 (PFA-100) can be used as a measure of function. Qualitative dysfunction (ie, a problem in the structure/function of the platelet) is often caused by missing or defective proteins, either on the surface or granules of the platelet, that prevent events in aggregation and clotting. The manifestations are presented as easy bruising, nosebleeds, bleeding of the mouth or gums, heavy menstrual bleeding (periods), postpartum (after child birth) bleeding, and bleeding following dental work, surgical, or invasive procedures.

Bleeding Time

Bleeding time is evaluated as a measure of the time until bleeding stops after a 1 mm slit is made in the skin. Normal times range from 7 to 9 minutes. Although not very specific for ruling in a dyscrasia, bleeding time is used in conjunction with thrombin time, which measures the conversion of fibrinogen to fibrin. The normal range is less than 10 seconds. Other adjunctive tests for suspected bleeding dyscrasias include liver panels, hepatitis panels, complete blood count screening tests for HIV, and genetic testing.

EPIDEMIOLOGY OF BLEEDING DYSCRASIAS

It is estimated that up to 1% of the general population has a congenital bleeding disorder and as such, it is more likely than not any practicing dental surgeon will at 1 point have occasion to manage this patient population.[6] The epidemiology of bleeding disorders has their basis within the molecular breakdown of protein defects in the plasma. These proteins are directly responsible for how the blood coagulates.[6–8] Congenital hemophilia, both A and B, von Willebrand disease, and inherited qualitative platelet defects constitute the bulk of these disorders, with the rest distributed between much rarer conditions.[6,7] The most common coagulation defects involve factor VIII, IX, XI, and von Willebrand. Hemophilia A (factor VIII deficiency) is the most common X-linked genetic disease, with a worldwide incidence rate of 1 case per 5000 males and one-third prevalence of 20.6 cases per 100,000.[6,7] Hemophilia B (factor IX deficiency) is less common and evident in 1 case per 25,000 to 30,000 male births and a prevalence of 5.3 per 100,000 males. Of all the cases of hemophilia, 80% to 85% are of the A group, and 14% are type B. von Willebrand disease (factor VIII c) is the second most common factor deficiency. Although males and females are affected equally with von Willebrand disease, the incidence rate is 125 persons per million population with severe disease affecting 0.5 to 5 persons per million.[6–9] Hemophilia C (factor XI deficiency) occurs in 1 case per 100,000. Although females are most often carriers since Hemophilia is x-linked, they may exhibit a mild form of the disease. The etiologies of these diseases are discussed with respect to perioperative treatment strategies (see below).

ACQUIRED BLEEDING DYSCRASIAS

Acquired bleeding disorders can develop because of systemic conditions like liver disease, renal dysfunction, nutritional deficiencies (ie, vitamin K deficiency), and medication adverse effects that create iatrogenic coagulation abnormalities.[5] Treatments for cardiovascular diseases such as heart valve replacement, atrial fibrillation, and venous thromboembolism have become more common, and millions of patients receive anticoagulant and antiplatelet therapies to reduce thrombosis and life-threatening sequela (ie, ischemic events in the heart, lungs, and brain).[10] The medical and dental communities have sought to craft a wide variety of strategies during the perioperative period to modify anticoagulants and antiplatelet agents to prevent hemorrhagic events during and after dental surgery.

The general algorithm for managing patients on either direct/indirect anticoagulant/antiplatelet medications is to first characterize the severity of bleeding based on the procedure that is planned and whether it will pose a significant risk. Routine dental procedures such as localized periodontal scaling or single tooth extraction may be considered low risk and as such not require a change in anticoagulating doses. As the complexity of the procedure increases and surgical time increases, so does the potential for hemorrhage. For elective procedures, one might consider staging procedures to decrease risk (ie, limiting the number of extractions per visit or conservative flap design). In general, the risk of thromboembolism increases transiently as anticoagulants are discontinued, so careful planning of elective procedures will benefit the patient. The following sections discuss the perioperative management of dental patients who require either direct anticoagulant or antiplatelet therapy for management of their medical issues.

Anticoagulants: Vitamin K Antagonists/Heparin/Direct Anticoagulants

Anticoagulants, which are agents that hinder the formation of blood clots, are the mainstay of treatment for many thromboembolic disorders including pulmonary embolism and stroke from atrial fibrillation and deep vein thrombosis. An estimated 30 million prescriptions are written annually in the United States for the anticoagulant warfarin alone.[1] Anticoagulants fall into 3 major categories: vitamin K antagonists, heparins, and direct anticoagulants (direct thrombin inhibitors/direct factor Ax inhibitors). The anticoagulant that requires the most attention in regard to outpatient dental procedures is warfarin, a vitamin K antagonist, as it is the most widely prescribed and requires close monitoring. However, newer anticoagulants such as the direct thrombin inhibitors are gaining attention because of their broad therapeutic window. **Box 2** describes a stepwise approach developed by Hasalszynki for perioperative workup of patients prescribed anticoagulants.[11]

Vitamin K antagonists

The oral anticoagulants most often seen in practice are derivatives of Coumadin (warfarin) or vitamin K antagonists, which act by inhibiting vitamin K epoxide reductase, the enzyme needed for cyclic interconversion of vitamin K.[12] Warfarin (Coumadin, Bristol-Meyers Squibb, New York, New York), which is derived from 4-hydroxycoumarin, is a competitive inhibitor of vitamin K and blocks the function of the vitamin K epoxide reductase complex in the liver. This inhibits the action of vitamin K-dependent factors II, VII, IX, and X and proteins C and S. Warfarin is metabolized in the liver by the cytochrome P450 system, and is administered in doses to achieve an INR of 2.0 to 3.0 for most clinical indications except in patients with mechanical heart valves and deep venous thromboses (DVT), where a higher INR is recommended (2.5–3.5).[11] Warfarin is absorbed rapidly from the gastrointestinal (GI) system and has a peak activity at 90 minutes with a half-lie of 36 to 42 hours.[13] The patients who are

Box 2
A stepwise workup of a patient on anticoagulant therapy

Step 1. Consider whether or not the anticoagulant medication can be discontinued or be maintained without interruption prior to the surgical procedure.

Step 2. Decide on the time period for discontinuation needed if the practitioner chooses to take the patient off the anticoagulant.

Step 3. Define a risk-to-benefit ratio with respect to risk of a thrombotic event if the anticoagulant is stopped during the perioperative period.

Step 4: If the patient is at high risk for a thromboembolic event, consider a bridging therapy protocol during the perioperative period of patient treatment.

Data from Halaszynski TM. Administration of coagulation-altering therapy in the patient presenting for oral health and maxillofacial surgery. Oral Maxillofac Surg Clin North Am. 2016:28(4):443–60.

prescribed warfarin must be carefully evaluated, as dosing can be affected by diet, drug-drug interactions, and other chronic illnesses. As such, the assessment of perioperative bleeding involves an understanding of these risk predictors when considering invasive oral health care intervention. The HAS-BLED score was crafted as a decision-making strategy for patients who required anticoagulation for atrial fibrillation (AF).[14] This pneumonic accounts for a history of hypertension, abnormal renal and liver function, stroke, bleeding predisposition, labile INR, elderly, and use of alcohol.[11,14] It also accounts for decisions on whether bridging should be considered to avoid thrombotic events.[15] The CHAD52 and CHA2DS2-VASc scores are other models (congestive heart failure, hypertension, age >65, diabetes, and stroke/TIA) that predict increase risk of thrombotic events. The CHADS2 more precisely predicts whether bridging therapy needs to be initiated for those taking warfarin and requires a discontinuation of anticoagulation.[14,15]

Debate continues with respect to risk of altering dosing in patients who are on warfarin. Several studies have suggested that anticoagulation can continue without interruption. High-risk procedures, however, lack a consensus statement with respect to continuation of therapy. van Diermen and colleagues[16] recommend discussion with the patient's physician if the INR is greater than 3.5 and complicated oral surgery is planned. Other studies did not confirm the association of increased risk of bleeding and a high INR. Bajkin and colleagues[12,17] studied 54 patients with INR values 3.5 to 4.2 who had up to 3 teeth extracted and recorded postoperative bleeding at 3.7% (2 of 54 patients). Scully and Wolff found that uncomplicated extraction of 3 teeth was safe if the INR is less than 3.5, while Chugani suggested that periodontal flaps, implant placement, and apicoectomy were not recommended in patients with INR ranges of 3.0 to 4.0.[18,19] Several studies mentioned that along with INR values and surgical trauma, an important risk predictor that influences postoperative bleeding is inflammation of the dental tissue environment, which is associated with a greater chance of significant bleeding.[19,20] Ward and Smith reviewed the literature in comparison with current practice by oral and maxillofacial surgeons who perform dentoalveolar procedures for the anticoagulated patient. They concluded that for moderate-to-high-risk procedures, warfarin discontinuation is recommended to minimal therapeutic levels as determined by the INR.[21] Future prospective trials are required, however, for stronger management guidelines in this population of patients.

The normal INR for a patient not on anticoagulation ranges from approximately 0.8 to 1.4. The target range of INR in the anticoagulated patient is 2.5, ranging from 2 to 3; however, some conditions such as the presence of an artificial heart valve require a higher target INR of 3 (range 2.5–3.5).[5,11,22] As a general rule, anticoagulation should not be discontinued prior to low-risk procedures, such as a simple dental extraction, if the INR on the day of surgery is within the therapeutic range, or less than 3.5. INR should be measured within 24 hours of surgery or within 72 hours for an INR stable patient. If the INR is above 3.5, then low-risk procedures are contraindicated as significant bleeding can occur.[11,22] Values greater than 3 warrant holding of warfarin for up to 5 days and retesting the INR.[5,22] Decisions to discontinue medication should always be done in conjunction with the patient's physician. Warfarin can be discontinued 5 days prior to surgery, with an INR drawn up to 24 hours prior. INR is then rechecked on the day of surgery to ensure that it is normal or less than 1.4. **Box 3** suggests the range of INR based on the condition being treated.[5,11,17,22] The practitioner must also check for concurrent medications affecting hemostatic mechanisms such as antiplatelet drugs, ASA and NSAIDS that can hamper hemostasis and cause hematoma formation.[11,22,23] Postoperatively, warfarin can usually be restarted 12 to 24 hours following the procedure as long as the risk of significant postoperative

Box 3
Recommended international normalized ratios for surgical procedures

1. INR Goal of 2.5 with a range from 2 to 3
   a. Venous thrombosis prophylaxis
   b. Treatment of pulmonary embolism
   c. Prevention of systemic embolism
   d. Tissue heart valves
   e. Acute myocardial infarction
   f. Atrial fibrillation
2. INR goal of 3 with a range from 2.5 to 3.5
   a. Most mechanical prosthetic heart valves
   b. Prevention of recurrent myocardial infarction

Data from Bajkin BV, Vujkov SB, Milekic BR, Vuckovic BA. Risk factors for bleeding after oral surgery in patients who continued using oral anticoagulant therapy. J Am Dent Assoc. 2015;146(6):375–81.

hemorrhage has passed. Because warfarin takes approximately 5 to 10 days to reach therapeutic levels, patients with high risk of thromboembolism might require bridging therapy in which an anticoagulant with a shorter onset and offset is used perioperatively.[24] Bridging therapy refers to anticoagulation using a short-acting blood thinner like low molecular weight heparin (LMWH) for 10 to 12 days around the time of the surgical intervention when warfarin is interrupted and the effect is outside of the therapeutic range. This will prevent the patient from risk of developing blood clots. Warfarin is stopped usually 5 to 6 days prior to surgery and restarted 24 hours after.[11,22,24]

Post-myocardial infarction patients with high risk of thromboembolism may also be taking low-dose antiplatelet medication. These patients on high-intensity anticoagulation have a fivefold greater risk for bleeding compared with low-intensity anticoagulation. Warfarin can be reversed with fresh-frozen plasma (10–15 mg/kg) as well as with a slow infusion of vitamin k (5–10 mg). The US Food and Drug Administration (FDA) is evaluating a 4-factor prothrombin complex concentrate containing factors II, VII, IX, X.[25] Warfarin therapy can be resumed within 12 to 24 hours after procedure if hemostasis is well-controlled. If bridging was required, then this approach may be altered. The American College of Chest Physicians (ACCP) recommends the administration of an oral prohemostatic agent (eg, 5 mL tranexamic acid rinse 5–10 minutes before surgery and 3 or 4 times daily for the next 1–2 days), which is associated with a low risk (<5%) of a major bleeding event.[26]

Heparin: unfractionated heparin/low molecular weight heparin

Heparin is a glycosaminoglycan found in the secretory granules of the mast cells. It serves as an anticoagulant that is activated by antithrombin, which binds to a 5-saccharide sequence on heparin, which then activates an antithrombin enzyme that will bind to factor Xa. Thrombin (factor II) inhibition will occur when antithrombin and thrombin both bind to sites on heparin. The heparin will then act as a catalyst, contributing to thrombin inhibition by activating antithrombin III.[27] Unfractionated heparin is comprised of heterogeneous heparin molecules not degraded by the enzyme glucuronidase in the mast cells. It activates thrombin III and can be monitored with use of aPTT with a prolongation time 2 to 3 as therapeutic. Low molecular weight heparin (LMWH) activates thrombin III and inhibits factor Xa. It does not require monitoring of aPTT to be therapeutic. Fondaparinux is a synthetic derivative of the 5-chain binding sequence found on heparin. It selectively causes inhibition of factor Xa and similar to LMWH. Like LMWH, it is given subcutaneously once daily at a dose of 5.0 to 10.0

based upon weight (in kilograms), and it also does not respond to laboratory monitoring. Its half-life is 17 hours, and it is cleared by the kidneys.[11,27]

Heparin can be administered either by intravenous or subcutaneous approaches. Unfractionated heparin is often indicated as a bridging therapy (in the event that warfarin needs to be stopped) or as an inpatient anticoagulation therapy for thromboembolism, because the onset is immediate. Bridging can also be accomplished with LMWH, and either unfractionated heparin or LMWH can be initiated 24 to 48 hours after warfarin cessation with INR monitoring to a normal range.[11,27] Unfractionated heparin is discontinued at 6 to 8 hours prior to surgical intervention, and LMWH is administered at 50% of the dose 12 to 24 hours before surgery. Several local hemostatic measures can be applied to prevent hemorrhage; however, careful monitoring involves the extent of surgical exposure and systemic risks such as cerebral infarcts and acute coronary syndrome.[11,27,28] Other prophylactic approaches for hemostasis include external compression stockings in patients with high-risk criteria such as obesity, malignancy, immobility, smoking, and hypercoagulability. The perioperative management of patients who are on fondaparinux is less well studied. Recommendations include a discontinuation for 2 half-life time periods prior to minimal surgical intervention and a 3- to 4-day discontinuation period prior to major procedures. The drug is resumed 24 hours after.[27]

Several contraindications of heparin-based therapy need to be addressed. Patients are often on several drugs at the same time, and as such they can affect hemostasis. Antiplatelet and other fibrinolytic agents can increase the risk of hemorrhage with subsequent need for transfusions. Other factors such as liver disease susceptibility to thrombocytopenia can cause adverse events during the perioperative period of treatment. The latter is a result of a heparin-induced thrombocytopenic (HIT) caused by antibodies that activate platelets in the presence of heparin.[11,27] Type I HIT is a nonimmunological-mediated response that usually appears within the first 2 to 3 days after the initiation of heparin treatment. It typically causes a mild and transient thrombocytopenia (rarely <100, 000/mm3), which occurs because of a direct interaction with platelets and heparin that causes clumping and is not associated with an increased risk of thrombosis. HIT type II, however, is associated with an immunologic response and does have an increased risk of thrombosis and can be detected via laboratory testing (heparin-induced platelet aggregation [HIPA] and the serotonin release assay). The treatment is immediate cessation of heparin therapy and monitoring until thrombocytopenia resolves.[29]

The half-life of heparin and its coagents is short. In the event of a major bleeding episode, it can be neutralized with protamine sulfate (PS). PS binds to heparin as a complex that neutralizes the anticoagulant effect. 1 mg dosing of PR can neutralize 100 units of heparin. LMWH is partially neutralized by PS at the antifactor Xa portion of the protein chain. PS can elicit an adverse event because of its causation of histamine release and risk of a resultant anaphylactic event. Careful slow dosing intravenously should not exceed 50 mg.[11,27,28]

Direct anticoagulants:/thrombin inhibitors

The dynamic of thromboprophylaxis with anticoagulants is of the utmost importance in managing patients who are at risk for systemic embolization and catastrophic events. Newer anticoagulants have gained popularity over direct vitamin K antagonists because of their more predictable anticoagulation.[11,30] These direct thrombin inhibitors (DOAs) have broad therapeutic windows, allow fixed dosing, and lack interaction with cytochrome P450 enzymes, which eliminate the need for frequent monitoring. Their targets are enzymes that affect thrombin and factor Xa; they have shorter half-lives and as such are easier to discontinue and resume rapidly.[22] These agents, however, were thought to lack a specific antidote, which raises concern for emergent management of patients who require hemostatic control (ie, maxillofacial trauma patients or those who require full mouth extractions prior to cardiothoracic intervention) and increased risk of a thromboembolic event (see below). The newer oral anticoagulants, whether they be direct thrombin inhibitors or antifactor Xa, have a peak anticoagulant effect within 2 to 3 hours that will potentially reduce the need for temporary bridging.

Thrombin inhibitors These medications interrupt the proteolysis of thrombin by inactivating fibrin bound to thrombin and target factor IIa to cause direct inhibition of thrombin. Direct thrombin inhibitors prevent thrombin from cleaving fibrinogen to fibrin, which is involved in the formation of clots. This effect is exerted on the soluble and fibrin-bound forms of thrombin. Additionally, thrombin activates factors V, VIII, XI and XIII and binds to thrombomodulin and activating protein C.[31] The term hirudins refers to a class of antithrombotic agents structurally derived from the medicinal leech salivary protein hirudin. These proteins prevent deep venous thrombosis and are often prescribed for patients who have had hip replacements who are at risk for deep vein thrombosis (DVT) or PE. Their half-life is 30 minutes to 3 hours, and they can be monitored using the aPTT, which is prolonged for thromboprophylaxis.[11,32] Dabigatran (PRADAXA, Boehringer-Ingelheim, Ridgefield, Connecticut) is the only widely available oral direct thrombin inhibitor, but parenteral drugs in this class are available and include lepirudin, desirudin, bivalirudin, and argratroban. They are currently approved for use in the prevention of venous thromboembolism and stroke in nonvalvular atrial fibrillation.[11,32]

The risk of perioperative bleeding in patients who are taking direct thrombin inhibitors is comparable to those on warfarin (ie, warfarin,4.6%; dabigatran, 5.1%).[33] Monitoring. however, can be challenging, as no laboratory value can determine risk of bleeding with dabigatran, and as such a careful assessment of risk with surgical intervention is required. Several studies have characterized rare bleeding events in patients who were on dabigatron and received dental extractions, while other studies find it prudent to stop the medications except in those oral procedures that may result in minimal bleeding.[11,33] When on direct thrombin inhibitors, the risk of hemorrhage is comparable to anticoagulation with warfarin, with an INR of 2.0 to 3.0. When the risk of hemorrhage is significant, and anticoagulation needs to be discontinued, renal function should be considered, as 80% of the drug is excreted unchanged in urine; therefore, a patient with reduced creatinine clearance will require a longer drug hiatus prior to surgery.[34] For low risk of bleeding, dabigatran can be held for 24 hours prior to surgery. For high risk of bleeding, it can be held 48 to 72 hours or longer if renal function is diminished. Postoperatively, because of its fast onset, dabigatran can be restarted once hemostasis is achieved or within 24 hours after a low-risk procedure and within 48 to 72 hours if the procedure is of high risk.[35]

Bleeding complications from an interventional procedure such as nerve blocks and soft tissue procedures can result in hematomas, and subcutaneous ecchymosis require a formal risk assessment as described previously with the treating physician as to the need for altering the patient's anticoagulant therapy when necessary. Patients who present emergently from maxillofacial trauma should have therapy discontinued and be placed on supportive measures to prevent hemorrhage. Laboratory values can be applied if they are on warfarin or dabigatran that will serve only to indirectly measure whether the drugs are in their system. Idarucizumab (Praxbind) is an antidote for patients taking Dabigatran and used against the risk of major bleeding in this patient group.[34,35]

Direct factor Xa inhibitors The direct factor Xa inhibitors are a new group of anticoagulants that are being considered as substitutes for both vitamin K antagonists and LMWH in certain patient populations.[11] These xabans (inhibitors) include rivaroxaban (XARELTO, Janssen Pharmaceuticals, Titusville, New Jersey, apixaban ELIQUIS, Pfizer, New York, New York), edoxaban (Savaysa), and Betrixaban (in development). Their monitoring is less needed because of quick onset and fewer drug and food interactions, thereby providing consistency in therapeutic blood levels.[11,22,36] Factor Xa inhibitors prevent the cleaving of prothrombin to thrombin. The inhibition of factor Xa is important and provides a robust response, because 1 molecule of factor Xa can cleave approximately 1000 molecules of prothrombin to thrombin. Additionally, factor Xa exists in both circulating and clot-bound forms, and direct Xa inhibitors are able to act on both. This is advantageous, as these inhibitors do not require a cofactor, act at a single step in coagulation, and are metabolized in the liver and kidney, which will prevent liver accumulation of the drug and prevent hepatic insufficiency.[11,22]

Generally speaking, dentoalveolar procedures that are simple; that is, extraction of up to 3 teeth require no monitoring of factor Xa. It is prudent, however, to know the level of anticoagulation in circumstances of trauma and the high-risk surgical patient. Rivaroxaban should be discontinued 48 hours in advance of a high-risk procedure and restarted as soon as hemostasis has been achieved (or in 48–72 hours if there is high risk of postoperative bleeding). For lower-risk bleeding procedures, rivaroxaban can be stopped as little as 1 day prior if renal function is normal. Moderate- to high-risk patients on apixaban (Eliquis) in the perioperative period should be managed individually. Apixaban is recommended to be discontinued 3 to 5 days in advance of a high-risk procedure in those with normal renal function. In low-risk procedures such as dental extractions (excluding multiple tooth extraction), apixaban can be continued.[35] For patients who experience minor bleeding, consider local hemostatic measures (suturing, placement of gelatin sponge, and tranexamic acid rinse). In moderate-to-severe bleeding, mechanical compression, fluid replacement, hemodynamic support, oral charcoal (if recent ingestion <2 hours to remove the pro-drug from the gastrointestinal tract) or hemodialysis may be appropriate. In situations where there is major life-threatening bleeding, administration of a 4-factor prothrombin complex concentrate (factors II, VII, IX, X) is recommended (see section on postoperative hemostatic measures).[34,37] **Table 1** lists the most recent guidelines for continuance/discontinuance of anticoagulant therapy.

Antiplatelet Agents: Aspirin/Adenosine Diphosphate Inhibitors/Phosphodiesterase Inhibitors

The antiplatelet medications are categorized based on mechanism of action. The 3 most common agents seen in oral health care practice are aspirin, adenosine diphosphate inhibitors, and phosphodiesterase inhibitors.

Aspirin (acetylsalicylic acid); thromboxane/cyclooxygenase inhibitors

Salicylic acid, the active ingredient of aspirin, suppresses the action of prostaglandins and thromboxane. Dosing varies, and low-dose ASA (40–100 mg) irreversibly blocks thromboxane A2 on platelets with a resultant inhibition on platelet aggregation. At higher doses, ASA inhibits the synthesis of A2, as well as cyclooxygenase 1 and 2.[38] These characteristics of ASA make it advantageous in reducing cardiovascular events in the acute phase of a myocardial infarction

Table 1
Antiplatelet and anticoagulant crugs

Anticoagulants (DOAC)				
Generic	**Proprietary**	**Mechanism of Action**	**Renal Function Cr/Cl/min**	**Discontinue (D/C) or not (N)**
Warfarin Half-life: 20–60 h	Coumadin	Antagonist of vitamin K, and affecting II,VII,IX,X	>80 mL/min: Hold 48 h 50–80 mL/min: Hold 72 h	D/C based upon INR (If >4 no surgery)
Dabigatran Half-life: 12–17 h	Pradaxa	Inhibitor of free thrombin Thrombin bound to fibrin; inhibits activity of IIa (INR not required)	≥80 mL/min	N based upon number of teeth to be removed (>2 discuss with physician)
Rivaroxaban Half-life: 9–13 h	Xarelto	Selective factor Xa inhibitors (INR not required)	≥50 mL/min	N based on the number of teeth (ie, >2–3)
Apixaban Half-life: 9–14 h	Eliquis	Selective factor Xa inhibitors (INR not required)	≥50 mL/min	N based on the number of teeth (ie, >2–3)
Heparin (LMWH) enoxaparin Half-life: 4.5 h Dalteparin Half-life: 2.2 h	Lovenox Fragmin	Inhibit activity of Xa and IIa		Used for bridging to avoid undue thromboembolic events

Antiplatelet Medication (NOAP/Others)				
Generic	**Proprietary**	**Mechanism of Action**	**Renal Function CR/Cl/ min**	**Discontinue (D/C) or Not (N)**
Acetyl salicylic acid Half-life:15–20 min	Aspirin, BioPak, Adira	Inhibits TXA_2 and platelet aggregation		D/C depends upon dosing: 325 mg vs. 81 mg
Dipyridamole	Persantine	Blocks adenosine transport in platelets, erythrocytes and endothelial cells; acts on platelet A2-receptors increasing cAMP and blocks platelet aggregation		Works with ASA and not usually used alone; short half-life D/C based upon dual effects with other antiplatelet drugs

(*continued on next page*)

Table 1
(continued)

Antiplatelet Medication (NOAP/Others)				
Generic	**Proprietary**	**Mechanism of Action**	**Renal Function CR/Cl/ min**	**Discontinue (D/C) or Not (N)**
Clopidogrel bisulfate Half-life: 7–9 h	Plavix, Iscover	Inhibit platelet aggregation by blocking ADP binding to platelet receptors (P_2Y_{12}) and activation of GPIIb-IIIa complex		Do not D/C up to 1 y; after 1 y check with physician prior to D/C based on complexity of procedure
Ticlopidine hydrochloride	Ticlid, Ticlodone	Inhibits platelet binding to ADP-fibrinogen as well as platelet aggregation		D/C 10–14 d prior to elective surgery
Cilostazol	Pletal	Prevents platelet aggregation and indices vasodilatory effects		Must D/C 10–14 d prior to elective surgery
Prasugrel Half-life: 7 h	Effient	A thieno-pyridine that binds irreversibly to P_2Y_{12} platelet receptors		N: do not D/C for elective surgery
Ticagrelor Half-life: 7–9 h	Brilique	A thieno-pyridine that binds irreversibly to P_2Y_{12} platelet receptors		N: do not D/C for elective surgery

(MI), stroke and vascular diseases at a dosing regimen of 75 to 325 mg.[38,39] The oral health care practitioner routinely sees patients in his or her practice who are on ASA at varying doses. Numerous studies agree that it is unnecessary to withhold ASA for dental extractions, because most surgical bleeding is resolved with local hemostatic methods.[40,41] A recent consensus statement from the American Heart Association, American College of Surgeons, and the American Dental Association recommends discontinuing ASA therapy for minor oral surgery procedures in patients with coronary stents or delaying major procedures until the initial regimens of antiplatelet therapy are completed.[42] Other studies agree that antiplatelet treatment with ASA shows no clinical significant increases in the frequency of intraoperative and/or postoperative bleeding complications during dentoalveolar surgery. Major oral and maxillofacial surgery, however, may require closer monitoring because of the likelihood of large hematoma formation in repairs of the midface and orbit.[38] For more invasive noncardiac surgery such as full mouth extractions, the recommendation is to discontinue aspirin 5 to 10 days prior to surgery and resume when the risk of major bleeding has resolved.

Adenosine diphosphate inhibitors

There are 2 classes within this group of antiplatelet medications: thienopyridines consisting of ticlopidine, clopidogrel, and prasugrel; and cyclopentyltriazopyrimidine (CPTP), consisting of ticagrelor.

Thienopyridines Ticlopidine was one of the initial medications in this group and provided antiplatelet protection against stroke. Its adverse effect of causing thrombotic thrombocytopenic purpura (TTP) has resulted in its unavailability in the United states.[38] Clopidogrel inhibits the P2Y12 receptor on the ADP platelet cellular membrane. Dosing is at 75 mg daily, and the most common adverse event is bleeding if dual therapy with ASA is prescribed.,[38] TTP is a rare occurrence. Prasugrel also binds to the same receptor as clopidogrel but works more efficiently than clopidogrel. Side effects are similar to the factors already mentioned.

Cyclopentyltriazopyrimidine Ticagrelor blocks the P2Y12 receptor that is different than the ADP, and the binding is reversible. It is not activated by the liver, and it is superior to clopidogrel for reducing cardiovascular death. Adverse effects are bleeding and dyspnea.

Phosphodiesterase inhibitors

Cilostazol is a type-3 phosphodiesterase inhibitor that increases cAMP with subsequent platelet aggregation and vasodilatation. It is avoided in patients susceptible to congestive heart failure, and patients need to avoid grapefruit juice in their diet because of its effect on prolongation of the drug action.[38,43] Other intravenous antiplatelet drugs exist for patient treatment and the reader is referred to the bibliography for references.

Surgeons are faced with the same dilemma of whether to discontinue antiplatelet therapy during perioperative dental and oral and maxillofacial surgical intervention, as this period is associated with an increased risk of a thrombotic and/or hemorrhagic event. The latter is predicated upon the timing of pharmacologic therapy (ie, when the angioplasty/stenting took place). Rebound platelet activity has the potential for a severe thrombotic event.[38,44] Studies suggest a discontinuation 5 to 7 days prior to surgical therapy, and patients at high risk should undergo a bridging regimen with either unfractionated or LMWH.[38] Patients who are on combination medicine regimens require special consideration. The most common combinations consist of antiplatelet agents and nonsteroidal anti-inflammatory drugs (NASAIDS), as well as herbal supplements such as garlic, gingseng, fish oil and gingko. Aspirin and NAIDS may be discontinued at the discretion of the practitioner. The antiplatelet medications such as ticlopine/clopidogrel and other GPIIb/IIIa antagonists are still being studied. For most outpatient procedures, continuation of antiplatelet therapy outweighs risk of discontinuation. It is prudent, however, to consult with the patient's cardiologist and cardiac surgeon, as their expertise is as rigorous as ours with respect to level A evidence. **Table 1** lists the most recent guidelines for continuance/discontinuance of antiplatelet and anticoagulant therapy.

HEREDITARY BLEEDING DYSCRASIAS

Oral and dentoalveolar surgery can be complicated, with a significant degree of morbidity in patients with inherited bleeding disorders. The severity of the event depends upon both the invasiveness of the surgery, as well as systemic manifestations that the disorder produces. Many disorders seen are congenital in nature and often result in barriers to treatment because of the patient's access to care, as well as fear of bleeding, lack of dental provider experience, and in some cases long waiting times to access dental care in hospitals. The following common congenital bleeding dyscrasias are discussed with respect to etiology and treatment options that can be applied for best practice in the oral health care setting.

Hemophilia A and Hemophilia B

Hemophilia A is the most common congenital bleeding disorder seen in the oral health care arena. It is x-linked, exhibited by a deficiency in factor VIII. The incidence rate is 1 case per 5000 male births with no racial or geographic predilection.[6,45] Concerns for adverse catastrophic bleeding include soft tissue bleeding into the neck and retropharyngeal region with its impingement on the airway, intracranial bleeding, and death, as well as bleeding into the retroperitoneal region and resultant shock.[45] These events depend on the clinical expression of factor VIII (normal: 50%–100%), which can be mild (5%–40%), moderate (1%–5%), or severe (less than 1%).[46] Another form of hemophilia A is acquired A (AHA), which manifests itself as an autoimmune disorder with autoantibodies (immunoglobulin G [IgG]) that inhibit factor VIII. The epidemiology is 0.2 to 1.5 patients per 1 million population with a bimodal distribution in an age from 20 to 40 and age greater than 60, most of whom are young pregnant females and/or those who exhibit collagen vascular diseases, reactions to antibiotics and NSAIDS, and idiopathic dermatologic disease.[45,47] Although pregnancy-related AHA can resolve, other causation requires immunosuppressive therapy.

Patients who exhibit mild hemophilia A do not bleed spontaneously but only when invasive therapy is undertaken. Moderate cases will be characterized by an excess bleeding after surgery such as dental extractions, as well as injuries to muscles and joints that increase in severity as the factor VIII decreases. **Fig. 1** depicts where factor VIII (made in the liver and reticuloendothelial system) acts as a cofactor of factor IXa, followed by factors X to Xa. A deficiency of factors VIII and/or IX will impede thrombin and clot formation. Those who suffer from the severe form will be susceptible to increased risk of bleeding beginning in their first year of life with concomitant bruising; hematoma formation in muscles, knee joints, ankles, shoulders, and elbows; and occurrence of painful hemarthroses leading to joint dysfunction.

Hemophilia B, referred to as Christmas disease is also an x-linked recessive disorder that affects the cascade of factor IX to IXa in the clotting pathway. It exhibits an incidence rate of 1 case per 30,000 patients and one-third of all cases occur through a spontaneous mutation.[6,45] Clinically, hemophilia A and hemophilia B appear similar, and laboratory testing is uniform using an increased partial thromboplastin time (aPTT) as an indicator. Hemophilia B is 4 times less common than hemophilia A with mild (6%–49%), moderate (1%–5%), and severe (<1%) presentations. The most common symptoms at presentation relate to bleeding into the joints, with inflammation leading to deformities and rare findings of abdominal pseudotumours.[6,45]

The perioperative management of the patient requires an approach that includes an understanding of the mechanism by which hemophilia exerts its pathologic effects and severity of disease expression. This mechanism has its basis in the formation of inhibitors that are immunoglobulins, which develop against factors VIII and IX.[48] The influence of IgG inhibition is more severe in hemophilia A than B. The severity of IgG in hemophilia B, however, is significant systemically with resultant renal damage, as well as risk of anaphylaxis because of its influence on inhibitor activation.[49] Studies suggest that the influence of inhibitor activity lies in repeated exposures of factor concentrates used for patient protection. Some authors have postulated the effect of ethnicity, while other studies produced conflicting findings.[6,50] In general, the treatment of inhibitor adverse events is based on immune tolerance induction (ITI) that will prevent active bleeding during surgery. Patients who suffer from hemophilia A or B can receive high doses of factor VIII or IX, respectively, to override the inhibitor's ability to produce enough IgG as a causation for increased bleeding. This requires an initial measurement of the levels of inhibitors already present. Levels of inhibitors at 5 BU/mL (Bethesda units) or less are referred to as low responders and good candidates for high levels of factor replacement, while those greater than 5 BU/mL are considered as high responders of inhibitors and are treated with other factor products.

ITI approaches are often applied in patients with hemophilia A, as ITI helps to eliminate inhibitory activation. ITI must be utilized at an early age, and various protocols can be applied including immunopheresis techniques, as well as pharmacologic agents such as dexamethasone, cyclophosphamide, and other immunosuppressive drugs.[6,51] Treatment success will be predicated upon plasma factor peak serum levels measured over a time period of 30 minutes, with factor recovery at 66% better than predicted, and inhibitor titers less than 20%.

Perioperative management of bleeding

As stated previously, the management of a patient with hemophilia is based on the severity, history of inhibitor levels, and previous surgical intervention. A hematological workup and prior consultation with the patient's hematologist will make the perioperative course easier to manage. In general, the goal is to raise factor levels at 70% to 80% preoperatively based upon the depth of surgical intervention (ie, dentoalveolar surgery requires 50% to 70% factor present before and 50% 5 to 7 days postoperatively).[6,52] Factor VIII has a half-life of 6 to 16 hours, while Factor IX has a half-life of 14 to 27 hours. This will determine the degree of factor replacement required, and as such there are specific guidelines that have been developed.[52] The World Federation of Hemophilia recommends treating the factor deficiency with the specific concentrate and that factor levels be maintained in the normal range prior to surgical intervention.[53,54] Rasaratnam and colleagues[55] (2017) developed a risk management assessment tool (DeBRATT) to enable a risk-based approach for the management of dental procedures to aid in the interdisciplinary consults required prior to surgery in patients suffering from hemophilia. Their results supported a comprehensive approach to decrease the anxiety for both patients and hematology colleagues when facilitating safe management in this patient population.

The specific guidelines for factor replacement suggest a dose of 1.0 IU/kg of factor VIII to increase factor VIII by 2%. Factor IX requires 1.0 IU/kg to increase by 1%. A dose of 50 IU/kg of factor VIII and 1000 IU/kg of factor IX concentrate is required for major surgery.[56] The administration of factor concentrate requires a window of 10 to 20 minutes to avoid decreased effectiveness and as such, repeated dosing every 12 hours in hemophilia A and 24 hours in hemophilia B patients is required.[6,56] Patients susceptible to inhibitory IgG should be screened in order to support the factor concentrates needed perioperatively and intraoperatively. Low inhibitory responders will require higher dosing of VIII or IX. Those with high IgG should be treated with factor VIII inhibitor bypass agent (FEIBA).[6,51] Patients with low or moderate levels of IgG inhibitor can be treated alternatively with desmopressin (DDAVP), a synthetic analog of vasopressin. Dosing can be given either through an intravenous, intranasal, or subcutaneous route every 12 hours. Patients who receive DDAVP, however, may develop a tolerance because of tachyphylaxis, as well as a hyponatremia because of the action of DDAVP as an antidiuretic.[57]

von Willebrand Disease

von Willebrand Disease is an inherited or drug/disease induced condition first described in 1926 by von Willebrand.[58] He referred to this bleeding dyscrasia as "hereditary pseudo hemophilia" with no gender predilection and severe prolongation of bleeding time. von Willebrand disease is the most common bleeding disorder, with 1% of the population affected most who are asymptomatic because of its incomplete penetrance.[59] von Willebrand factor is on the gene off chromosome 12 and is synthesized in endothelial cells and megakaryocytes. von Willebrand factor serves to bind and stabilize factor VIII so that factor VIII activates factor X to eventually form a fibrin clot. Three variants are characterized: type 1 as a partial quantitative deficiency of normal von Willebrand factor; type 2 (qualitative defects in von Willebrand factor); and type 3 (almost complete quantitative deficiency of von Willebrand factor).[9] The age at which symptoms begin vary from young childhood crawling with joint pain and bleeding to patients who have no symptoms until exposed to trauma and/or surgery. Epistaxis and bleeding after dental extractions to heavy menses and excessive postpartum bleeding are leading presentations. von Willebrand factor can slow down the turnover of factor VIII and present analogous to hemophiliac patients (ie, bleeding, muscle hemarthroses, and ecchymotic expansive lesions).

Perioperative management of bleeding

Perioperative treatment for von Willebrand factor is predicated on the type of severity presented. DDAVP elicits the release of von Willebrand factor and factor VIII from endothelial cells in patients with type 1 disease, as well as certain type 2 variants.[60] DDAVP is ineffective in type 3 patients, and so type 2 and type 3 patients are better managed with von Willebrand factor replacement agents that are plasma based and contain factor VIII, three of which are approved by the US Food and Drug Administration (FDA) (Humate B; wilate, and Alphanate).[9,60] Alphanate, however, is not approved under cases of major surgical intervention in type 3 patients.[9] Single dosing of von Willebrand factor is given before surgery and continued 5 to 7 days postoperatively. The initial dosing is 50 U/kg body weight with repeated dosing every 12 to 24 hours, as the half-life of von Willebrand Factor is 12 hours. Ristocetin, a cofactor usually measured to determine levels of von Willebrand factor, can be determined as an additional calculator of von Willebrand factor dosing.

Antifribinolytic agents are also recommended to help maintain the clot. Transexamic acid or epsilon-aminocaproic acid is used prophylactically before surgery and continued 5 to 7 days postoperatively. Concomitant local measures for hemostasis are also applied during the first week of postoperative healing. Transexamic acid and epsilon-aminocaproic acid can be used in an oral rinse form to control postoperative hemostasis in patients after dentoalveolar surgery. 10 mL of a 5% solution of transexamic acid or epsilon-aminocaproic acid can be held in the mouth for 2 min/2 h interval up to 6 to 10 times per day and continued for 5 days postoperatively.

HEMOSTATIC AGENTS

The maintenance of hemostasis is paramount in any surgical procedure but especially of significance when treating patients with acquired and/or hereditary bleeding disorders. With the advent of technological advances in hemostasis there are numerous topical agents that can be of benefit to patients who are unusually susceptible to increased postoperative bleeding. Postextraction hemorrhage can be classified as primary, reactionary, and secondary. Primary postextraction hemorrhage occurs at the time of surgery, Secondary postextraction hemorrhage occurs 2 to 3 hours postoperatively, often as a result of a cessation of vasoconstriction, and reactive postextraction hemorrhage can occur up to 2 weeks postoperatively, often as a result of infection.[61] For many simple low-risk oral and maxillofacial surgical procedures, direct gauze pressure applied for a few minutes to up to a few hours over the surgical site will allow for blood clot formation and cessation of bleeding. Abnormal postextraction bleeding may occur as a result of local and/or systemic factors. Local bleeding can come from soft tissues or bone. This can be caused by a traumatic extraction leading to lacerations of capillary, venous, or arterial blood vessels. Bone bleeding can come from nutrient canals or central vessels. Local inflammation or infection at the surgical site can be associated with persistent postoperative bleeding.[62] First-line measures for more-than-normal bleeding may consist of local injection of local anesthetic with epinephrine or topical agents such as ferrous sulfate or silver nitrate for small areas of bleeding. Suturing flaps and packing bleeding sockets are generally effective for persistent postextraction bleeding.

The surgical literature has reevaluated the variety of topical hemostatic agents available, and Vezeau[63] has classified them according to their mechanism of action.[63] Hemostatic agents often used in packing bleeding sockets and other defects can generally be classified as passive agents and active agents. More specifically, these are further separated into scaffold/matrix, biologic, stypic, tissue adhesive, occlusive, sealant, and vasoconstrictive.[62–64] There are few contraindications to the use of topical hemostatic agents, such as not being applied intravascularly because of the risk of a thrombotic event. In addition, most of the hemostatic agents are contraindicated in contaminated wounds.[62,63] **Table 2** summarizes these agents.

SUMMARY/FUTURE DIRECTIONS

The oral health care provider, regardless of specialty, is faced with the management of medically compromised patients whose systemic illnesses require not only surgical skills but skills of a medicine specialist. Patients who present with either acquired or congenital coagulopathies require an interdisciplinary collaboration whose level of communication accounts for a mutual understanding of surgical principle, as well as

Table 2
Local hemostatic agents

Passive Hemostatic Agents	Source	Action	Remarks
Collagen-based			
Micro fibular collagen Avitene, Colla-plug, Colla-tape, Colla-Cote	Purified bovine collagen	Stimulates aggregation of platelets to form thrombus	Thrombin not effective with this product because of pH Adsorbed in 10–14 d Effective in moderate to severe capillary, venous or small arterial bleeding
Absorbable collagen hemostatic sponge Helistat	Freeze-dried bovine tendon	Causes aggregation of platelets Mechanical obstruction to bleeding Forms 3-dimensional matrix strengthening clot	Promotes wound protection and control of oozing and bleeding from clean oral wounds Contraindicated in infected or contaminated wounds
Cellulose-based			
Surgicel	Oxidized regenerated plant-based cellulose	Absorbable physical matrix for clotting initiation Expands 7–10 times Hemostasis by mechanical pressure	Thrombin not effective with this product because of pH More bacterial static than other agents Use dry Absorption in 4–8 wk May delay bone regeneration
ActCel, Gelitacel	Treated, sterilized cellulose mesh	Acts biochemically on intrinsic pathways enhancing platelet aggregation Physically aids in clot stabilization Expands 3–4 times	Dissolves in 1–2 wk Does not affect wound healing Hypoallergenic Bacteriostatic Gelitacel absorbs in as fast as 4 d
Gelatin-based			
Gelfoam	Purified pork skin gelatin	Absorbs 40 times weight Expands 2 times volume Provides clotting framework	Little tissue reaction Absorbs in4–6 wk Do not use in contaminated or infected wounds

Active hemostatic agents			
Thrombin	Bovine plasma, human plasma or recombinant DNA	Converts fibrinogen to fibrin	Used as a dry powder, solution mixed with gelatin sponge or as a spray Used to treat moderate to severe bleeding Avoid injection into bloodstream or use near large open vessels
FloSeal	Bovine-derived gelatin granules coated in human-derived thrombin	Swells 10%–20% Mechanically seals bleeding site Activates common pathway of the coagulation cascade	Resorption in 6–8 wk Can be used in irregular spaces Effective in hard and soft tissues
Sealants			
Fibrin sealant			
Tisseel	Natural of synthetic combination of hemostatic agent and tissue adhesive	Forms a barrier impervious to the flow of most liquids Impacts tissue angiogenesis and wound healing	Can be used in bone grafting, especially sinus lift surgery Can be used in patients with insufficient fibrinogen Can be used on patients receiving heparin Not effective in vigorous bleeding
Newer hemostatic agents			
Chitosan-based			
HemCon	Positively charged polysaccharide derived from crustacean shells	Attracts negatively charged RBCs forming a cellular lattice forming an artificial clot	Clot formed is independent of intrinsic or extrinsic pathways Effective for patients on anticoagulant meds Does not cause adverse reactions in shell-fish sensitive patients
Hemostatic solutions			
Tannic acid	Similar to plant polyphenol tannin	Causes local vasoconstriction	

(continued on next page)

Table 2
(continued)

Passive Hemostatic Agents	Source	Action	Remarks
Tranexamic acid		Inhibits plasminogen Stabilizes clots	Can be used as a perioperative mouthwash or rinse Helpful in minor oral surgical procedures in patients with bleeding diatheses or who are on anticoagulant meds
Epsilon aminocaproic acid			Less potent than tranexamic acid
Hemocoagulase botroclot	Derived from snake venom	Accelerates conversion of prothrombin to thrombin Causes transformation of fibrinogen to fibrin monomer	Contraindicated in conditions with risks of thrombosis formation
Bone hemostats			
Bone wax	Water-insoluble beeswax, paraffin, and a softening agent	Physically tamponades localized medullary bone bleeding	Nonresorbable Interferes with localized bone healing Use with caution in future bone graft sites
Ostene	Water-soluble alkyelene oxide copolymer	Used much like bonewax	Eliminated from body in 48 h Does not cause infections, inflammatory reactions or interference with bone healing

Data from Kumar S. Local hemostatic agents in the management of bleeding in oral surgery. Asian J Pharm Clin Res. 2016;9(3):35–41.

risk of hemorrhage from pharmacologic interventions and how to balance the risk-to-benefit ratio when considering the standard of care and best practice for patient safety. Advantages now exist so that the alteration of anticoagulant and antiplatelet therapeutics may not be necessary for decreasing intra- and postoperative risks of bleeding. Safe effective perioperative management strategies are also available for patients with hereditary bleeding diatheses as long as thoughtful coordination among the team exists to adequately prepare and carefully follow their patients during the early postoperative period. Finally, the ever-expanding development and application of topical agents provide well tested evidence-based techniques that induce hemostasis in patients who are at risk for postoperative hemorrhage. Future directions include the application of precision medicine by the patient's physician in order to refine their pharmacologic dosing based on the systemic disease. The application of more rigorous trials to confirm the risk of bleeding and timing of pharmacotherapy during dentoalveolar surgical procedures is also of necessity, as the algorithms given may not fit every size of patient.

DISCLOSURE

The authors have nothing to disclose.

ACKNOWLEDGMENT

The authors thank D4 student Yuliya Petokhova for the artwork of figure 1 in this article.

REFERENCES

1. Beirne RO. Anesthetic considerations for patients with bleeding disorders. In: Bosack RC, Lieblich S, editors. Anesthesia complications in the dental office. Iowa: John Wiley and Sons, Inc; 2014. p. 103–11.
2. Norris LA. Blood coagulation. Best Pract Res Clin Obstet Gynaecol 2003;17:369–83.
3. Haghighi AG, Finder RG, Bennett JD. Systemic disease and bleeding disorders for the oral and maxillofacial surgeon. Oral Maxillofac Surg Clin North Am 2016;28:461–71.
4. Hirsh J, Poller L. The international normalized ratio: a guide to understanding and correcting its problems. Arch Intern Med 1994;154:282–8.
5. Maimquist JP. Complications in oral and maxillofacial surgery: management of hemostasis and bleeding disorders in surgical procedures. Oral Maxillofac Surg Clin North Am 2011;23:307–94.
6. Smith JA. Hemophilia: what the oral and maxillofacial surgeon needs to know. Oral Maxillofac Surg Clin North Am 2016;28:481–9.
7. Schramm W. The history of Hemophilia: a short review. Thromb Res 2014;134:54–9.
8. Franchini M. The modern treatment of hemophilia: a narrative review. Blood Transfus 2013;11:178–82.
9. Swami A, Kaur V. von Willebrand disease: a concise review and update for the practicing physician. Clin Appl Thromb Hemost 2017;23(8):900–10.
10. Bruno EK, Bennett JD. Platelet abnormalities in the oral and maxillofacial surgery patient. Oral Maxillofac Surg Clin North Am 2016;28:473–80.

11. Halaszynski TM. Adminstration of coagulation-altering therapy in the patient presenting for oral health and maxillofacial surgery. Oral Maxillofac Surg 2016;28: 443–60.
12. Bajkin BV, Urosevic IM, Stankov KM, et al. Dental extractions and risk of bleeding in patients taking single and dual antiplatelet treatment. Br J Oral Maxillofac Surg 2015;53(1):39–43.
13. Daniels PR. Peri-procedural management of patients taking oral anticoagulants. BMJ 2015;351:h2391.
14. Roldan V, Marin F, Manzano-Fernandez S, et al. The HAS-BLED score has better prediction accuracy for major bleeding than CHADS2 VASc scores in anticoagulated patients with atrial fibrillation. J Am Coll Cardiol 2013;62:199–204.
15. Apostolakis S, Lane DA, Buller H, et al. Comparison of the CHADS2, CHAD2DS2-VASc and HAS-BLED scores for the prediction of clinically relevant bleeding in anticoagulated patients with atrial fibrillation: the AMADEUS trial. Thromb Haemost 2013;110:1074–9.
16. Van Diermen DE, van der Waal I, Hoogstraten J. Management recommendations for invasive dental treatment in patients using oral antithrombotic medication, including novel oral anticoagulants. Oral Surg Oral Med Oral Pathol Oral Radiol 2013;116(6):709–16.
17. Bajkin BV, Vujkov SB, Milekic BR, et al. Risk factors for bleeding after oral surgery in patients who continued using oral anticoagulant therapy. J Am Dent Assoc 2015;146(6):375–81.
18. Scully C, Wolff A. Oral surgery in patients on anticoagulant therapy. Oral Surg Oral Med Oral Pathol Oral Radiol Endod 2002;94(1):57–84.
19. Chugani V. Management of dental patients on warfarin therapy in a primary care setting. Dent Update 2004;31(7):279–382.
20. Yan S, Shi Q, Liu J, et al. Should oral anticoagulant therapy be continued during dental extraction? A meta-analysis. BMC Oral Health 2016;16:1–9.
21. Ward BB, Smith MH. Dentoalveolar procedures for the anticoagulated patients: literature recommendations versus current practice. J Oral Maxillofac Surg 2007;65(8):1454–60.
22. Steed MB, Swanson MT. Warfarin and newer agents: what the oral surgeon needs to know. Oral Maxillofac Surg Clin North Am 2016;28:151–521.
23. Lip G. Perioperative management of patients receiving anticoagulants. 2017. Available at: https://www.uptodate.com/contents/perioperative-management-of-patientsreceivinganticoagulants?search=anticoagulation%20and%20surgery&source=search_result&selectedTitle=1~150&usage_type=default&display_rank=1#H6446132. Accessed July 10, 2019.
24. Cushman M, Lim W, Zakai N. Clinical practice guide on anticoagulant dosing and management of anticoagulant associated bleeding. American Society of Hematology 2011;8:1–3.
25. Milling TJ, Refael MA, Goldstein JN, et al. Thromboembolic events after vitamin K antagonist reversal with 4-factor prothrombin complex concentrate: analyses of two randomized, plasma controlled studies. Ann Emerg Med 2016;67(1):96–105.
26. Douketis JD, Spyropoulos AC, Spencer FA, et al. Perioperative management of antithrombotic therapy: antithrombotic therapy and prevention of thrombosis, 9th ed: American College of Chest Physicians evidence-based clinical practice guidelines. Chest 2012;141(2 Suppl):e326S–50S.
27. Di Pasquale LD, Ferneini EM. Heparin and Lovenox: what the oral and maxillofacial needs to know. Oral Maxillofac Surg Clin North Am 2016;28:507–13.

28. Farr DR, Hare AR. The use of thromboembolic prophylaxis in oral and maxillofacial surgery. Br J Oral Maxillofac Surg 1994;32(3):161–4.
29. Ahmed I, Majeed A, Powell R. Heparin induced thrombocytopenia: diagnosis and management update. Postgrad Med J 2007;83(983):575–82.
30. Eriksson BI, quinlan DJ, Weitz JL. Comparative pharmacodynamics and pharmacokinetics of oral direct thrombin and factor Xa inhibitors in development. Clin Pharmacokinet 2009;48(1):1–22.
31. Leung L, Mannuccio Mannucci P, Tirnaur J. Direct oral anticoagulants and parenteral direct thrombin inhibitors: dosing and adverse effects. 2017. Available at: https://www.uptodate.com/contents/direct-oral-anticoagulants-and-parenteral-direct-thrombin-inhibitors-dosing andeffects?search=Direct%20oral%20anticoagulants%20and%20parenteral%20direc&source=search_result&selectedTitle=1~150&usage_type=default&display_rank=1. Accessed February 6, 2018.
32. Greinacher A, Lubenow N. Recombinant hirudin in clinical practice : focus on lepirudin. Circulation 2001;103(10):1479–84.
33. Dinkova AS, Atanasov DT, Vladmirova-Kirova LG. Dabigatran and dental extractions: case report. J IMAB 2017;23(2):1536–40.
34. Davis C, Robertson C, Shivakumar S, et al. Implications of dabigatran, a direct thrombin inhibitor, for oral surgery practice. J Can Dent Assoc 2013;79:d74.
35. Sunkara T, Ofori E, Zarubin V, et al. Perioperative management of direct oral anticoagulants (DOACs): a systemic review. Health Serv Insights 2016;9(Suppl 1): 25–36.
36. Barnes GD, Ageno W, Ansell J, et al. Recommendation on the nomenclature for oral anticoagulants: communication from the SSC of the ISTH. J Thromb Haemost 2015;13:1154.
37. Garcia D, Crowther M. Management of bleeding in patients receiving direct oral anticoagulants. Up to date. 2017. Available at: https://www.uptodate.com/contents/management-of-bleeding-in-patients-receiving-direct-oral-anticoagulants?source=see_link. Accessed January 14, 2018.
38. Ghantous AE, Ferneini EM. Aspirin, Plavix, and other antiplatelet medications: what the oral and maxillofacial surgeon needs to know. Oral Maxillofac Surg Clin North Am 2016;28:497–506.
39. Collaborative overview of randomized trials of antiplatelet treatment, 1: prevention of vascular death, MI, stroke by prolonged antiplatelet therapy in different categories of patients. Antiplatelet Trialists Collaboration. Br Med J 1994;308:235–46.
40. Canigral A, Silvestre FJ, Canigral G, et al. Evaluation of bleeding risk and measurement methods in dental patients. Med Oral Patol Oral Cir Bucal 2010; 15(6):e863–8.
41. Brennan MT, Wynn RL, Miller CS. Aspirin and bleeding in dentistry: an update and recommendations. Oral Surg Oral Med Oral Pathol Oral Radiol Endod 2007;104(3):316–23.
42. Grines CL, Bonow RE, Casey DE Jr, et al. Prevention of premature discontinuation of dual antiplatelet therapy in patients with coronary artery stents: a science advisory from the American Heart Association, American college of Cardiology, Society for Cardiovascular Angiography and Interventions, American College of Surgeons and American Dental Association with representations from the American College of Physicians. Circulation 2007;1159(6):813–8.
43. Aniguchi K, Ohtani H, Ikermoto T, et al. Possible case of potentiation of the antiplatelet effect of cilostazol by grapefruit juice. J Clin Pharm Ther 2007;32(5): 457–9.

44. Mauer P, Conrad-Hengerer I, Hollstein S, et al. Orbitalk hemorrhage associated with orbital fractures in geriatric patients on antiplatelet or anticoagulant therapy. Int J Oral Maxillofac Surg 2013;42(12):1510–4.
45. Zimmerman B, Valentino LA. Hemophilia: in review. Pediatr Rev 2013;34(7): 289–95.
46. Pavlova A, Oldenburg J. Defining severity of hemophilia: more than factor levels. Semin Thromb Hemost 2013;39:702–10.
47. Webert K. Acquired hemophilia A. Semin Thromb Hemost 2012;38:735–41.
48. Kreuz W, Ettingshausen CE. Inhibitors in patients with haemophilia A. Thromb Res 2014;134:S22–6.
49. DeFrates SR, McDonagh KT, Adams VR. The reversal of inhibitors in congenital hemophilia. Pharmacotherapy 2013;33(2):157–64.
50. Gomez K, Klamroth R, Mahlangu J, et al. Key issues in inhibitor management in patients with haemophilia. Blood Transfus 2014;12(Suppl1):s319–29.
51. Francini M, Coppola A, Tagliaferri A, et al. FEIBA versus novoseven in hemophilia patients with inhibitors. Semin Thromb Hemost 2013;39:772–8.
52. Ljung R, Andersson NG. the current status of prophylactic replacement therapy in children and adults with haemophilia. Br J Haematol 2015;169:777–86.
53. Srivastava A, Brewer AK, Mauser-Bunschoten EP, et al. Guidelines for the management of hemophilia. Haemophilia 2012;19:e1–47.
54. Ramos EA, Diamante M, Caruso D, et al. Outpatient minor oral surgery in patients with hemophilia: a case series of 23 patients. J Clin Exp Dent 2019;11(5):395–9.
55. Rasaratnam L, Chowdary P, Pollard D, et al. Risk-based management of dental procedures in patients with inherited bleeding disorders: development of a dental bleeding risk assessment and treatment tool (DeBRATT). Haemophilia 2017;23: 247–54.
56. Fijnvandraat K, Cnossen MH, Leebeek FW, et al. Diagnosis and maangement of hemophilia. BMJ 2012;344:1–5.
57. Mensah PK, Gooding R. Surgery in patients with inherited bleeding disorders. Anaesthesia 2015;70(Suppl 1):112–20.
58. Leebeek FWG, Eikenboom JCJ. Von Willebrand's Disease. N Engl J Med 2016; 375:2067–80.
59. Sadler JE, Mannucci PM, Berntop E, et al. Impact, diagnosis and treatment of von Willebrand disease. Thromb Haemost 2000;84(2):160–74.
60. Federici AB, Mazurier C, Berntop E, et al. Biologic response to desmopressin in patients with severe type 1 and type 2 von Willebrand disease: results of a multicenter European study. Blood 2004;103(6):2032–8.
61. Ria B, Wates E, Ria S. A review of haemostasis following minor oral surgery procedures. J Dent Health Oral Disord Ther 2017;7(1):246–9.
62. Kumbargere Nagraj S, Prashanti E, Aggarwal H, et al. Interventions for treating post-extraction bleeding. Cochrane Database Syst Rev 2018;(3):CD011930.
63. Vezeau PL. Topical hemostatic agents: what the oral and maxillofacial surgeon needs to know. Oral Maxillofac Surg Clin North Am 2016;28:523–32.
64. Kumar S. Local hemostatic agents in the management of bleeding in oral surgery. Asian J Pharm Clin Res 2016;9(3):35–41.

Soft-Tissue Grafting Solutions

Romeo Minou Luo, DMD[a,*], David Chvartszaid, DDS, MSc (PROSTHO), MSc (PERIO), FRCD(C)[b], Sang Woo Kim, DDS[a], Jason Eli Portnof, DMD, MD, FICD[c]

KEYWORDS

- Soft-tissue graft • Gingival graft • Subepithelial palatal • Platelet-rich plasma
- Platelet-rich fibrin • Periodontal surgery • Soft-tissue augmentation

KEY POINTS

- Functional and esthetic status of both natural dentition and implants is largely influenced by surrounding keratinized attached gingiva.
- Aside from the obvious final esthetic advantage, keratinized attached gingiva also provides a stable background for the prosthetic phase and facilitates oral hygiene care.
- Numerous solutions are available in soft-tissue grafting, each with their own advantages and shortcomings, which a skilled practitioner can apply to appropriate clinical scenarios. These solutions are explored within the content of this article.

ANATOMY AND BIOLOGY OF ORAL SOFT TISSUES

To achieve proficiency and mastery of intraoral soft-tissue grafting, the surgeon must have a strong grasp in understanding the anatomy and biological processes that occur during the maturation and modification of oral soft tissues. Oral mucosa can be identified and classified under 3 primary entities: masticatory mucosa, oral mucous membranes, and specialized mucosa covering the dorsum of the tongue. Implant surgeons, in particular, are most concerned with the masticatory mucosa, which includes the gingiva as well as the mucosal component of the hard palate. The gingival complex, while sharing an essential esthetic responsibility, also serves a crucial protective and structural function within the periodontium and peri-implant tissues. For these reasons, defects of the gingiva can be particularly devastating to the status of the dentition and endosseous implants.

[a] Department of Oral & Maxillofacial Surgery, Nova Southeastern University College of Dental Medicine, 3200 South University Drive, Davie, FL 33328, USA; [b] Prosthodontics, Faculty of Dentistry, University of Toronto, 124 Edward Street, Toronto, ON M5G 1G6, Canada; [c] Private Practice, 9980 North Central Park Boulevard Suite 113, Boca Raton, FL 33428, USA
* Corresponding author. Department of Oral and Maxillofacial Surgery, 3200 South University Drive, Davie, FL 33328, USA.
E-mail address: Romeoluo1@gmail.com

Dent Clin N Am 64 (2020) 435–451
https://doi.org/10.1016/j.cden.2019.12.008
dental.theclinics.com

Periodontal Soft Tissues

The periodontium consists of 4 intimately collaborating structural components: periodontal ligament, cementum, alveolar bone, and gingiva. Although the cellular composition, foundational architecture, and biochemical mechanisms are extraordinarily diverse between the components, traumatic and pathologic insults to any of these 4 individual units have deleterious effects on the entire periodontal complex. The periodontal ligament is a vascular fibrous connective tissue that bridges the tooth root to the alveolar bone and measures 0.15 to 0.21 mm on average.[1] The principal purpose of the periodontal ligament is to resist occlusal force impact, provide protection to nerve and vascular structures from mechanical insult, and communicate occlusal forces to bone. Cementum is the calcified outer covering of the anatomic root that is attached to Sharpey's fibers of the periodontal ligament to transmit occlusal forces. The alveolar process is the portion of the maxilla and mandible that forms the tooth sockets. Although it is not the goal of this article to delve into an extended discussion of the individual anatomic and biochemical components of the periodontium, the gingival component is discussed in closer detail to build a foundation for the remainder of the article.

The gingiva can be classified into marginal, attached, and interdental areas and serves to protect against both mechanical and microbial insults. Evidence exists that gingival epithelium participates actively in states of infection.[2] Marginal gingiva is the border that surrounds the dentition in a collar-like fashion. Typically it measures less than 1 mm in thickness and in its apicocoronal dimensions. On the tooth side of the marginal gingiva, the gingival sulcus is found. In healthy adult human gingiva, this sulcus is shallow and is typically measured to be an average of 1.8 mm with variations from 0 to 6 mm.

The attached gingiva is coronally continuous with the marginal gingiva. It receives its name from its tight attachment with the underlying periosteum of the alveolar bone and terminates apically at the mucogingival junction. In the esthetic zone, the attached gingiva retains its greatest dimensions, between 3.5 to 4.5 mm, while being much narrower in the posterior segments. The loss of width of attached gingiva is primarily attributed to changes in the position of the gingival margin as the mucogingival junction remains stationary in the adult anatomy.

Interdental gingiva is found in the interproximal space beneath tooth contacts and embodies the gingival embrasure. The presence of an adequate papilla depends on the presence of interproximal contact between the adjacent teeth and the distance of this contact from the alveolar crest.

Histologically, gingiva is composed of a highly cellular stratified squamous epithelium overlying a central compartment of connective tissue. Within the connective tissue, collagen fibers and ground substance are found. Keratinocytes constitute the primary cellular makeup of the gingival epithelium and alongside these cells, Merkel cells, Langerhans cells, and melanocytes are observed within the epithelium. Variations of this histologic makeup occur at different sites of the gingiva. Oral epithelium is keratinized and covers the outer surface of the marginal gingiva and the surface of the attached gingiva. On the other hand, sulcular epithelium that lines the gingival sulcus is nonkeratinized and extends from the coronal dimension of the junctional epithelium to the crest of the gingival margin. Sulcular epithelium can keratinize if exposed to the oral cavity,[3] and the outer oral epithelium can "dekeratinize" once in contact with the dentition.[4]

Biologic Width

Moving apically from the base of the gingival sulcus, the junctional epithelium is encountered, followed by connective tissue. The "biologic width" (also known as supracrestal tissue attachment according to the 2017 Classification of Periodontal and Peri-Implant Diseases and Conditions)[5] encompasses these 2 tissue layers. The biologic width holds responsibility in establishing a seal around the tooth. Junctional epithelium forms a tight connection to afibrillar cementum and root cementum via an hemidesmosome attachment within the internal basal lamina.[6] This tight attachment forms a physiologic barrier against penetration of oral pathogens to the subgingival tooth surface while providing an avenue for immunologic host defense components to gingival sulcus.[7,8] This barrier is often penetrated during periodontal probing, especially in the setting of gingival inflammation.[9,10] The cells of the junctional epithelium are characterized by a rapid rate of cellular turnover and a distinct ability to spread across both tooth and implant surfaces after mechanical postsurgical insults.[11,12]

The gingival connective tissue is principally composed of organized groups of collagenous fibers that insert into the cementum, bone, and soft gingival tissues. In close association with these fibers is an extracellular matrix of ground substance interspersed with fibroblasts, vessels, and nerves. Epithelial and connective tissue attachments around teeth were analyzed on cadaver specimen in a classic study, in which Gargiulo and colleagues[13] found that the average width of the junctional epithelium was 1.07 mm and the connective tissue component measured on average of 0.97 mm with average biologic width of 2.04 mm. As with any average, there are physiologic individual variations to these measurements, with greater variation in the junctional epithelial component than the connective tissue. Infringement upon the biologic width has been theorized to cause gingival inflammation, alveolar bone loss, and eventual periodontitis.[14,15] Given these dimensions, it is recommended that restorations must allow for at least 3.0 mm to exist between the alveolar crest and the margin of the restoration.[6,15,16]

Gingival Biotype

Gingival biotype (more recently known as gingival phenotype according to the 2017 Classification of Periodontal and Peri-Implant Diseases and Conditions)[17] is defined as the thickness of gingiva in the faciopalatal or faciolingual dimension. Accurate diagnosis of the gingival biotype is essential to both esthetic dentistry and implant planning. In 1989, Seibert and Lindhe[18] introduced the categories of "thick-flat" and "thin-scalloped" gingival biotypes. Periodontal probe visibility has been held as the clinical gold standard to identify thick from thin gingival biotype. As such, difficulty arises in the subjective interpretation of what defines visibility, and studies have since attempted to quantify gingival thickness in lieu of subjective analysis.[19]

Thin-scalloped biotype is distinguished by small contact dimension and is located near the incisal edge of the tooth, scarce attached gingiva, a highly scalloped soft tissue and bone architecture, and thin underlying osseous form.[20,21] This is clinically significant because thin biotype is subjected toward a tendency to gingival recession, apical migration of attachment, loss of underlying alveolar volume, dehiscence, and fenestration after surgical or prosthetic manipulation or after sustaining irritation. Removal of supracrestal implant abutments often results in immediate collapse of peri-implant soft tissue. In this biotype, every effort must be made to use minimally traumatic surgical techniques. Some investigators advocate a conservative approach to preserve circulation and soft-tissue volume at implant sites. Flapless surgery techniques such as a tissue punch or U-shaped peninsula are recommended for these patients.[22] Despite the use of minimally invasive techniques, patients with this biotype should still be warned of increased risk of soft-tissue loss, and consideration for soft-tissue grafting procedures should be given. However, studies have shown that gingival biotype does not have significant influence in surgical root coverage results associated with connective tissue grafting,[23] nor does it have significant effects on hard-tissue augmentation results.[24]

Thick-flat biotype is characterized by broader contact areas located closer to the gingiva accompanied by distinct cervical convexities, dense fibrotic tissue, and often a thick underlying osseous form (**Box 1**). In contrast to the thin-scalloped biotype, patients with this characteristic gingival biotype are more resistant to recession but more susceptible to development of scarring after implant therapy.

Peri-Implant Soft Tissues

Biologic width must also be considered for implant-supported restorations. Multiple studies have revealed that the peri-implant soft tissues closely mimic those of natural dentition. In comparison with the biologic width around implants and teeth, the major equivalence between natural teeth and implants is the junctional epithelial attachment,[9] whereas the chief disparity is the absence of collagenous supracrestal connective tissue fiber insertions into the implant and lack of periodontal ligament fiber attachments within alveolar bone.[17] After surgical interruption of the gingiva, the cut edge of remaining attached gingiva rapidly differentiates and reattaches to the surface of a clean, uncontaminated implant to form the junctional epithelial attachment.

This brings us to the discussion of importance of attached gingiva around an implant site. Stable peri-implant mucosa is necessary for the preservation of bone around an implant. However, there is much debate in the literature regarding the necessity of peri-implant keratinized attached gingiva versus nonkeratinized mucosa. Some clinicians warn of an increased risk for peri-implant mucosal recession and attachment loss when surrounded by inadequate keratinized attached mucosa,[25] whereas others report that there is no difference in peri-implant bone levels when placed in alveolar mucosa.[26,27] Most studies do agree, however, that aside from the obvious final esthetic advantage, keratinized attached gingiva also provides a stable background for the prosthetic phase and facilitates oral hygiene care.[28–33] Inadequate keratinized tissue can impede proper oral hygiene and result in increased plaque accumulation. Subsequently, gingival inflammation results and may potentially lead to peri-implantitis.[30–33] Thus, the peri-implant soft-tissue seal provided by attached peri-implant soft tissues can simplify oral hygiene care and facilitate a "prosthetic-friendly" environment that is essential for long-term implant success.

INDICATIONS FOR SOFT-TISSUE GRAFTING

Marginal Tissue Recession

When marginal soft tissue is displaced in an apical direction away from the cementoenamel junction with resultant exposure of the tooth root surface, it is referred to as

Box 1
Seibert and Lindhe: periodontal biotypes

Thin-Scalloped	Thick-Flat
• Highly scalloped gingival architecture • Contact located near the incisal edge of the interproximal • Thin, narrow interdental papilla • Minimal attached soft tissue • Associated with narrow, triangular teeth • Thin underlying bone • Prone to gingival recession • Less resistant to traumatic insults	• Less scalloped, flat gingival architecture • Thick, wide interdental papilla • Minimal attached soft tissue • Associated with wide, square teeth • Thick, dense underlying bone • Prone to pocket formation • More robust and resistant to traumatic insults

Data from Seibert JL, Lindhe J. Aesthetics and periodontal therapy. In: Lindhe J, editor. Textbook of clinical periodontology. 2nd ed. Copenhagen: Munksgaard; 1989. p. 477–514.

marginal tissue recession.[34] The term gingival recession is also often used interchangeably, but a study by Maynard and Wilson[35,36] in 1979 suggested that marginal tissue may originally have been alveolar mucosa rather than gingiva. The exposure of a tooth root may be associated with hypersensitivity to extremes in temperature, exposure of root surfaces to potentially carious microbiota, and pronounced esthetic defects. The primary causes of marginal tissue recession are inadequate oral hygiene that leads to plaque accumulation and subsequent inflammation, orthodontic tooth movement, and mechanical, thermal, and chemical insults.[37–39] Patients who are especially susceptible to gingival recession include those with thin gingival biotype and those with reduced or absent keratinized tissue.[40,41]

Proper identification and classification of marginal tissue recession is essential to preoperative evaluation for periodontal plastic surgical procedures on tooth-borne defects and for implant planning to decide whether soft-tissue grafting is indicated in conjunction with implant therapy. Several classification systems exist to classify the amount of marginal tissue recession.[42,43] In 1968, Sullivan and Atkins[42] introduced a system that organized defects into "shallow-narrow," "shallow-wide," "deep-narrow," and "deep-wide" categories based on the width and length of the recession defect. These categories were used to predict the success of tissue-grafting procedures.

Subsequently, in 1985 Miller[43] proposed an expanded classification system (**Box 2**) that correlates the location of the apicalmost aspect of the marginal tissue defect with the location of the mucogingival junction while taking account of the degree of interdental hard-tissue and soft-tissue loss. He considered that many cases of recession were impossible to identify using the classification system developed by Sullivan and Atkins. Based on the Miller classification, prognosis of soft-tissue grafts used for root coverage could be systematically predicted. Class I and class II defects resulted in 100% root coverage. Partial root coverage could be expected in class III defects, and the amount of root coverage could be predicted by the surgeon by

Box 2
Miller's classification system of marginal soft-tissue recession

Class I:
- Recession does not extend to mucogingival junction
- There is no loss of interproximal clinical attachment
- 100% root coverage can be anticipated

Class II:
- Recession extends to or beyond mucogingival junction
- There is no loss of interproximal clinical attachment
- 100% root coverage can be anticipated

Class III:
- Recession extends to or beyond mucogingival junction
- Presence of interproximal clinical attachment loss
- Presence of malpositioned teeth
- Partial root coverage can be anticipated

Class IV:
- Recession extends to or beyond mucogingival junction
- Presence of severe interproximal clinical attachment loss
- Presence of severe malpositioning of teeth
- No root coverage is attainable

Data from Miller PD. A classification of marginal tissue recession. Int J Periodontics Restorative Dent 1985;5:9.

placing a periodontal probe horizontally at the midfacial tissue level of the 2 adjacent teeth to the tooth exhibiting recession. No root coverage is often anticipated in class IV defects.

Most recently, in 2017, the American Academy of Periodontology agreed to undertake the 2017 World Workshop classification system of periodontal and peri-implant diseases and conditions as the new classification system for periodontal conditions around teeth and edentulous ridges. This new system incorporates a multidimensional staging and grading system for the classification of periodontitis. The system also incorporates a novel classification for peri-implant diseases and conditions.

Peri-Implant Soft-Tissue Dehiscence

It has been well established in the literature that the dental implant success rate is more than 95% when measured in terms of osseointegration.[35] However, esthetic and biological implant complications are relatively abundant.[44] Apical migration of the peri-implant soft tissues is often referred to as soft-tissue dehiscence, mucosal recession, or mucosal dehiscence. There is no agreed classification of mucosal recession around implants, and most investigators advocate the use of exposure of the metallic implant or abutment surface as a reference point, or the adjacent levels of the mucosal margins surrounding natural dentition.[45] Lack of adequate dimensions of keratinized tissue paired with inadequate oral hygiene routines has been shown to increase plaque accumulation around implants and increase the potential for peri-implant inflammation.[46]

PRINCIPLES OF ORAL SOFT-TISSUE GRAFTING

Recipient Site

There are several principles in oral soft-tissue grafting that must be strongly considered and adhered to for graft success. The primary concern is the sufficient nourishment of the newly placed graft. Soft-tissue grafts initially survive by plasmic imbibition and later on through neovascularization. To achieve this, firstly the recipient site must be vascularized. Second, recipient sites must facilitate rigid immobilization and intimate adaptation of the donor tissue. Excess movement of the graft precludes angiogenesis and plasmic imbibition, thus starving the site of adequate nutrition. In large areas of decreased vascularity such as a tooth root surface or implant abutment, treatment planning should include the use of a pedicled graft rather than free grafts. An intimate adaptation of the soft tissues will decrease the distance over which plasmic diffusion and capillary development will occur. In addition, hemostasis must be achieved at the recipient site. Blood products and active hemorrhage will prevent the ability of the graft to properly adapt to the recipient site. Loss of delivery of nutrition to the graft site often leads to the sloughing and inevitable loss of the graft. Consideration of these principles explains why periosteum is widely considered as an excellent recipient site for oral soft-tissue grafts. It is characterized by an abundant vasculature, is immobile, and can facilitate rigid and intimate adaptation of donor tissue.

Donor Site

With strong understanding of the essential features of a suitable recipient graft site, one would realize the necessity for proper planning and delicate harvesting of the graft from the donor site. The harvested graft should have a uniform thickness to facilitate intimate adaptation and immobilization to the recipient site which, in turn, would enable efficient angiogenesis and nutrient diffusion. Secondary contracture is often a concern when considering the thickness of a harvested graft. Thin grafts are highly subject to this phenomenon, whereas thicker grafts are better able to maintain their physical dimensions. Thicker grafts are generally preferred because they must have dimensions even after contracture.

SOFT-TISSUE GRAFTING OPTIONS

Although it is not the purpose of this article to cover the techniques involved in all the options of soft-tissue grafting procedures, free gingival grafts (FGGs) and subepithelial connective tissue grafts are covered in depth to provide the reader with a procedural foundation in this topic and to demonstrate the clinical application of the previously discussed concepts. Other techniques, such as vascularized interpositional periosteal-connective tissue grafts, modified palatal roll, and epithelialized palatal grafts, are heavily covered in detail within the current existing literature.

Free Gingival Graft

The FGG technique was first described by Björn in 1963 and was used to enhance zones of attached gingiva.[47,48] The primary indication for free gingival grafting is to prevent peri-implantitis and facilitate oral hygiene through keratinized attached gingiva augmentation in both tooth-borne and peri-implant sites. As stated previously, keratinized tissue has been shown to form a more stable environment around implant abutments, which would limit biofilm development on an implant interface. However, the primary flaw of free gingival grafting is that the harvested graft retains the tissue characteristics of the donor site. This eliminates FGG as a treatment option in the esthetic zone. In addition, postsurgically the donor site is left with a soft-tissue defect that must heal by secondary intention. This increases the amount of discomfort experienced by the patient and delays healing time at the donor site.

Surgical Technique

Recipient-site preparation

The recipient site is prepared by creating a horizontal incision at the existing mucogingival junction using a #15 blade (**Fig. 1**). This facilitates the blending of any surgical scar into the existing mucogingival line. It is important not to disturb the periosteum during the initial incision because this layer will facilitate the intimate adaptation and immobilization of the graft. If 2 vertical incisions are to be incorporated into the recipient site, they should be made to be 2-times the width of the intended augmentation to allow for contracture during the healing phase.

Donor-site graft harvest

The palate is the usual site from which the split-thickness keratinized mucosal graft is harvested. The harvested graft should be approximately the same size as the prepared recipient site and, hence, the desired dimension of soft-tissue augmentation. Although some experienced surgeons free-hand this harvest, it is recommended to use some form of template (eg, metal foil) to be as conservative and efficient as possible.[49] In this method, the metallic foil that is cut in the silhouette of the recipient site and then used for transfer forms an outline that a #15 blade can trace. The initial outline incision should be shallow. It is important to remember that this is to be a partial-thickness graft. Burying the depth of the scalpel deep into the periosteum should be avoided because this will impede a smooth harvest as well as donor-site healing. Also, one should be wary of possible damage to the palatal arteries. After creating the outline, one edge of the graft is elevated with tissue forceps or with well-placed sutures for retraction, and is gently lifted away from the site while continuing to separate the graft with the blade. If one does opt to place retraction

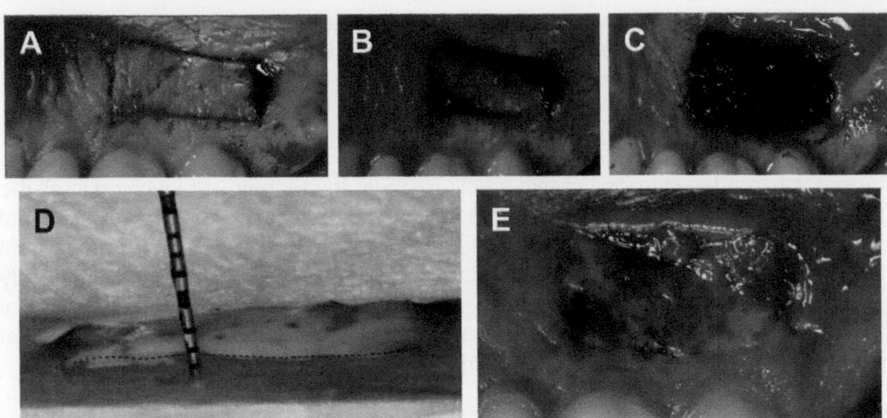

Fig. 1. Harvest of the free gingival graft. (*A*) Outline of the donor tissue harvest made with a #15 blade. (*B*) Soft-tissue defect left in hard palate after harvest. (*C*) Donor site packed with absorbable hemostat for hemostasis and patient comfort. (*D*) Measured thickness of FGG 1.5 mm. (*E*) Donor-site healing at 1-week follow-up revealing proper granulation. (*Courtesy of* Teresa Yang, DMD, Resident, Division of Periodontics, Columbia University College of Dental Medicine, New York, NY.)

sutures, they may remain in place to facilitate tissue transfer. Ideally, graft thickness should be 1.0 to 1.5 mm, keeping in mind that thicker grafts may be more difficult to immobilize and vascularize while a graft that is too thin may be subject to excessive shrinkage or necrosis.[50] After transfer and immobilization of the graft, it is essential to cover the donor site to facilitate patient comfort. A variety of materials have been used for this purpose, including periodontal dressing (eg, Coe-Pak), oxidized regenerated cellulose (Surgicel), fast-drying butyl cyanoacrylate tissue adhesive (PeriAcryl), and palatal stent.

Graft transfer and immobilization

Transfer of the newly harvested tissue must proceed in a delicate fashion. Preferably, minimal pressure should be used to avoid trauma to the graft. The recipient site must be cleared of clots, but care must be taken to obtain adequate hemostasis. As stated previously, clots and hemorrhage will impede the intimate adaptation required for plasmic imbibition and neovascularization to occur. The graft must be in direct contact with the recipient site because the presence of intervening clots, hemorrhage, and dead space will impede plasmic imbibition and subsequent neovascularization. Several techniques have been described to secure the FGG to the recipient site, including interrupted sutures, continuous sutures, and the use of fast-drying butyl cyanoacrylate tissue adhesive (PeriAcryl). Some surgeons also advocate the use of periodontal dressing (eg, Coe-Pak). The key aspect is achieving graft immobilization.

Subepithelial Connective Tissue Autograft

Subepithelial connective tissue grafts (SCTGs) have gained tremendous popularity since their conception in 1980 by Langer and Calagna.[51] This is an impressively versatile technique that is used to enhance esthetic gingival appearance, obtain root coverage, and correct uneven gingival margins. Of note, SCTGs maintain color match and esthetics unmatched by FGGs.[51] In addition, SCTGs can be used to increase the gingival width and modify the biotype to cover metallic show-through in implant sites with thin gingival phenotype in esthetic zones. Harvesting the subepithelial connective tissue graft from the palate can be accomplished with various techniques, all of which result in a palatal pouch that can be primarily reapproximated, eliminating much of the discomfort with the open wound that was experienced by patients receiving free gingival autografts and facilitating donor-site healing.

Surgical technique

Recipient-site preparation: overview

There are 2 primary options available for the recipient-site preparation steps for a subepithelial connective tissue graft. Consideration should be made regarding whether the surgeon would like to proceed with an open technique versus a closed technique whereby no releasing incisions are necessary. Both of these techniques require the surgeon to keep the dissection in a supraperiosteal plane. The closed technique preserves circulation by avoiding vertical releasing incisions. However, it may be limited in its ability in apical repositioning of the graft, and also is much more technically taxing when trying to ensure that the graft is uniformly placed. An open technique allows for direct visualization of the site and thus allows for ease of access for the surgeon. It has the obvious drawback of requiring vertical incision(s) that sacrifice circulation and can be esthetically concerning.

Recipient-site preparation: closed technique

After adequate anesthesia has been administered, a #15 blade is used to create a 1-mm deep, partial-thickness sulcular incision along the periphery of the soft-tissue defect (**Fig. 2**). A horizontal incision is then extended mesially and distally to the defect to facilitate supraperiosteal dissection. It has been recommended that the area of supraperiosteal dissection should be roughly 3-times the area of the soft-tissue defect to ensure adequate peripheral circulation is available to the region, and this plane can be created by inserting the scalpel parallel into the pouch created, with extreme care not to perforate buccally through the gingiva. This pouch can then be explored with the blunt end of a periosteal elevator to ensure that a uniform recipient site was prepared.

Recipient-site preparation: open technique

The open technique for recipient-site preparation is a standard elevation of a buccal flap in a supraperiosteal plane, incorporating vertical releasing incisions similar to those previously discussed in for FGGs.

Donor-site graft harvest: overview

The most common location for harvest of a subepithelial connective tissue graft is from the masticatory mucosa located on the patient's hard palate between the mesial line angle of palatal root of the first molar and the distal line angle of the canine, as this is where the thickest tissue can be found.[53] Care must be taken not to injure the greater palatine artery, which arises from the greater palatine foramen. This is located at the junction of the horizontal and vertical shelves of the palatine bone, often apical to the third molar. As the neurovascular bundle courses anteriorly, they are often found between 7 and 17 mm from the cementoenamel junction of the maxillary premolars and molars. The bundle then courses anteriorly to meet the incisive foramen. It is recommended not to extend the donor-site incision past the lateral incisors to avoid damage to the bundle, leading to postsurgical bleeding and altered sensation. Any bleeding that is experienced in this area can be addressed with immediate and direct application of pressure, injection of local anesthesia with vasoconstrictor, placement of sutures proximally to the bleed, and ligation of the vessel.[52]

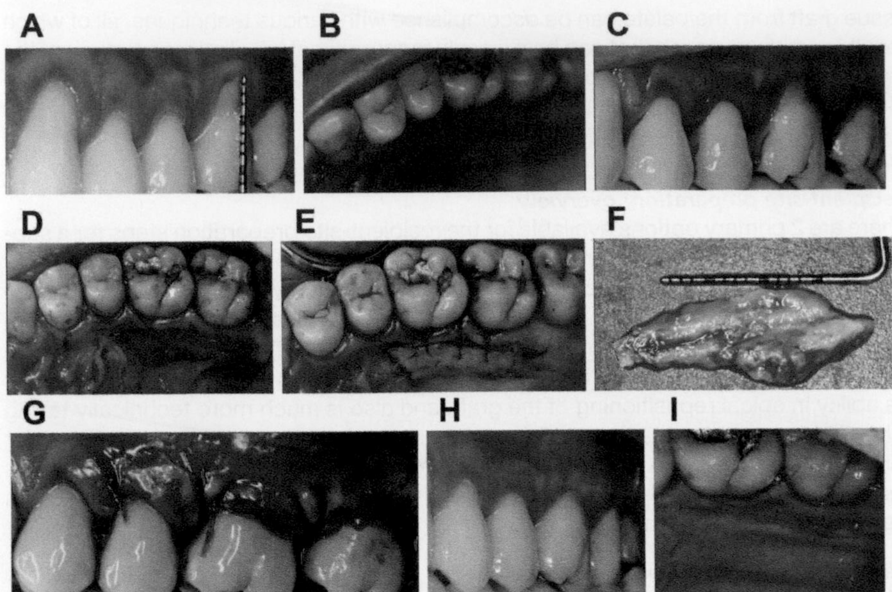

Fig. 2. Subepithelial connective tissue graft. (*A*) A 4-mm Class I Miller defect at the mesial root of tooth #14. (*B*) Donor site. (*C*) Closed tunneling technique used for preparation of recipient site. (*D*) Harvest of subepithelial connective tissue graft via L-shaped incision with an anterior vertical release. (*E*) Primary closure of the donor site. (*F*) Harvested donor tissue (measured 1.5 mm in thickness, not shown). (*G*) Application and immobilization of the harvested graft into recipient site. (*H*) An 8-week follow-up with 100% root coverage. (*I*) Donor-site healing at 8 weeks. (*Courtesy of* Teresa Yang, DMD, Resident, Division of Periodontics, Columbia University College of Dental Medicine, New York, NY.)

Donor-site graft harvest: dual-incision technique

After local anesthetic with vasoconstrictor has infiltrated the area, the surgeon should palpate the palate to identify the bony palatal groove in which the neurovascular bundle lies. This is key for identifying the apical boundary for the donor-site incisions. A full-thickness incision is made 2 to 3 mm apical to the palatal gingival margin from the first molar to the canine. A second partial-thickness incision is then made 1 to 2 mm apical to the first incision at a depth of at least 1 mm. This allows for adequate thickness of the flap for primary closure to prevent sloughing and necrosis, which would lead to significant postoperative discomfort. A rectangular pouch is then formed by turning the scalpel parallel from the second incision, extending further apically while being wary of the location of the previously identified palatal groove and neurovascular bundle. Once this is satisfactory, full-thickness incisions are made mesial and distal to the graft, with only the apical portion of connective tissue still keeping it attached to the donor site. Coronally directed traction can then be placed with forceps and the entire graft is detached with a full-thickness horizontal incision at the apical base of the graft. The dual-incision technique harvests the graft with a thin sliver of epithelium from the 1 to 2 mm of palatal tissue between the 2 incisions. This epithelium should be removed after harvest and before immobilization within the recipient site. The harvested tissue can then be placed aside briefly after moistening with saline while the palate is sutured. Primary closure is not always attainable with this technique, and dressing of the donor site or use of a palatal stent is highly advisable.

Donor-site graft harvest: single-incision technique

The single-incision technique is very similar to that of the dual incision but is slightly more technique sensitive. It does, however, provide the benefit of a guaranteed primary closure that provides added comfort for the patient and decreased probability of prolonged bleeding. A slightly beveled full-thickness incision is made 2 to 3 mm apical to the palatal gingival margins between the first molar and canine. With the scalpel still in contact with bone, it is withdrawn slightly, leaving the cutting edge 1 mm from the epithelial surface. The blade is then reoriented parallel to the palatal surface to create a rectangular pouch. The rest of the surgical approach is completed in the same manner as for the dual-incision technique. The palatal flap can then be sutured to achieve primary closure.

Donor-site graft harvest: other techniques

Many harvest techniques have been discussed and suggested in the literature, all of which have their advantages and disadvantages. For example, the anterior vertical release technique begins with the horizontal incision parallel to the gingival margin and then proceeds to make a vertical anterior releasing incision. This allows for increased visibility and access to the site. However, poor operator technique can damage the palatal neurovascular bundle.

Graft immobilization

Graft placement and immobilization is significantly more technique sensitive when the closed technique is used. It is essential to place the graft so that no overfolding or bunching occurs. A suture can be introduced at the apical aspect of the supraperiosteal pouch from the mucosal side and, without penetrating periosteum, should be expressed from the sulcular opening. The needle is then introduced into the connective tissue side of the donor tissue and back through the periosteum side a few millimeters away near the border of the tissue. This suture needle is reintroduced into the pouch and then re-expressed through the apical aspect of the pouch. This suture is then used in conjunction with a blunt instrument to guide the graft uniformly and apically into the supraperiosteal pouch and subsequently tied. The covering flap is then approximated with sutures without piercing the underlying graft. Coronal advancement can be attempted, but it is likely that the graft material will remain uncovered at the coronalmost aspect of the defect.

The open approach is much less technique sensitive. The graft is secured with periosteum side against recipient periosteum and sutured in place through the mesial papilla. The graft should then be slightly stretched and secured at the papilla moving distally. Grafts are then secured to the periosteum laterally and apically. Much care must be taken to avoid tearing either the graft or periosteum. The cover flap is then repositioned and secured.

Grafting Options Avoiding Secondary Surgical Sites

Allografts and xenografts have become viable and widely incorporated options for soft-tissue augmentation around both teeth and implants: they offer the appeal of soft-tissue regeneration without the necessity of creating a secondary surgical donor site. Although autografts have been shown to result in higher keratinized tissue and attachment regeneration and increased defect coverage, nonautogenous grafts offer the appeal of significant soft-tissue regeneration without the necessity of creating a secondary surgical donor site.[53,54] These options eliminate the excruciating postoperative discomfort that can be experienced from donor sites that must heal via secondary intention, such as from the defect in the palate that remains after harvesting an FGG. They also eliminate the risk of multiple donor-site postoperative complications such as delayed wound healing, necrosis, tissue sloughing, hemorrhage, development of soft-tissue cysts, and altered sensation.[55,56]

Allografts

The AlloDerm acellular dermal matrix (ADM) was originally manufactured and introduced for the treatment of burn wounds starting in the 1994 and is currently the most heavily researched and used soft-tissue allograft on the market. This product's versatility has enabled its use in numerous fields including breast reconstruction, hernia repair, esophageal leak repair, and dural and meningeal repair.[57–62] Since its inception, the ADM allograft has been introduced into periodontal plastic surgery as an alternative to autograft harvest. This allograft is a freeze-dried dermal matrix from which the cellular components have been removed. The collagen bundles and elastic fibers are the primary components of the structurally integrated basement membrane complex and extracellular matrix. The key function of this allograft is to serve as an active scaffold for the migration of fibroblasts, epithelial cells, and endothelial cells while predictably integrating into the host tissue.[63] This ADM provides many advantages to both the surgeon and patient in its use for soft-tissue grafting. Use of this product has the obvious benefit of avoiding a secondary surgical site for graft harvest, an "unlimited" supply of graft material, a guaranteed uniform thickness that is easy to trim and adapt, decrease in postoperative pain and postoperative complications, and better esthetics and color blend with surrounding tissues[53] compared with free gingival grafting. AlloDerm is not without its disadvantages, however, because shrinkage has been shown to be noticeably higher in AlloDerm versus traditional autogenous free gingival grafting. This is associated with the lack of ability in epithelial differentiation. The amount of time required for incorporation of the graft is also higher because vasculature or cells are not present at the time of graft immobilization.[64] AlloDerm placement is very technique sensitive and must be fully submerged under the recipient tissue. Premature AlloDerm exposure leads to a prolonged unesthetic poor healing response. Despite these drawbacks, AlloDerm remains a valuable option in periodontal reconstruction, especially in patients who are concerned with additional morbidity from a donor site or in those who have insufficient harvest content for a large defect.

Puros Dermis (Zimmer) is another example of an allograft. It uses a patented Tutoplast sterilization process that inactivates and removes pathogens, cells, and other unwanted materials.

Xenografts

Several soft-tissue xenografts have recently been introduced as an alternative to the soft-tissue autografts and allografts. Mucoderm (Biotiss Biomaterials) is a porcine-derived ADM. Biotiss uses a highly porous native collagen structure to facilitate increased revascularization and tissue integration rates.[65] Geistlich also recently released their version of a porous, porcine, resorbable collagen matrix, known as Fibro-Gide. A study by Pabst and colleagues[65] in 2014 revealed no cytotoxic effects of the porcine ADM and subsequently demonstrated significant revascularization within its collagen structure after subcutaneous implantation. This is a quickly developing field, and more products are likely to be introduced in the future. Research is ongoing to clarify the indications for each of these materials.

Platelet-Rich Plasma/Platelet-Rich Fibrin

Platelet-rich plasma (PRP) has become an effective and broadly used material for enhancement of wound healing. This autologous concentration of platelets is harvested from the patient's plasma easily through standard phlebotomy techniques to acquire a small amount of blood that is mixed with an anticoagulant. This blood is then centrifuged to isolate the platelets from the plasma. This isolate contains multiple biologically active components and growth factors that are highly conducive to wound healing including fibrin, fibronectin, vitronectin, the 3 isomers of platelet-derived growth factor (PDGF-$\alpha\alpha$, -$\beta\beta$, and -$\alpha\beta$), transforming growth factor β, vascular endothelial growth factor, and epithelial growth factor.[66] PRP has been extensively studied, and successful applications include its use in temporomandibular joint disorders, treatment of skin ulcers and alopecia, orthopedic sports medicine rehabilitation, sinus augmentations, and treatment of periodontal defects and peri-implantitis.[67–72]

After harvesting, nonactivated PRP solution is applied to soft-tissue or hard-tissue graft sites. Application of calcium chloride and thrombin results in the formation of a PRP blood clot within 60 to 90 seconds. The contact and stabilization of this blood clot to bone, implant surfaces, and soft tissue facilitates the migration of regenerator cells. For soft-tissue grafting, nonactivated PRP can be applied before immobilization and can an also be used topically after immobilization as a wound dressing.

Platelet-rich fibrin (PRF) is a second-generation modification of PRP, designed for increased operator convenience by eliminating the need for thrombin application for clot formation. PRF is constituted by a natural fibrin framework through which growth factors can maintain their activity for an extended period of time to allow for adequate cell migration, tissue regeneration, and wound healing.[73,74] PRF has been shown to sustain release of growth factors for between 7 and 28 days.[75,76]

DISCLOSURE

The authors have nothing to disclose.

REFERENCES

1. Baron M, Hudson M, Dagenais M, et al. Relationship between disease characteristics and oral radiologic findings in systemic sclerosis: results from a Canadian oral health study. Arthritis Care Res (Hoboken) 2016;68:673–80.
2. Dale BA. Periodontal epithelium: a newly recognized role in health and disease. Periodontol 2000 2002;30:70–8.
3. Bral MM, Stahl SS. Keratinizing potential of human crevicular epithelium. Periodontol 2000 1977;48:381.
4. Caffesse RG, Nasjleti CE, Castelli WA. The role of sulcular environment in controlling epithelial keratinization. Periodontol 2000 1979;50:1.
5. Jepsen S, Caton JG, Albandar JM, et al. Periodontal manifestations of systemic diseases and developmental and acquired conditions: consensus report of workgroup 3 of the 2017 World Workshop on the Classification of Periodontal and Peri-Implant Diseases and Conditions. J Periodontol 2018;89(Suppl 1):S237–48.
6. Listgarten MA. Electron microscopic study of the gingivo-dental junction of man. Am J Anat 1966;119(1):147–77.
7. Pollanen MT, Salonen JI, Uitto J. Structure and function of the tooth-epithelial interface in health and disease. Periodontol 2000 2003;31:12.
8. Eggert ME, Levin L. Biology of teeth and implants: the external environment, biology of structures, and clinical aspects. Quintessence Int 2018;49(4):301–12.
9. Fowler C, Garrett S, Crigger M, et al. Histologic probe position in treated and untreated human periodontal tissues. J Clin Periodontol 1982;9:373–85.
10. Skougaard M. Turnover of the gingival epithelium in marmosets. Acta Odontol Scand 1965;23:623–43.

11. Salonen JI, Persson GR. Migration of epithelial cells on materials used in guided tissue regeneration. J Periodontal Res 1990;25:215–21.
12. Berglundh T, Lindhe J, Ericsson I, et al. The soft tissue barrier at implants and teeth. Clin Oral Implants Res 1991;2:81–90.
13. Gargiulo AW, Wentz FM, Orban B. Dimensions and relations of the dentogingival junction in humans. Periodontol 2000 1961;32:261.
14. Parma-Benfenati S, Fugazzotto PA, Ruben MP. The effect of restorative margins on the postsurgical development and nature of the periodontium. Part I. Int J Periodontics Restorative Dent 1985;6:31.
15. Herrero F, Scott JB, Maropis PS, et al. Clinical comparison of desired versus actual amount of surgical crown lengthening. Periodontol 2000 1995;66:568.
16. Smukler H, Chaibi M. Periodontal and dental considerations in clinical crown extension: a rational basis for treatment. Int J Periodontics Restorative Dent 1997;17:465.
17. Caton J, Armitage G, Berglundh T, et al. A new classification scheme for periodontal and peri-implant diseases and conditions—introduction and key changes from the 1999 classification. J Periodontol 2018;89(Suppl 1):S1–8.
18. Seibert JL, Lindhe J. Aesthetics and periodontal therapy. In: Lindhe J, editor. Textbook of clinical periodontology. 2nd edition. Copenhangen (Denmark): Munksgaard; 1989. p. 477–514.
19. Frost NA, Mealey BL, Jones AA, et al. Periodontal biotype: gingival thickness as it relates to probe visibility and buccal plate thickness. J Periodontol 2015;86(10): 1141–9.
20. Kao RT, Pasquinelli K. Thick vs. thin gingival tissue: a key determinant in tissue response to disease and restorative treatment. J Calif Dent Assoc 2002;30:521–6.
21. Olsson M, Lindhe J. Periodontal characteristics in individuals with varying form of the upper central incisors. J Clin Periodontol 1991;18:78–82.
22. Sclar A. Soft tissue and esthetic considerations in implant therapy. Hanover Park (IL): Quintessence Publishing; 2003. p. 24.
23. Khan S, Almeida RA, Dias AT, et al. Clinical considerations on the root coverage of gingival recessions in thin or thick biotype. Int J Periodontics Restorative Dent 2016;34(3):409–15.
24. Verdugo F, Simonian K, Frydman A, et al. Long-term block graft stability in thin periodontal biotype patients: a clinical and tomographic study. Int J Oral Maxillofac Implants 2011;26(2):325–32.
25. Lin GH, Chan HL, Wang HL. The significance of keratinized mucosa on implant health: a systematic review. J Periodontol 2013;84(12):1755–67.
26. Linkevicius T, Apse P, Grybauskas S, et al. The influence of soft tissue thickness on crestal bone changes around implants: a 1-year prospective controlled clinical trial. Int J Oral Maxillofac Implants 2009;24(4):712–9.
27. Cairo F, Pagliaro U, Nieri M. Soft tissue management at implant sites. J Clin Periodontol 2008;35(Suppl 8):163–7.
28. Maynard JG Jr, Wilson RD. Physiologic dimensions of the periodontium significant to the restorative dentist. J Periodontol 1979;50:170–4.
29. Stetler KJ. Significance of the width of keratinized gingiva on periodontal status of teeth with submarginal restorations. J Periodontol 1987;58(10):696–700.
30. Schrott AR, Jimenez M, Hwang JW, et al. Five-year evaluation of the influence of keratinized mucosa on peri-implant soft-tissue health and stability around implants supporting full-arch mandibular fixed prostheses. Clin Oral Implants Res 2009;20:1170–7.

31. Crespi R, Capparè P, Gherlone E, et al. A 4-year evaluation of the peri-implant parameters of immediately loaded implants placed in fresh extraction sockets. J Periodontol 2010;81:1629–34.
32. Gobbato L. The effect of keratinized mucosa width on peri-implant health: a systematic review. et al. Int J Oral Maxillofac Implants 2013;28:1536–45.
33. Chung DM. Significance of keratinized mucosa in maintenance of dental implants with different surfaces et al. J Periodontol 2006;77:1410–20.
34. Genco RJ, Newman MG. Consensus report mucogingival therapy. Ann Periodontol 1996;1:702–6.
35. Maynard JG, Wilson RD. Attached gingiva and its clinical significance. In: Prichard JF, editor. The diagnosis and treatment of periodontal disease in general dental practice. Philadelphia: WB Saunders; 1979. p. 138.
36. Smith DE, Zarb GA. Criteria for success of osseointegrated endosseous implants. J Prosthet Dent 1989;62:567–72.
37. Serino G, Wennstrom J, Lindhe J, et al. The prevalence and distribution of gingival recession in subjects with a high standard of oral hygiene. J Clin Periodontol 1994;21:57–63.
38. Rawal SY, Lewis CJ, Kalmar JR, et al. Traumatic lesions of the gingiva: a case series. J Periodontol 2004;74:762–9.
39. Holmstrup P. Non-plaque-induced gingival lesions. Ann Periodontol 1999;4:20–9.
40. Ishikawa I, McGuire M, Mealey B, et al. Consensus report: mucogingival deformities and conditions around teeth. Ann Periodontol 1999;4:101.
41. Baker DL, Seymour GJ. The possible pathogenesis of gingival recession. A histological study of induced recession in the rat. J Clin Periodontol 1976;3:208–19.
42. Sullivan HC, Atkins JH. Free autogenous gingival grafts. III. Utilization of grafts III. Utilization of grafts in the treatment of recession. J Periodontol 1968;6:153.
43. Miller PD. A classification of marginal tissue recession. Int J Periodontics Restorative Dent 1985;5:9.
44. Kordbacheh C, Finkelstein J, Papapanou PN. Peri-implantitis prevalence, incidence rate, and risk factors: a study of electronic health records at a U.S. dental school. Clin Oral Implants Res 2019;30(4):306–14.
45. Mazzotti C, Stefanini M, Felice P, et al. Soft tissue dehiscence coverage at peri-implant sites. Periodontol 2000 2018;77:256–72.
46. Chung DM, Oh TJ, Shotwell JL, et al. Significance of keratinized mucosa in maintenance of dental implants with different surfaces. J Periodontol 2006;77:1410e20.
47. Bjorn H. Free transplantation of gingiva propria. Swed Dent J 1963;22:684–9.
48. Karring T, Ostergaard E, Löe H. Conservation of tissue specificity after heterotopic transplantation of gingiva and alveolar mucosa. J Periodontal Res 1971;6:282–93.
49. Nabers JM. Free gingival grafts, Periodontics 1966;4:243.
50. Mormann W, Schaer F, Firestone AC. The relationship between success of free gingival grafts and transplant thickness. Periodontol 1981;52:74.
51. Langer B, Calagna L. The subepithelial connective tissue graft. J Prosthet Dent 1980;44(4):363–7.
52. Reiser GM, Bruno JF, Mahan PE, et al. The subepithelial connective tissue graft palatal donor site: anatomic considerations for surgeons. Int J Periodontics Restorative Dent 1996;16(2):130–7.
53. Agarwal C, Tarun AB, Mehta DS. Comparative evaluation of free gingival graft and AlloDerm® in enhancing the width of attached gingival: a clinical study. Contemp Clin Dent 2015;6(4):483–8.

54. Hirsch A, Goldstein M, Goultschin J, Boyan BD, Schwartz Z. A 2-year follow-up of root coverage using sub-pedicle acellular dermal matrix allografts and subepithelial connective tissue autografts. J Periodontol 2005;76(8):1323–8.
55. Griffin TJ, Cheung WS, Zavras AI, et al. Postoperative complications following gingival augmentation procedures. J Periodontol 2006;77(12):2070–9.
56. Vastardis S, Yukna RA. Gingival/soft tissue abscess following subepithelial connective tissue graft for root coverage: report of three cases. J Periodontol 2003;74(11):1676–81.
57. Breuing KH, Warren SM. Immediate bilateral breast reconstruction with implants and inferolateral AlloDerm slings. Ann Plast Surg 2005;55:232–9.
58. Yim H, Cho YS, Seo CH, et al. The use of AlloDerm on major burn patients: AlloDerm prevents post-burn joint contracture. Burns 2010;36:322–8.
59. Buinewicz B, Rosen B. Acellular cadaveric dermis (AlloDerm): a new alternative for abdominal hernia repair. Ann Plast Surg 2004;52:188–94.
60. Warren WL, Medary MB, Dureza CD, et al. Dural repair using acellular human dermis: experience with 200 cases: technique assessment. Neurosurgery 2000;46:1391–6.
61. Clark JM, Saffold SH, Israel JM. Decellularized dermal grafting in cleft palate repair. Arch Facial Plast Surg 2003;5:40–4.
62. Bozuk MI, Fearing NM, Leggett PL. Use of decellularized human skin to repair esophageal anastomotic leak in humans. JSLS 2006;10:83–5.
63. Jhaveri HM, Chavan MS, Tomar GB, et al. Acellular dermal matrix seeded with autologous gingival fibroblasts for the treatment of gingival recession: a proof-of-concept study. J Periodontol 2010;81:616–25.
64. Vieira Ede O, Fidel Junior RA, Figueredo CM, et al. Clinical evaluation of a dermic allograft in procedures to increase attached gingiva width. Braz Dent J 2009;20: 191–4.
65. Pabst AM, Happe A, Callaway A, et al. In vitro and in vivo characterization of porcine acellular dermal matrix for gingival augmentation procedures. J Periodontal Res 2014;49(3):37–81.
66. Marx RE, Carlson ER, Eichstaedt R, et al. Platelet-rich plasma: growth factor enhancement for bone grafts. Oral Surg Oral Med Oral Pathol Oral Radiol Endod 1998;85:638–46.
67. Bousnaki M, Bakopoulou A, Koidis P. Platelet-rich plasma for the therapeutic management of temporomandibular joint disorders: a systematic review. Int J Oral Maxillofac Surg 2018;47(2):188–98.
68. Conde Montero E, Fernández Santos ME, Suárez Fernández R. Platelet-rich plasma: applications in dermatology. Actas Dermosifiliogr 2015;106(2):104–11.
69. Okuda K, Tai H, Tanabe K, et al. Platelet-rich plasma combined with a porous hydroxyapatite graft for the treatment of intrabony periodontal defects in humans: a comparative controlled clinical study. J Periodontol 2005;76:890–8.
70. Piemontese M, Aspriello S, Rubini C, et al. Treatment of periodontal intrabony defects with demineralized freeze-dried bone allograft in combination with platelet-rich plasma: a comparative clinical trial. J Periodontol 2008;79:802–10.
71. Consolo U, Zaffe D, Bertoldi B, et al. Platelet-rich plasma activity on maxillary sinus floor augmentation by autologous bone. Clin Oral Implants Res 2007;18: 252–62.
72. Petrungaro PS. Treatment of the infected implant site using platelet-rich plasma. Compend Contin Educ Dent 2002;23:363–6, 368, 370 passim; [quiz: 378].

73. Dohan DM, Choukroun J, Diss A, et al. Platelet-rich fibrin (PRF): a second-generation platelet concentrate. Part II: platelet-related biologic features. Oral Surg Oral Med Oral Pathol Oral Radiol Endod 2006;101:e45–50.
74. Dohan DM, Choukroun J, Diss A, et al. Platelet-rich fibrin (PRF): a second-generation platelet concentrate. Part I: technological concepts and evolution. Oral Surg Oral Med Oral Pathol Oral Radiol Endod 2006;101:e37–44.
75. Choukroun J, Diss A, Simonpieri A, et al. Platelet-rich fibrin (PRF): a second-generation platelet concentrate. Part V: histologic evaluations of PRF effects on bone allograft maturation in sinus lift. Oral Surg Oral Med Oral Pathol Oral Radiol Endod 2006;101:299–303.
76. Choukroun J, Diss A, Simonpieri A, et al. Platelet-rich fibrin (PRF): a second-generation platelet concentrate. Part IV: clinical effects on tissue healing. Oral Surg Oral Med Oral Pathol Oral Radiol Endod 2006;101:56–60.

Bone Regeneration

Properties and Clinical Applications of Biphasic Calcium Sulfate

Amos Yahav, DMD[a], Gregori M. Kurtzman, DDS[b,*],
Michael Katzap, DDS[c], Damian Dudek, DDS[d], David Baranes, DDS[e]

KEYWORDS

- Calcium sulfate • Biphasic calcium sulfate • Graft • Bone cements
- Sinus augmentation • Socket preservation • Ridge augmentation
- Osseous defect repair

KEY POINTS

- Biphasic calcium sulfate has a complete conversion to host bone over a period of 4 to 6 months.
- The material sets hard, acting like a "bone cement" and has been used for decades in orthopedics.
- Minimal flap reflection; flap closure is done under tension by stretching without releasing incisions to induce a tension-free flap.
- No membrane is required, with primary closure not mandatory; when gaps in the soft tissue of 3 mm or less are present, the soft tissue migrates across to close the gap over a short period without inflammation.
- Various grafting applications are achievable with biphasic calcium sulfate at a more cost-effective material cost and similar clinical results can be achieved as with other grafting products used in dental surgery.

INTRODUCTION

Clinically, there are situations in dental treatment that require osseous grafting. Pathologic voids (defects) or those surgically created during treatment may require grafting to restore the osseous anatomy. Conversely, resorption of the osseous contours may requiring grafting to place implants or augment around those implants to contain the entire implant within bone.

[a] Augma Biomaterials, Hadagan 15 Street, Katzir 37861, Israel; [b] Private Practice, 3801 International Drive, Suite 102, Silver Spring, MD 20906, USA; [c] Private Practice, 62-54 97th Pl, Rego Park, NY 11374, USA; [d] Artmedica Oral surgery department, Szosa Chelminska 166 street, Torun 87100 Poland; [e] Private Practice, Hatzadik Mishtefneshet 39 Street, Jerusalem 91000, Israel
* Corresponding author.
E-mail address: drimplants@aol.com

Dent Clin N Am 64 (2020) 453–472
https://doi.org/10.1016/j.cden.2019.12.006
0011-8532/20/

Various osseous grafting materials have been used clinically and reported in dental surgical applications. These include autografts, allografts, xenografts, and nonbiological-derived products (both synthetic and mineral based). Osseous grafts essentially act as a scaffold, maintaining the volume while allowing native bone formation over time. Some materials will resorb fully, whereas others never fully resorb. Autografts and allografts will resorb and, depending on mineralization and compaction if cortical, cancellous or a mixture resorbs quickly (cancellous) or takes longer (cortical). Xenografts, specifically bovine materials do not fully resorb and residual particles remain long term.[1] Synthetic graft materials, depending on their chemistry, may be replaced by conversion to host bone or remain partially or fully. The goal of grafting is conversion to native host bone that has vascularity that will remain in the long term, restoring the area to function; thus, selection of the material to be used is important to achieve that goal.

With those goals in mind, calcium sulfate, a natural mineral and one of the oldest biomaterials, has been used as a bone void filler, binder, grafting material, and as a delivery vehicle for pharmacologic agents and growth factors for more than 120 years, having a longer history of clinical use than most currently available biomaterials.[2] The material has been used in a wide range of clinical applications in orthopedic, plastic surgery, oncologic, and maxillofacial applications in the treatment of osseous voids and traumatic or inflammatory bone deficiencies. Calcium sulfate exists in 3 different forms; calcium sulfate anhydrate, calcium sulfate dehydrate, and calcium sulfate hemihydrate. The difference between these chemical species is represented by the amount of water molecules residing within a single molecule unit. The crystalline structure defines its physical, mechanical, and dissolution properties. The hemihydrate state of hydration exists as either an α or a β form, both of which are found in medical-grade calcium sulfate products. When this hemihydrate is mixed with water, a dehydrate is formed in a mild exothermic reaction with crystallization taking place, and the material sets and hardens.[3] Calcium sulfate as an augmentation material was first reported by Dressman in 1892 to obliterate bone cavities caused by tuberculosis.[4] Later, in the 1920s and 1930s, Nystrom,[5] and Edberg[6] reported results on the use of calcium sulfate plaster of Paris as bone filler without any reported postoperative complications. An extensive review in 1966 regarding the use of calcium sulfate reported the material as a simple, inexpensive substance that offers many advantages as a graft material for bone filling.[7] Studies have demonstrated that calcium sulfate is resorbable and is well tolerated by the tissues, acting primarily as a space filler, restoring morphologic contour, and preventing soft tissue ingrowth into the defects during the healing phase.[8,9] Peltier and colleagues[10–12] confirmed the osteoconductive properties of calcium sulfate allowing ingrowth of blood vessels (angiogensis) and osteogenic cells. When calcium sulfate is implanted in the body, over time (short term) it completely dissolves leaving behind calcium phosphate deposits that stimulate bone growth.[13,14] Evidence has been reported that biphasic calcium sulfate not only serves as a 3-dimensional scaffold but also is able to promote osteoinduction.[15] Therefore, it is considered a bioactive material.

A study reported 26 patients who had been treated with calcium sulfate for unicameral bone cysts, with a follow-up of 1 to 20 years. Of the study participants, 24 had successful healing of the defect with bone formation in the cyst, without complications or the need for additional surgery.[16] Another study reporting on 110 patients treated with calcium sulfate, primarily for osseous defects in the skull and facial bones, concluded that calcium sulfate was an outstanding bone graft substitute that ensured bone formation and produced results comparable with, if not better than, autogenous bone graft.[17] Extensive research has accumulated during the past few decades confirming the effective and safe use of calcium sulfate in both orthopedic and dental applications, consistently reporting high biocompatibility. In dental (maxillofacial and periodontal) applications, calcium sulfate has been used in a variety of clinical applications, including periodontal defect repair, the treatment of osteomyelitis, radicular cyst defect repair, sinus augmentation, socket preservation, ridge augmentation, and as an adjunct to dental implant placement.[18,19] Following graft placement, it can be monitored radiologically; during its placement, it appears radiopaque, after 2 to 3 weeks it appears radiolucent, and it regains radiopacity after 12 weeks, reflecting the transformation of the material into newly formed uncalcified osteoid turning gradually to calcified young native bone.

Following placement, during the healing phase, calcium sulfate dissolves into its component elements naturally found in the body. When placed in direct contact with viable host bone, new bone growth occurs in apposition to the calcium of the graft material. Calcium sulfate bioresorption studies and clinical experience have shown consistent osteoconduction and complete resorption, replaced by newly formed bone that is ultimately remodeled.[20] Calcium ions activate platelets to release bone morphogenetic proteins and platelet-derived growth factors that stimulate proliferation and osteogenic differentiation of mesenchymal stem cells.[21,22] This makes this osseous graft material well tolerated and nonimmunogenic, with no adverse reactions or failure to heal being reported in the literature.[23,24]

Biphasic calcium sulfate acts as a cement, and its hard structure after fast setting prevents infiltration of epithelio-conjunctive cells into the material, acting as a barrier membrane. Yet, connective cells are able to proliferate over the surface of the material, promoting rapid healing of the overlaying soft tissue. Therefore, its related surgical protocols are less invasive compared with other grafting materials in which a tension-free flap and primary closure are mandatory. The opposite is found with biphasic calcium sulfate surgical protocols, indicating minimal flap reflection, and flap closure is done under tension with no releasing incisions to induce a tension-free flap,[25] taking advantage of the flexibility of the mobile mucosa to stretch the flap into place for closure. Thus, the flap and graft are not influenced by muscle movements during the healing phase. In addition, maximal closure with graft exposure of 3 mm is acceptable. The hardness and stability of the biphasic calcium sulfate placed into the defect being grafted means that no membrane or other intermediary barrier is needed. Biphasic calcium sulfate graft material has been shown not to compromise the desired results. Soft tissue cells at the flap margin proliferate over the exposed hardened graft, closing the flap margin fairly quickly over a few days to a week or so.

Calcium sulfate is considered to be one of the bone graft materials of choice in orthopedics due to its excellent osteoconductive bioactivity capacity.[26,27] It can be concluded that calcium sulfate is a biocompatible osteoconductive bioactive material that is well tolerated by the tissues when used for the treatment of osseous defects and guided tissue regeneration in animals and humans.

BIPHASIC CALCIUM SULFATE

In maxillofacial applications, however, difficulties with hardening calcium sulfate in the presence of saliva and bleeding have hampered its routine use. This obstacle to its use dentally was overcome in 2010 by Dr Amos Yahav by modifying the material behavior without changing its chemical structure or adding any additives making it biphasic. The biphasic calcium sulfate form allows the calcium sulfate to harden in the presence of saliva and blood, expanding its use in the maxillofacial arena. As

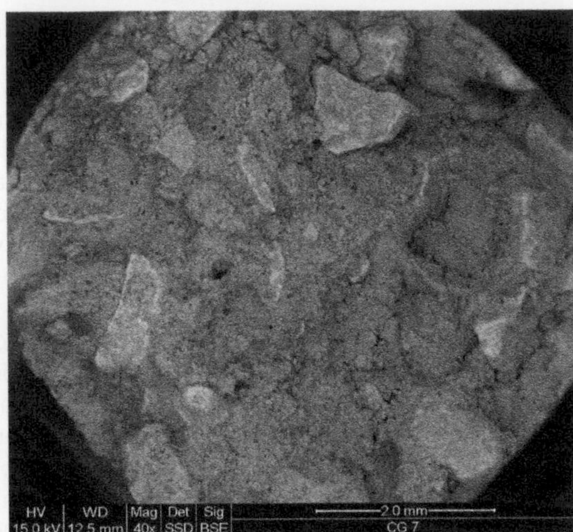

Fig. 1. HA consists of particles of different sizes and shapes incorporated within the biphasic calcium sulfate matrix (scanning electron microscopy).

calcium sulfate is a completely resorbable synthetic material with short-term space-maintaining abilities, in the case of large osseous defects, the use of biphasic calcium sulfate as a composite graft in a mixture slows the resorption time allowing space maintenance, and the host replaces it with early bone. This is available as an already-made composite graft product called Bond Apatite (Augma Biomaterials), a biphasic calcium sulfate composite bone graft cement containing an average of one-third hydroxyapatite in a controlled particle distribution. The hydroxyapatite particles are of various sizes and shapes of 90 μm to 1 mm (**Fig. 1**). On setting, the

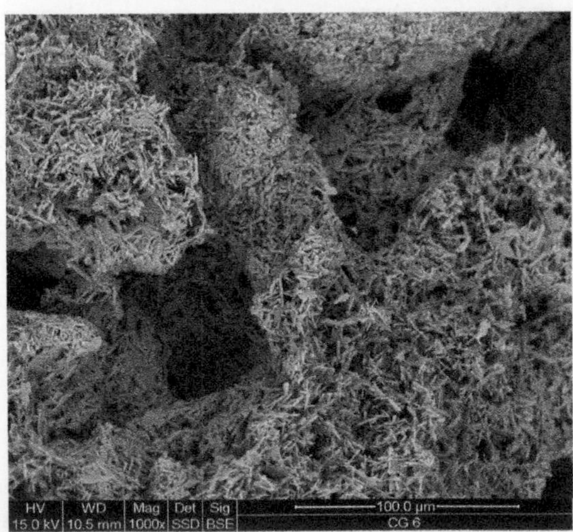

Fig. 2. Postsetting structure of biphasic calcium sulfate at higher magnification, which is composed of needle-like crystals presenting microporosity (1–50 μm) and macroporosity (300–800 μm) promoting growth factor infiltration angiogenesis formation and cell proliferation (scanning electron microscopy).

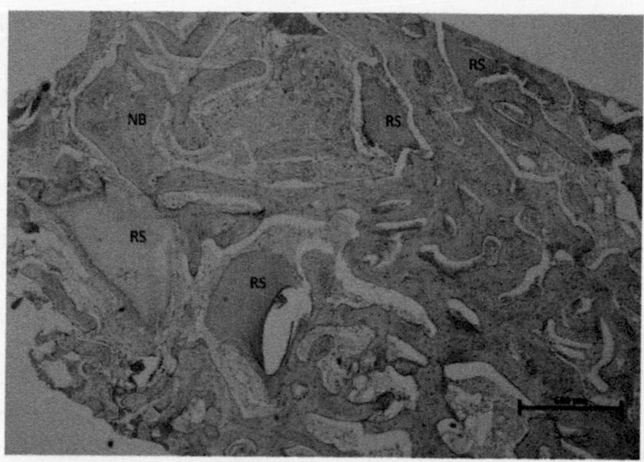

Fig. 3. Histology of Bond Apatite graft specimen at 3 months after graft placement showing residual graft scaffold (RS) and new bone (NB) within the sample studied.

material has a needle-like crystal structure (**Fig. 2**). This allows maintenance of the material in the defect for a much longer period, as the calcium sulfate component resorbs first, with later (slower) resorption of the hydroxyapatite component. This allows space maintenance of the defect while the host vascularizes the grafted area and develops bone, preventing soft tissue ingrowth. The cement has 2 resorption pattern mechanisms related to its components. The biphasic calcium sulfate portion has a resorption pattern of 4 to 10 weeks, which enables fast bone modeling and angiogenesis formation between the hydroxyapatite (HA) particles that act as a longer space maintainer to slow down the overall resorption of the graft. The small to middle-sized HA particles resorb completely after 3 to 5 months, then the larger particles, which are less than 10% by volume, remain for a longer period until complete resorption takes place. The resorption mechanism of the HA particles within the Bond Apatite cement is unique; the HA particles do not integrate with the newly formed bone. Instead, they become encapsulated by connective tissue where degradation occurs as the connective tissue undergoes ossification into a vital host bone.

Histologically, in samples taken at 3 months after graft placement, new bone can be observed in close approximation to remaining residual scaffold particles of Bond Apatite (**Fig. 3**). Analysis at this stage of healing demonstrates ~10% of residual graft particles surrounded by connective tissue. At 8 months after graft placement, histologically, little remains of the Bond Apatite and bone marrow is noted in the organizing new bone (**Fig. 4**). Some areas of connective tissue are also noted, indicating that the graft is maturing and the host is converting the graft material into native bone without any observed inflammatory process. Analysis at 8 months demonstrates the components of the sample to be 79% bone, 11% bone marrow, 7% connective tissue, and only 3% residual graft particles.

Bond Apatite is provided in a double-compartment syringe with one side containing the composite mixture of biphasic calcium sulfate powder with hydroxyapatite and the other compartment containing sterile saline solution. Advancing the syringe shaft until the first plunger on the syringe reaches the blue line marked on the syringe activates the material. The syringe cap is then removed, and the graft is ready for placement directly into the osseous defect. After placement into the defect, sterile gauze is pressed firmly over the graft for 3 seconds to remove residual moisture and harden the material, while compressing it to the

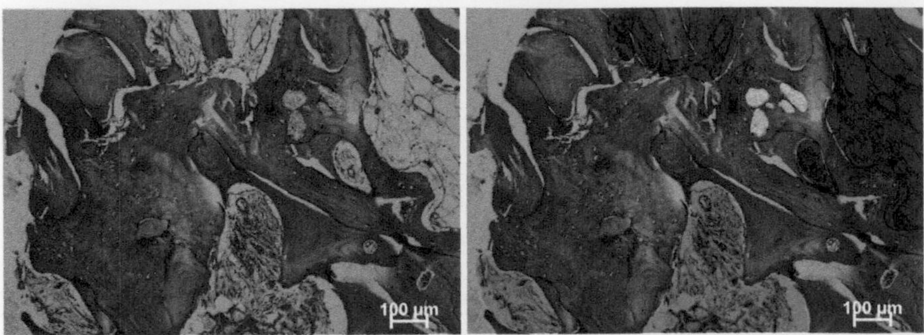

Fig. 4. Histology of Bond Apatite graft specimen at 8 months after graft placement showing (*right*) bone (*purple*), bone marrow (*blue*), connective tissue (*green*), and residual graft particles (*yellow*).

osseous bed. Soft tissue is then reapproximated by stretching, and sutures are placed to fixate the flap margins. The flap should be positioned in direct contact with the graft with tension and secured with sutures. A membrane is not required between the graft material and soft tissue. Exposure of the graft material of up to 3 mm does not require membrane coverage or mobilization of the soft tissue to achieve primary closure. Because of the biocompatible nature of the biphasic calcium sulfate and its set hardness, any minimal exposure will result in peripheral soft tissue migration to cover the material without loss of graft material in the interim period.

As a salt, the graft material has bacteriostatic qualities, which are induced by the presence of sodium chloride in the physiologic saline used to mix the powder with the liquid.[28] The cement obtained after mixing the biphasic calcium sulfate powder with the physiologic saline has bonding qualities. After mixing, it is deposited into the osseous defect in a dehydrated (wet) form. The material is then compressed with sterile gauze for 3 seconds to remove any residual liquid, resulting in a dehydrated crystallized form, which hardens and sticks to the osseous defect walls, thus forming a stable block unlike graft materials in granule or paste form. Bond Apatite may be used in small and large defects, such as socket grafting, periodontal defects, lateral ridge widening, and horizontal sinus augmentation (crestal and lateral approaches).

CLINICAL APPLICATIONS

Extraction Socket Preservation (Grafting)

Extraction socket grafting is often indicated to preserve the osseous crestal margins and prevent resorption during healing (**Fig. 5**). This may also be performed in anticipation of implant placement at a later date or simultaneous with the extraction. After extraction, the sockets are thoroughly curetted to remove any residual tissue or pathologic matter. Bond Apatite is mixed and placed into the extraction socket by injection from the syringe. It is not necessary to place a membrane over the graft material. However, exposure of several millimeters (>3 mm) of set material at the superior aspect of the crest requires a simple collagen sponge with average resorption of 7 to 10 days, which should be secured in place to cover and protect the exposed material during the first healing stage until soft tissue proliferation takes place above its surface; this does not affect the clinical results. Sutures are placed to help maintain the soft tissue margins with the collagen sponge in contact with the graft material during initial healing (**Fig. 6**). After 4 months

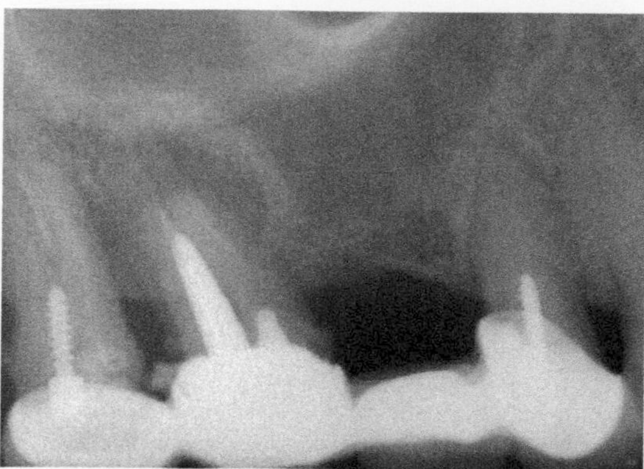

Fig. 5. Radiograph demonstrating failure of bridge abutments related to endodontic failure and periodontal bone loss.

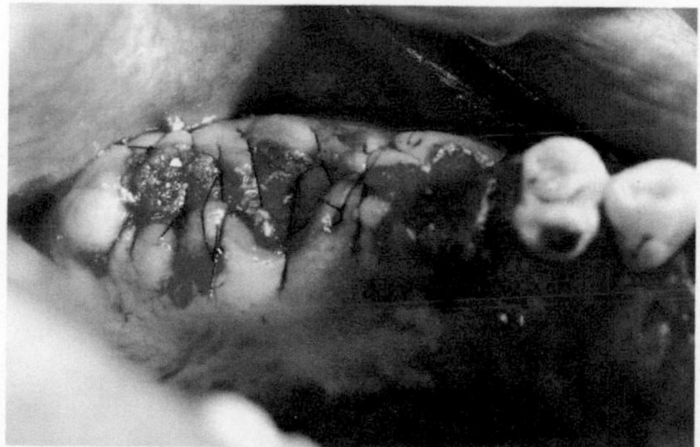

Fig. 6. After extraction of the bridge abutment teeth, the extraction sockets were curetted and filled with Bond Apatite, and exposed material over 3 mm was covered by a collagen sponge secured in place by sutures to help contain the graft material without primary closure of the soft tissue.

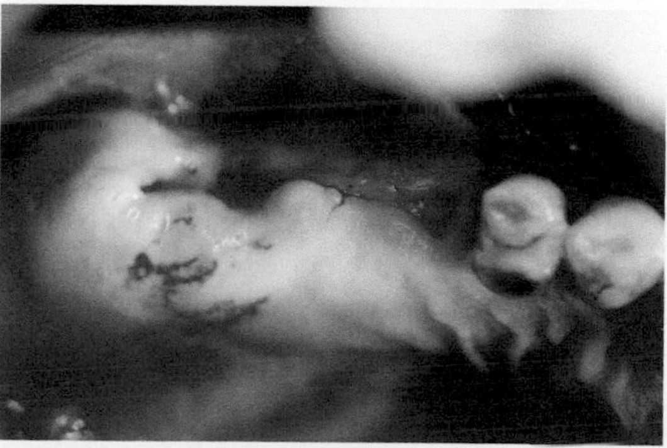

Fig. 7. Presentation at 4 months after surgery demonstrating complete coverage of the area with keratinized soft tissue and closure of the areas of Bond Apatite that had been left exposed at completion of the surgical appointment.

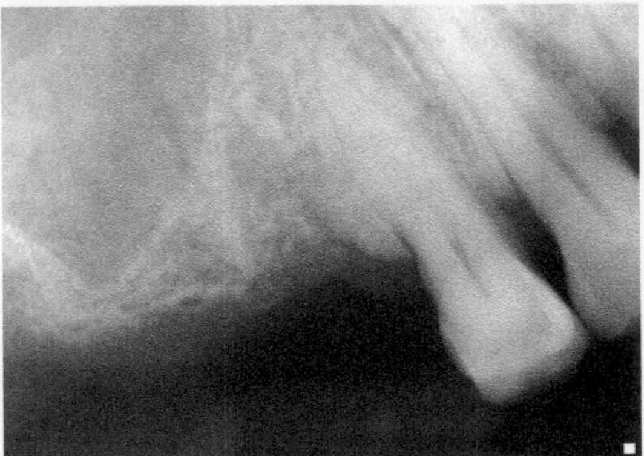

Fig. 8. Radiograph at 4 months after surgical placement of Bond Apatite demonstrating early bone fill and conversion of the graft material.

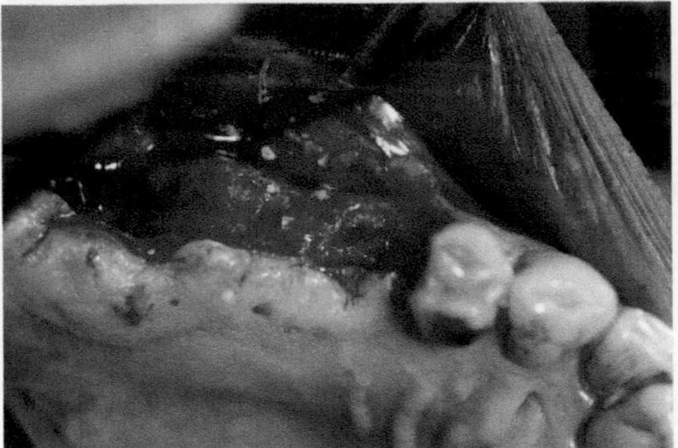

Fig. 9. Site was flapped at 4 months after surgical grafting demonstrating bone filling the extraction sockets previously grafted.

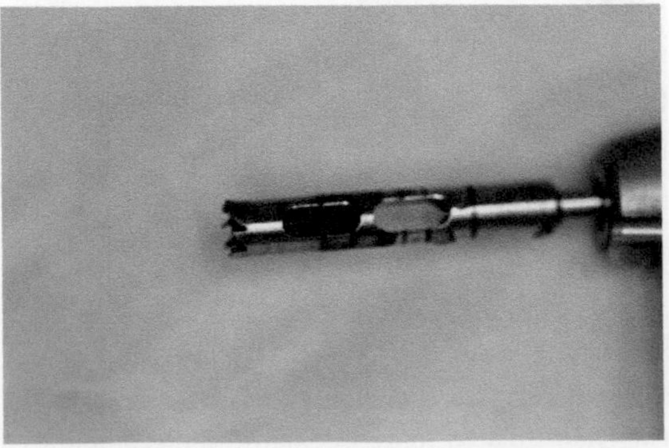

Fig. 10. Core sample retrieved with a trephine from a surgical site that had been grafted with Bond Apatite 4 months previously.

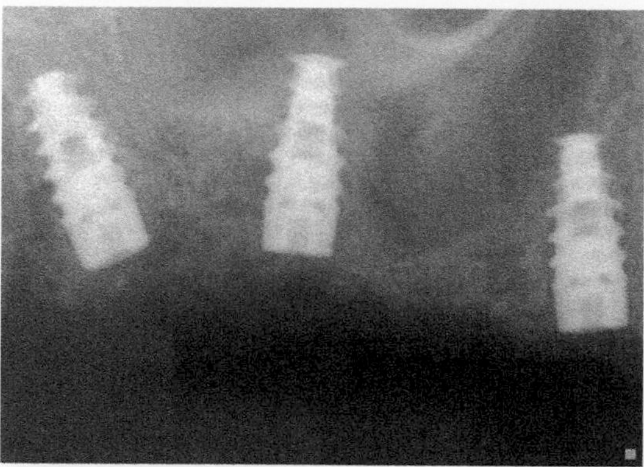

Fig. 11. Radiograph after implant placement at 4 months and socket grafting with Bond Apatite.

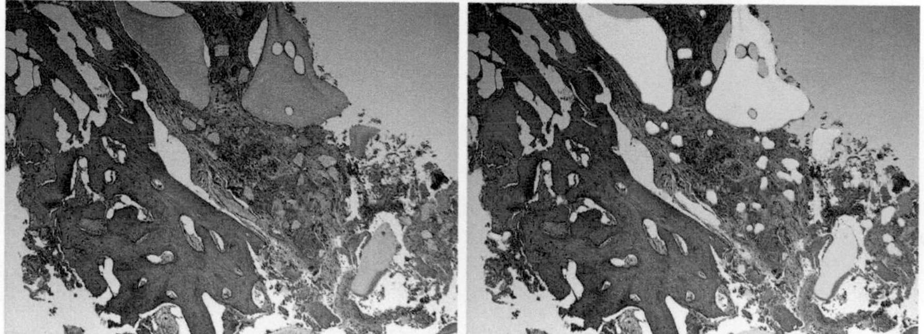

Fig. 12. Histologic evaluation of the core specimen at 40× demonstrating residual particles of Bond Apatite (*yellow, right side*) and young bone in proximity with the particles.

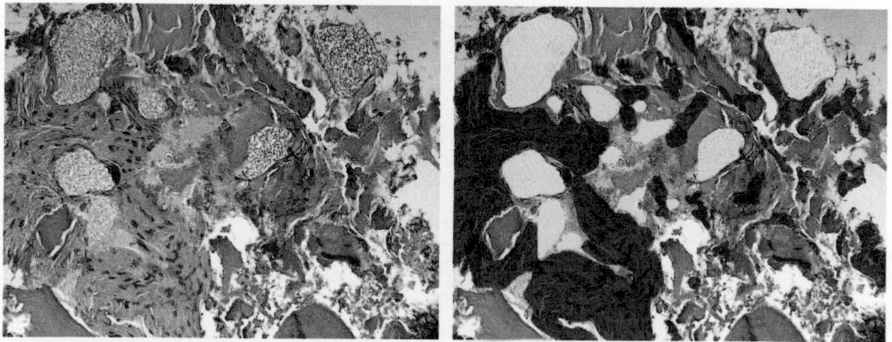

Fig. 13. Microscopic evaluation of the core specimen at 200× demonstrating residual particles of Bond Apatite (*yellow, right side*) and young bone (*blue, right side*) in proximity with the particles.

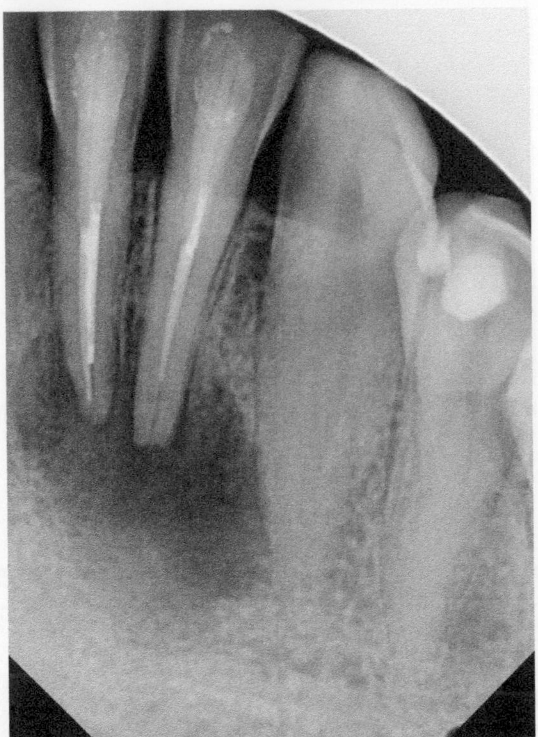

Fig. 14. Periapical radiograph with a lesion associated with previous endodontic treatment on the left mandibular lateral and central incisors.

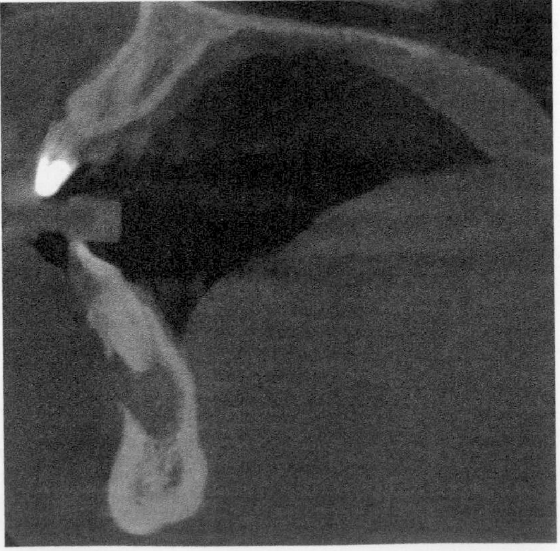

Fig. 15. Cone beam computed tomography cross-section demonstrating the size of the odontogenic cyst associated with failing endodontic teeth in the mandibular anterior, with lack of facial plate noted.

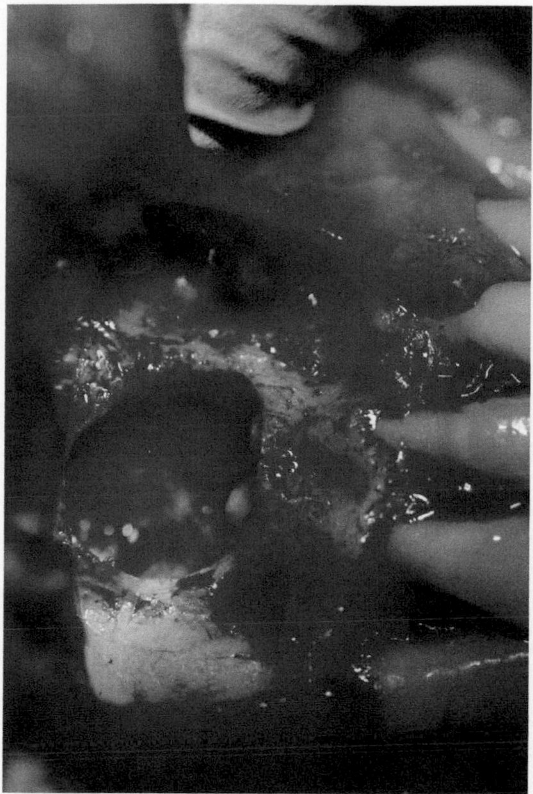

Fig. 16. Size of the defect after enucleation of the odontogenic cyst, root resection, and retrograde filling.

of site healing, the previously exposed areas at the superior aspect of the crest are covered with keratinized gingiva (**Fig. 7**). A radiograph confirms osseous fill of the extraction sockets (**Fig. 8**). The area is flapped for implant placement, demonstrating osseous fill of the sockets (**Fig. 9**), and a core sample is removed by trephine (**Fig. 10**). Implants are placed as planned and a radiograph is taken (**Fig. 11**). Histologic evaluation of the core specimen demonstrates residual particles of Bond Apatite with young bone in proximity with the few remaining particles (**Figs. 12** and **13**). The remaining graft particles will convert while the implants are integrating.

Radicular Cyst or Defect Grafting

An osseous defect resulting from pathologic lesions may necessitate surgical intervention to remove the source of the lesions (**Figs. 14** and **15**). The area is flapped and pathologic tissue is excised, leaving an osseous defect that will require grafting (**Fig. 16**). Bond Apatite is mixed and placed into the osseous defect until the graft material is flush with the exterior aspect of the ridge (**Fig. 17**). After a healing period, radiographs are taken to verify conversion of the graft material placed into host bone (**Figs. 18** and **19**). Histologic analysis via a trephined core sample of the site demonstrates some residual particles of Bond Apatite with new young bone formulation with the absence of an inflammatory reaction (**Fig. 20**). Immunohistochemical study (CD68, a surface antigen used for detection of bone cells)

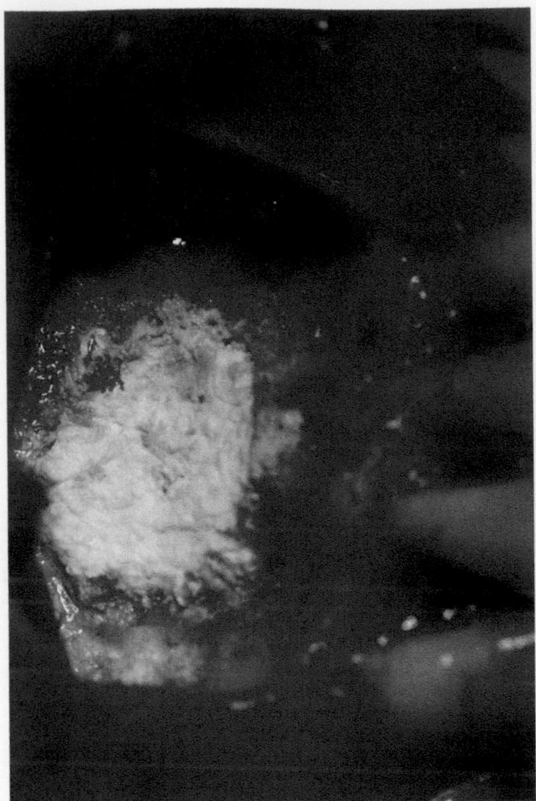

Fig. 17. Bond Apatite placement to fill a large osseous defect.

demonstrates active osteoblasts in the tissue and little remaining Bond Apatite (**Fig. 21**).

Sinus Elevation via a Crestal Approach

The osteotomy is prepared in anticipation for crestal sinus elevation. The sinus is elevated using Summers' technique. Bond Apatite is activated in its syringe and then injected into a sterile dish and left to harden for 3 minutes. Thereafter, the semi-hard material is reloaded back into the Bond Apatite syringe barrel or any other bone graft carrier and introduced into the osteotomy (**Fig. 22**). An osteotome is used to gently place the graft material into the elevated sinus area (**Fig. 23**). When the implant can be placed at that appointment, it is introduced into the site, a cover screw placed, and the site closed with a suture across. Should an implant not be able to be placed at that appointment, the entire osteotomy is filled with additional Bond Apatite, compressed with gauze, and the site closed with a suture over the socket. After a period of 4 months to allow the sinus augmentation graft to heal, implants were placed in the new available crestal height and further healing was allowed for implant integration (**Fig. 24**).

Sinus Elevation via a Lateral Approach

Conventional preparation of the lateral window for sinus elevation is performed after flap elevation and the sinus membrane is elevated (**Fig. 25**). Bond Apatite

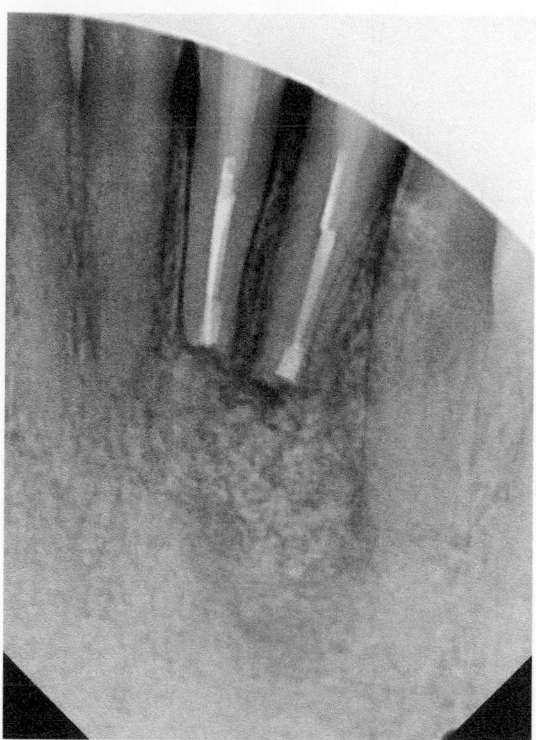

Fig. 18. Bond Apatite placement to fill a large osseous defect.

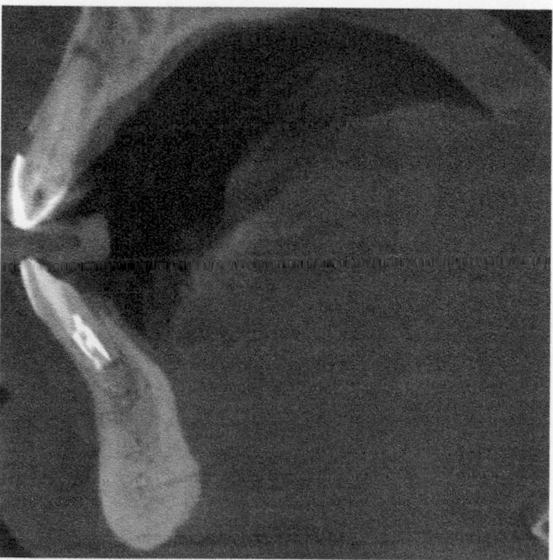

Fig. 19. Cone beam computed tomography cross-section at 6 months demonstrating replacement of the Bond Apatite with new host bone maintaining the facial contour of the mandible cortical plate that was affected by the lesion that was removed.

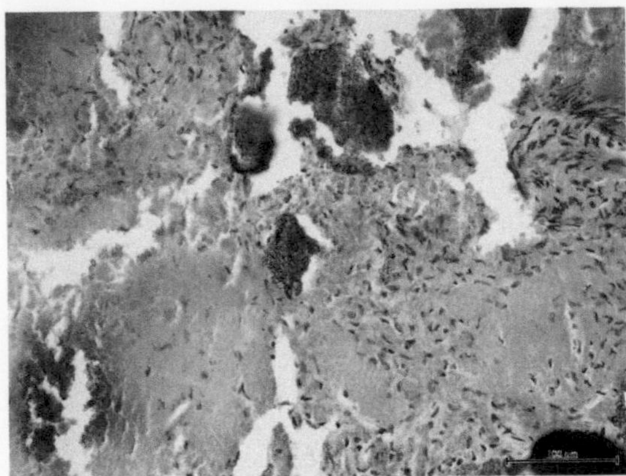

Fig. 20. Histology after 3 months, shown at 100× with visible new young bone formulation (*dark purple spots*) and residual Bond Apatite (*dark areas*) that is converting to bone with the absence of an inflammatory reaction.

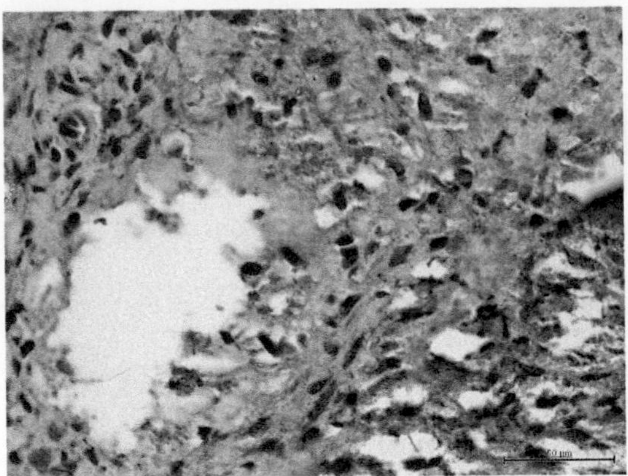

Fig. 21. Immunohistochemical study of CD68, a surface antigen used for detection of bone cells, demonstrates active osteoblasts in the tissue and little remaining Bond Apatite (*green*).

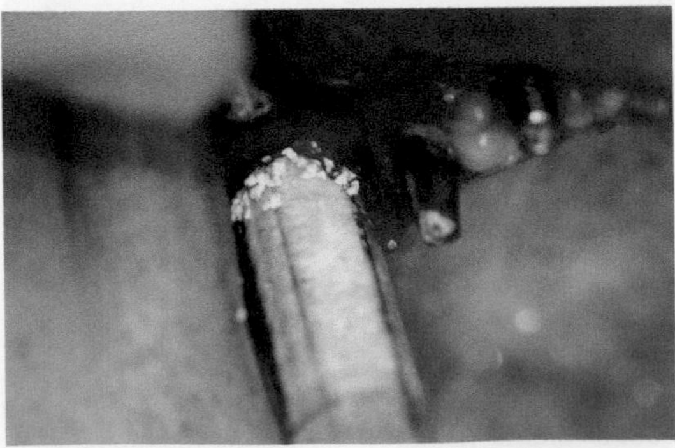

Fig. 22. Bond Apatite is introduced into the crestal sinus elevation with the syringe.

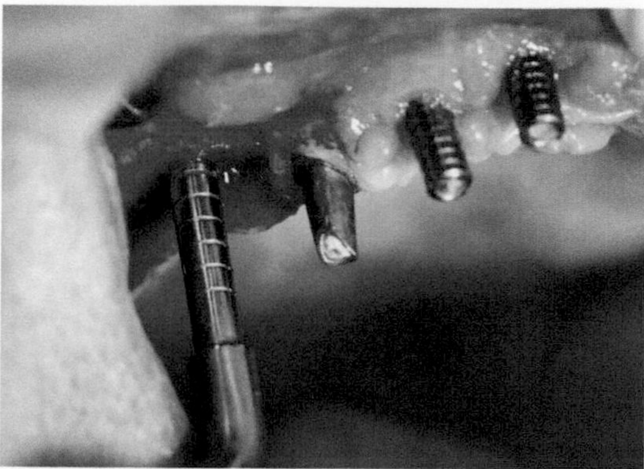

Fig. 23. An osteotome is used to compact the Bond Apatite graft material into the crestally elevated maxillary sinus before implant placement.

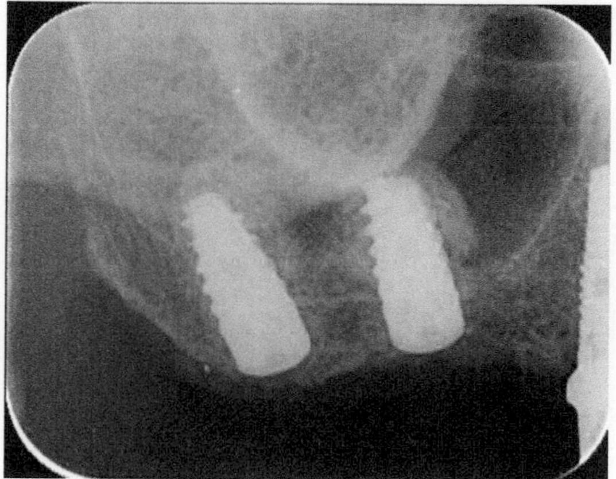

Fig. 24. After a healing period of 4 months to allow the sinus augmentation graft to heal, implants were placed in the new available crestal height and with further healing, allowed implant integration.

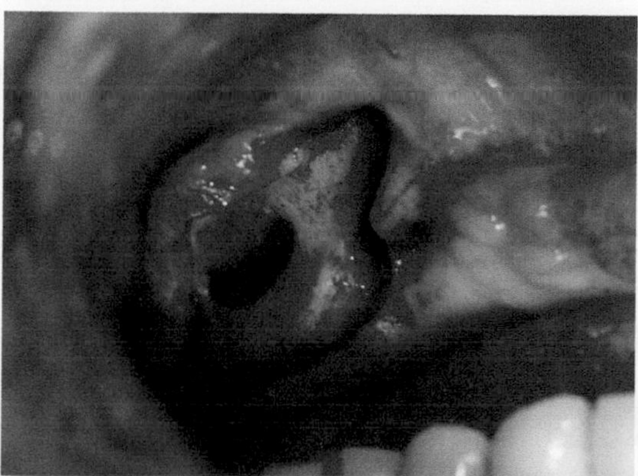

Fig. 25. A lateral osseous window has been created in the posterior maxilla as a prelude to sinus augmentation.

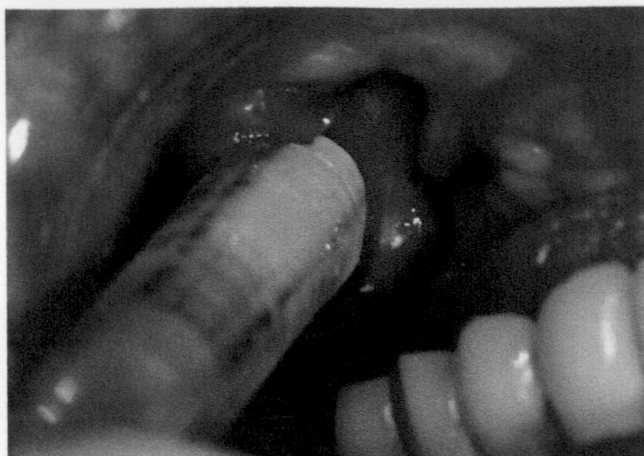

Fig. 26. Bond Apatite is mixed and a syringe is used to introduce the graft material into the elevated maxillary sinus.

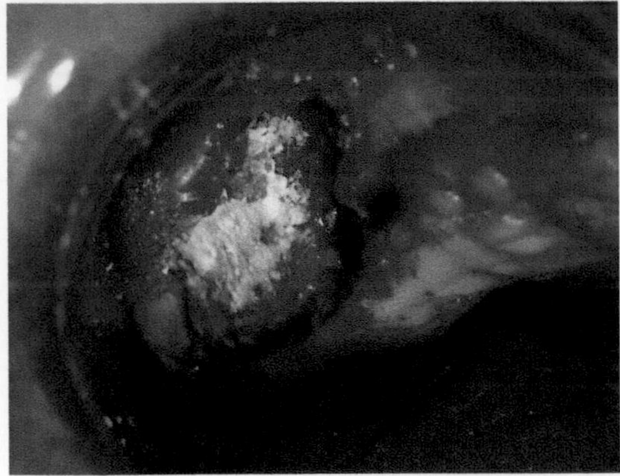

Fig. 27. The elevated maxillary sinus is filled with Bond Apatite graft material to the exterior contour of the lateral wall of the sinus.

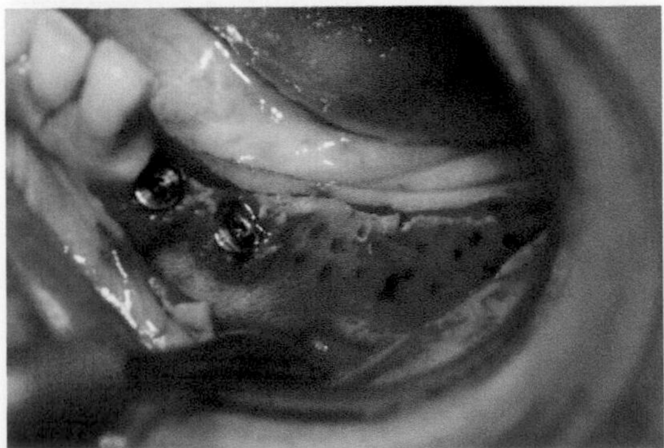

Fig. 28. Posterior mandible with insufficient width to accommodate implants has had the buccal aspect of the ridge perforated to create bleeding points in preparation for graft placement.

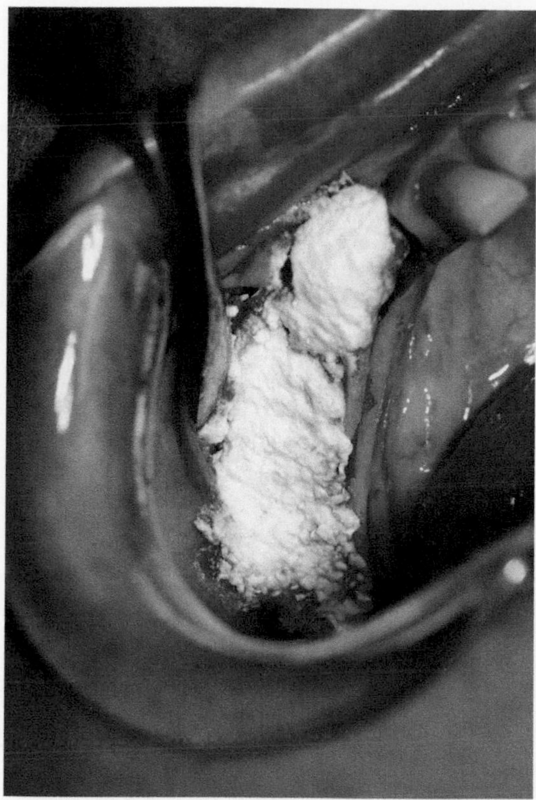

Fig. 29. The lateral aspect of the ridge has been grafted with Bond Apatite before flap closure.

is mixed and after a 1-minute waiting time, is injected into the sinus that was created by elevation of the sinus membrane (**Fig. 26**). The graft is dispersed in the sinus cavity first mesial, then distally, and finally in the center until two-thirds of the sinus is filled. During graft dispersion, the graft material should be compressed against the crest and the sinus walls and, if needed, dry sterile gauze is used to tap gently over the graft surface to absorb excess fluids and blood. When filling the last one-third and closing the sinus window, the last syringe of Bond Apatite is activated and immediately injected into the sinus, followed by pressing firmly for 3 seconds with dry sterile gauze. The augmentation is finished with graft material level with the buccal aspect of the bony window that was created (**Fig. 27**).

Lateral Ridge Grafting (Osseous Width Deficiency)

A full thickness flap extended 2 to 3 mm past the mucogingival line is reflected to visualize the site. If the crestal incision is long enough in the mesial distal direction, a vertical releasing incision may not be necessary and an envelope technique may be used. Decortication with a surgical carbide in a handpiece is performed on the buccal aspect of the ridge. This aids in providing stem cells for the graft to be placed (**Fig. 28**). Bond Apatite is activated in the syringe and placed over the buccal lateral aspect of the ridge, then compressed with gauze

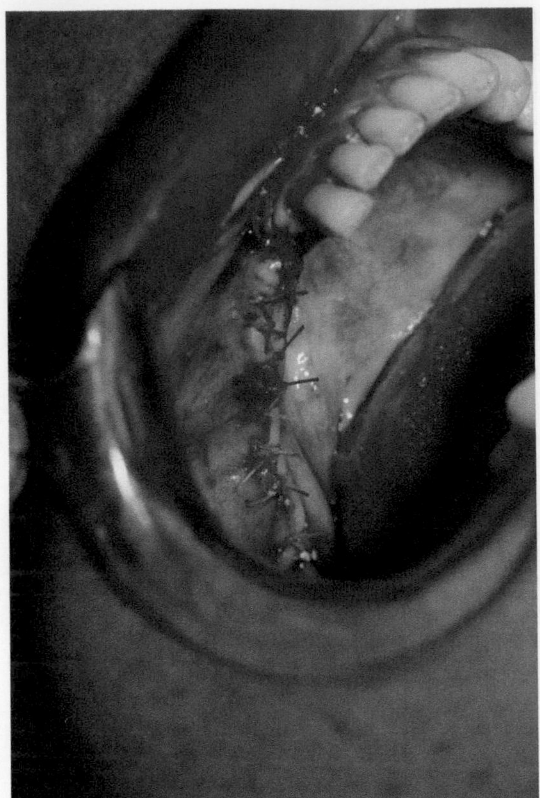

Fig. 30. The flap has been reapproximated over the graft and secured with sutures.

for 3 seconds (**Fig. 29**). The flap is repositioned directly on the graft under tension by stretching it for maximal closure over the graft. If primary closure cannot be achieved, 3 mm of graft exposure is acceptable and a membrane is not required to cover any of the exposed graft material. Sutures are placed to fixate the soft tissue (**Fig. 30**). After a 3- to 4-month healing period, the site is reflapped for implant placement, demonstrating ridge width that can accommodate

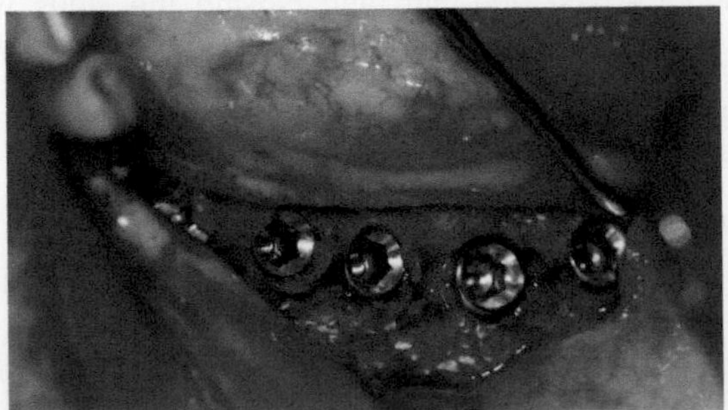

Fig. 31. At 3 months after grafting surgery, implants have been placed in the wider resulting ridge, with some particles of the Bond Apatite remaining that will finish conversion while the implants integrate.

the planned implants (**Fig. 31**). Residual graft particles may be noted at this phase and will fully convert as the implants integrate.

SUMMARY

The goal of osseous grafting is to maintain a space to provide a scaffold for the host to peripherally accomplish angiogenesis and replace the graft by host bone. To accomplish this, the graft material needs to be biocompatible and resorbable over time, but remain long enough to allow host conversion. Biphasic calcium sulfate provides a graft material with a long history in both orthopedic and maxillofacial applications. The addition of HA increases the resorption time and remains within the practical time frame for dental clinical applications with most of the graft material converting to young bone in a 3- to 6-month period and the remainder resorbing shortly thereafter. As outlined, these applications include elimination of osseous defects created either pathologically or as a result of surgical treatment and those clinical situations where osseous development is a prelude to implant treatment.

REFERENCES

1. Ohayon L. Histological and histomorphometric evaluation of anorganic bovine bone used for maxillary sinus floor augmentation: a six-month and five-year follow-up of one clinical case. Implant Dent 2014;23(3):239–44.
2. Thomas MV, Puleo DA. Calcium sulfate: properties and clinical applications. J Biomed Mater Res B Appl Biomater 2009;88(2):597–610.
3. Thomas MV, Puleo DA, Al-Sabbagh M. Calcium sulfate: a review. J Long Term Eff Med Implants 2005;15(6):599–607.
4. Dreesman H. Ueber knochenplombierung. Beitr Klin Chir 1892;9:804.
5. Nystrom G. Plugging of bone cavities with rivanol-plaster-porridge. Acta Chir Scand 1928;63:296.
6. Edberg E. Some experiences of filling osseous, cavities with plaster. Acta Chir Scand 1930;67:313–9.
7. Bahn SL. Plaster: a bone substitute. Oral Surg Oral Med Oral Pathol 1966;21(5): 672–81.
8. Pecora G, Andreana S, Margarone JE 3rd, et al. Bone regeneration with a calcium sulfate barrier. Oral Surg Oral Med Oral Pathol Oral Radiol Endod 1997; 84(4):424–9.
9. Kim CK, Kim HY, Chai JK, et al. Effect of a calcium sulfate implant with calcium sulfate barrier on periodontal healing in 3-wall intrabony defects in dogs. J Periodontol 1998;69(9):982–8.
10. Peltier LF, Bickel EY, Lillo R, et al. The use of plaster of paris to fill defects in bone. Ann Surg 1957;146(1):61–9.
11. Peltier LF. The use of plaster of paris to fill large defects in bone. Am J Surg 1959; 97(3):311–5.
12. Peltier LF. The use of plaster of Paris to fill defects in bone. Clin Orthop 1961; 21:1–31.
13. Yuan W, He X, Zhang J, et al. Calcium phosphate silicate and calcium silicate cements suppressing osteoclasts activity through cytokine regulation. J Nanosci Nanotechnol 2018;18(10):6799–804.
14. Urquia Edreira ER, Hayrapetyan A, Wolke JG, et al. Effect of calcium phosphate ceramic substrate geometry on mesenchymal stromal cell organization and osteogenic differentiation. Biofabrication 2016;8(2):025006.

15. Raina DB, Gupta A, Petersen MM, et al. Muscle as an osteoinductive niche for local bone formation with the use of a biphasic calcium sulphate/hydroxyapatite biomaterial. Bone Joint Res 2016;5(10):500–11.
16. Peltier LF, Jones RH. Treatment of unicameral bone cysts by curettage and packing with plaster-of-Paris pellets. J Bone Joint Surg Am 1978;60(6):820–2.
17. Coetzee AS. Regeneration of bone in the presence of calcium sulfate. Arch Otolaryngol 1980;106(7):405–9.
18. Strocchi R, Orsini G, Iezzi G, et al. Bone regeneration with calcium sulfate: evidence for increased angiogenesis in rabbits. J Oral Implantol 2002;28(6):273–8.
19. Intini G, Andreana S, Margarone JE 3rd, et al. Engineering a bioactive matrix by modifications of calcium sulfate. Tissue Eng 2002;8(6):997–1008.
20. Bagoff R, Mamidwar S, Chesnoiu-Matei I, et al. Socket preservation and sinus augmentation using a medical grade calcium sulfate hemihydrate and mineralized irradiated cancellous bone allograft composite. J Oral Implantol 2013; 39(3):363–71.
21. Huang TH, Kao CT, Shen YF, et al. Substitutions of strontium in bioactive calcium silicate bone cements stimulate osteogenic differentiation in human mesenchymal stem cells. J Mater Sci Mater Med 2019;30(6):68.
22. Ali Akbari Ghavimi S, Allen BN, Stromsdorfer JL, et al. Calcium and phosphate ions as simple signaling molecules with versatile osteoinductivity. Biomed Mater 2018;13(5):055005.
23. Robinson D, Alk D, Sandbank J, et al. Inflammatory reactions associated with a calcium sulfate bone substitute. Ann Transplant 1999;4(3–4):91–7.
24. Evaniew N, Tan V, Parasu N, et al. Use of a calcium sulfate-calcium phosphate synthetic bone graft composite in the surgical management of primary bone tumors. Orthopedics 2013;36(2):e216–22.
25. Baranes D, Kurtzman GM. Biphasic calcium sulfate as an alternative grafting material in various dental applications. J Oral Implantol 2019;45(3):247–55.
26. Hak DJ. The use of osteoconductive bone graft substitutes in orthopaedic trauma. J Am Acad Orthop Surg 2007;15(9):525–36.
27. Gitelis S, Piasecki P, Turner T, et al. Use of a calcium sulfate-based bone graft substitute for benign bone lesions. Orthopedics 2001;24(2):162–6.
28. Nuñez de Gonzalez MT, Keeton JT, Acuff GR, et al. Effectiveness of acidic calcium sulfate with propionic and lactic acid and lactates as postprocessing dipping solutions to control *Listeria monocytogenes* on frankfurters with or without potassium lactate and stored vacuum packaged at 4.5 degrees C. J Food Prot 2004;67(5):915–21.

Maxillofacial Bone Grafting Materials

Nabil Takahiro Moussa, DDS[a,*], Harry Dym, DDS[b]

KEYWORDS

- Bone graft • Allograft • Xenograft • Bone morphogenic protein
- Regenerative materials • Tissue engineering

KEY POINTS

- Bone is a dynamic composite structure that provides framework to the human body. The ultimate goal of bone grafting is to regenerate bone into well-vascularized bone that will undergo normal remodeling.
- Four basic types of bone grafting materials are available for use clinically: autologous bone, allogeneic bone, xenogenic bone, and alloplastic bone.
- Bone morphogenic protein is a family of osteoinductive proteins that stimulate endochondral and intramembranous bone formation from mesenchymal cells.
- The literature reports evidence of successful, clinically significant, bone regeneration with each respective grafting material. However, autologous bone grafting remains the gold standard.
- Autogenous bone grafts will most likely remain the gold standard of grafting materials. All four types of bone grafting material show good clinical evidence of bone regeneration in different degrees, respectively.

INTRODUCTION

The ultimate goal of bone grafting is to replace normal bone volume and structure with healthy, well-vascularized bone that will undergo normal remodeling. The ideal bone graft regardless of the purpose, whether it is to augment the alveolus for prosthetic reasons or reconstruct the mandible following enucleation of a cyst, is to achieve histology of bone with no distinguishing features from the original local tissue. The ideal bone will regenerate bone and not repair it. The purpose of this article is to cover the biology of bone grafting and provide an overview of the different grafting materials that are available.

[a] Department of Dentistry, Division of Oral and Maxillofacial Surgery, The Brooklyn Hospital Center, 121 DeKalb Avenue, Brooklyn, New York 11201, USA; [b] Dentistry and Oral & Maxillofacial Surgery, The Brooklyn Hospital Center, Outpatient Care Building - 1st Floor, 121 DeKalb Avenue, Brooklyn, NY 11201, USA
* Corresponding author.
E-mail address: moussanabil@gmail.com

Dent Clin N Am 64 (2020) 473–490
https://doi.org/10.1016/j.cden.2019.12.011 dental.theclinics.com

BIOLOGY OF BONE

Bone is a dynamic composite structure that provides framework to the human body. Bone is composed of cortical and lamellar bone originating from ectomesynchyme, an element of the developing embryo (**Table 1**). As the body grows mesenchymal cells are stimulated by growth factors and differentiate into osteoblasts and osteoclasts. As bone is deposited around osteoblasts, it becomes embedded in the matrix, becoming an osteocyte. The spaces that house the osteocyte are referred to as lacunae. In an adult immature bone cells referred to as osteoprogenitor cells linger in the periosteum and endosteum, which reserve the potential to differentiate into osteoblasts if the need arises. For example, osteoprogenitor cells will receive cytokine signals that induce differentiation into osteoblasts following bone fracture or during exercise where the bone loading is changed.

BONE HEALING BIOLOGY

Hard tissue heals through stages over the period of approximately 16 weeks. The stages when listed sequentially are the inflammatory, proliferative, and the remodeling phases. Initially the healing depends on formation of a hematoma and subsequently angiogenesis and vascular invasion from the surrounding periosteum and endosteum. Within 48 hours of surgery a hematoma forms with organizing soft tissue and collagen deposition. The decreased partial pressure of oxygen in the tissue induces release of growth factors and stimulates angiogenesis and osteogenesis. A fibrin mesh forms and acts as scaffolding for the fibroblasts and capillary buds. The addition of bone grafting provides the marginating osteoblasts and fibroblasts with a macrostructure to deposit new tissue.

After 4 days the soft tissue organizes with decreased fibrin content. The fibroblastic state depends on the migration of osteoprogenitor cells and fibroblasts

Table 1
Composition of bone

Type of Bone	Histologic Features
Organized matrix	40% of the dry weight of bone. Composed of 90% type 1 collagen, noncollagenous proteins, ground substance, water, proteoglycans, cytokines, and growth factors.
Cells	Osteoprogenitor cells Osteoblasts Osteocytes Osteoclasts
Vascular and nutrient distribution	Bone receives 5%–10% of cardiac output via arterial supply through the periosteum and endosteum. Extracellular fluid is drained through microcirculation, lymphatics, and venous return.
Neurologic	Bone is supplied by autonomic and neurosensory networks.
Marrow	Serves hematopoietic and osteogenic functions.
Periosteum	A source of osteoprogenitor cells, neurovascular distribution, and blood supply.
Endosteum	A source of osteoprogenitor cells.
Communication systems	A network including haversian and Volkmann canaliculi lacunae and extracellular fluid.

invading the tissue and depositing collagen matrix. The osteoprogenitor cells migrate from three sources: (1) periosteum, (2) endosteum, and (3) the mesenchymal cells in the bloodstream. Following a week of collagen deposition, islands of osteoid or immature and disorganized bone are found. Osteoblasts are found around the periphery of these spicules of bone formation with the absence of osteoclasts. The spicules of bone begin to coalesce and form larger blocks with osteoblasts housed within the bone structure. These units of osteoblasts within lacunae are referred to as osteocytes. Eight weeks mark the remodeling stage. There is evidence of Howship lacunae that form in the presence of osteocytes. This remodeling phase of bone healing is characterized by resorption and deposition of new bone. The remodeling of bone from immature and irregular osteoid to lamellar and organized bone is important in the formation of new trabecular and cortical bone. At 16 weeks mature bone formation is complete and bone reaches the necessary strength for normal functional loads.

In clinical practice bone formation depends largely on vascular supply. Angiogenesis and having adequate blood supply from the periphery is essential to maintain appropriate oxygen tension for the function of osteoblasts and osteoclasts. Mobility of the graft or pressure on the graft can easily compromise the vascular supply to the graft site. Poor vascularization means poor bone production. It is strongly recommended in patients when grafting to eliminate any potential sources of pressure on the graft site. This includes arresting the use of any dental prosthetic devices, such as complete or partial dentures and using the area for mastication. Additionally patients who smoke are at a significant risk for bone graft failure. The nicotine in smoke acts as a vasoconstrictor reducing the blood flow to the graft site. Carbon monoxide from the smoke binds, with 100 times the affinity, to hemoglobin forming carboxyhemoglobin. Increased levels of carboxyhemoglobin reduces availability of erythrocytes for oxygen transport and additionally shifts the hemoglobin curve to the left increasing the affinity of erythrocytes for oxygen and consequentially reducing the volume of oxygen released into the tissues.

BONE GRAFTING MATERIALS

Four basic types of bone grafting materials are available for use clinically to augment and reconstruct the maxillofacial skeleton (**Tables 2–4**).

Autologous Bone

Transplanted bone that is compromised of the individual's own tissue is referred to as an autologous bone graft. Historically, autologous bone graft harvested from the hip or tibia has been predictably used in orthopedics and reconstruction of the maxillofacial skeleton.[1] Other harvest sites commonly used in oral surgery are the ramus and

Table 2
Classes of Bone Graft Materials

Bone Type	Description
Autograft (autogenous)	Refers to a transplant of viable cortical or cancellous bone from one location of the body to another within the same patient.
Xenograft	Refers to a cross-species transplantation of tissue: the use of organic bovine bone or porcine collagen subjects.
Alloplast	Refers to implantation of synthetic material, such as apatite or tricalcium phosphate, bioactive glass, or polymers.

Table 3
Bone grafting material overview

Bone Graft	Structural Strength	Osteoconduction	Osteoinduction	Osteogenesis
Autograft				
Cancellous	No	+++	+++	+++
Cortical	+++	++	++	++
Allograft				
Cancellous				
Frozen	No	++	+	No
Freeze-dried	No	++	+	No
Cortical				
Frozen	+++	+	No	No
Freeze-dried	+	+	No	No

From Giannoudis PV, Dinopoulos H, Tsiridis E. Bone substitutes: an update. Injury. 2005;36(Suppl 3):S21; with permission.

symphysis of the mandible. For cranial reconstruction purposes the rib, calvarium, radius, and fibula may also be used. The hip, ramus, and symphysis provide a mixture of cortical and cancellous bone in block and particulate marrow forms. The cortical blocks are often used for its structural integrity. The graft provides volumetric support for the desired dimension of the grafted site. The marrow is often used for its handling properties, which make it ideal for filling defects and contouring. Autogenous bone is considered as the gold standard for bone grafting because of its osteoinductive, osteoconductive, and osteogenic properties.[2]

Table 4
Bone selection and properties

Type	Graft	Osteoconduction	Osteoinduction	Osteogenesis	Advantages
Bone	Autograft	3	2	2	Gold standard
	Allograft	3	1	0	Availability in many forms
Biomaterials	DBM	1	2	0	Supplies osteoinductive BMPs, bone graft extender
	Collagen	2	0	0	Good as delivery vehicle system
Ceramics	TCP, hydroxyapatite	1	0	0	Biocompatible
	Calcium phosphate cement	1	0	0	Some initial structural support
Composite grafts	β-TCP/BMA composite	3	2	2	Ample supply
	BMP/synthetic composite	—	3	—	Potentially limitless supply

Score: 0 (none) to 3 (excellent).

Abbreviations: BMA, bone marrow aspirate; BMP, bone morphogenetic protein; DBM, demineralized bone matrix; TCP, tricalcium phosphate.

From Giannoudis PV, Dinopoulos H, Tsiridis E. Bone substitutes: an update. Injury. 2005;36(Suppl 3):S22; with permission.

The major advantage of autologous graft is that it is the host's own tissue. Risks that may be encountered with allografts, such as disease transmission, are negligible (eg, human immunodeficiency virus and hepatitis B and C). Additionally, immunologic reactions, such as foreign body reactions, seen with alloplastic materials are not observed. The graft when transplanted, transplants vital tissues including the cellular components of bone. Finally, autologous bone graft is osteoconductive and osteoinductive. Because the graft material is harvested from live tissue, with appropriate handling during surgery, viable cells and their associated growth factors are transplanted along with the graft. Osteoprogenitor cells are present within the periosteum and endosteum, which when stimulated differentiate into osteoblasts and lay down new osteoid.

Some disadvantages of autologous bone grafting include donor site morbidities associated with the harvest site. Iliac crest bone graft harvest has been associated with a complication rate of 8.5% to 20%.[3–7] Hip grafts often used in sinus lifts have a significant risk of gait disturbance, which results in difficulty with ambulating. Other complications include hematoma formation, nerve injury, hernia formation, blood loss, ureteral injury fracture, pelvic instability, cosmetics defects, and some cases of chronic pain at the donor site. Harvesting from the symphysis of the mandible is often associated with temporary or permanent sensory changes of the lip and chin. It is prudent, as a surgeon, to weight the benefits to the risks of harvesting and make sure the patient understands completely the risks associated with the harvest. Finally, only a limited volume of bone is harvested from each site. In comparison, allograft is limited simply by the supply of bone that was purchased. Overall, faster and predictable bone grafting is expected when using autologous grafts.

Autogenous bone grafting is predictable and serves as a gold standard in bone augmentation. In a study completed by Fretwurst and colleagues[8] the crestal bone levels changes were observed around dental implant placed in augmented alveolus with the sole use of iliac crest bone graft (**Figs. 1** and **2**). The study followed 32 patients with edentulous ridges that required augmentation for implant placement. A standardized protocol was used to harvest and graft anterior iliac crest bone, which was grafted to the maxilla and the mandible. The study used corticocancellous bone blocks harvested from the crest. A total of 150 implants were placed and standardized radiographic documentation of the crestal bone was completed over a mean observation period of 69 months (12–165 months). Implant success rate was consistent with what is reported in the literature, 96% in the maxilla and 92% in the mandible. The mean crestal bone loss was 1.8 mm over a mean follow-up period of 10 years.[8]

In another example of autogenous grafting, Duttenhoefer and colleagues[9] investigated avascular fibula grafting for mandibular reconstruction. The fibula is a popular site for harvest for reconstruction of patients treated for head and neck cancer, specifically mandibular reconstruction. The graft is harvested as a vascular or avascular graft. The study showed fibular graft provided predictable results in augmenting an atrophic mandible for long-term stable integration of implants supporting a prosthesis with the use of an avascular fibular bone graft. Eight edentulous patients were augmented with avascular fibular graft with a follow-up to 15 years with stable results. Additionally, the study examined the histology of the grafted bone. The sampled bone showed a completely vascularized cortical bone structure (**Fig. 3**).[9] In a similar study Nelson and colleagues[10] observed 10 patients augmented with avascular fibular graft. The study showed good vascularization of the graft following a 3-month healing period. The patients were observed over a follow-up period of 6.25 years. A total of 7.2% of the grafted fibular height was lost in the first year, which then stabilized and did not show any further loss of bone height (**Fig. 4**).[10]

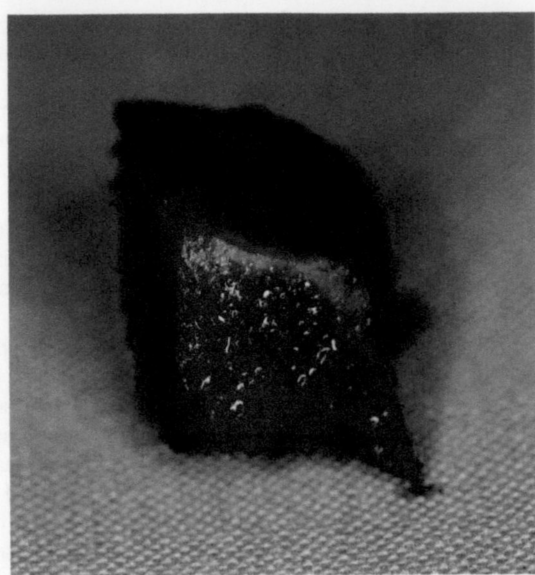

Fig. 1. Harvested iliac crest bone graft. (*From* Fretwurst T, Nack C, Al-Ghrairi M, et al. Long-term retrospective evaluation of the peri-implant bone level in onlay grafted patients with iliac bone from the anterior superior iliac crest. J Craniomaxillofac Surg. 2015;43(6):957; with permission.)

Allogeneic Bone

Allografts are those grafts that have been harvested from the same species. These grafting materials originate from cadaveric tissue and are processed for use. This type of graft has gained strong popularity in the medical field with a 15-fold increase in its use during its rise. In the year 2000 it accounted for one-third of the grafting material used in the medical community.[11] Before being transplanted allografts must be prepared using a rigorous process to ensure safety of the tissue. Often the method of processing the bone can change the properties of the bone. Examples of processed bone available are fresh, fresh frozen, freeze dried, and demineralized types of bone. When compared with mineralized bone grafting material, demineralized grafts have the advantage of being osteoinductive in addition to osteoconductive. Residual growth factors, such as bone morphogenic protein (BMP) found in allogeneic bone, can induce the differentiation of neighboring bone mesenchymal cells to differentiate into osteoblasts. The demineralization process removes the calcium phosphate and exposes the inherent BMPs contained in the bone matrix. This protein has effects that induce differentiation of progenitor cells to differentiate and deposit bone. The porous nature of the material facilitates movement of osteoblasts and osteoclasts into the graft material and promotes angiogenesis. The properties of BMP are not in the scope of this article.

There are two main types of allogenic bone available: mineralized bone graft and demineralized bone graft. The two materials differ in the processing of each tissue. Mineralized bone graft maintains the mineralized and collagen components of the materials. Demineralized grafts have been processed to remove the mineralized component and leave the collagenous matrix behind. A major disadvantage of allograft is that it has a risk, albeit minimal, of disease transmission. If any cellular components are remaining within the graft there is an additional risk of the host mounting an immunologic reaction to the graft material.

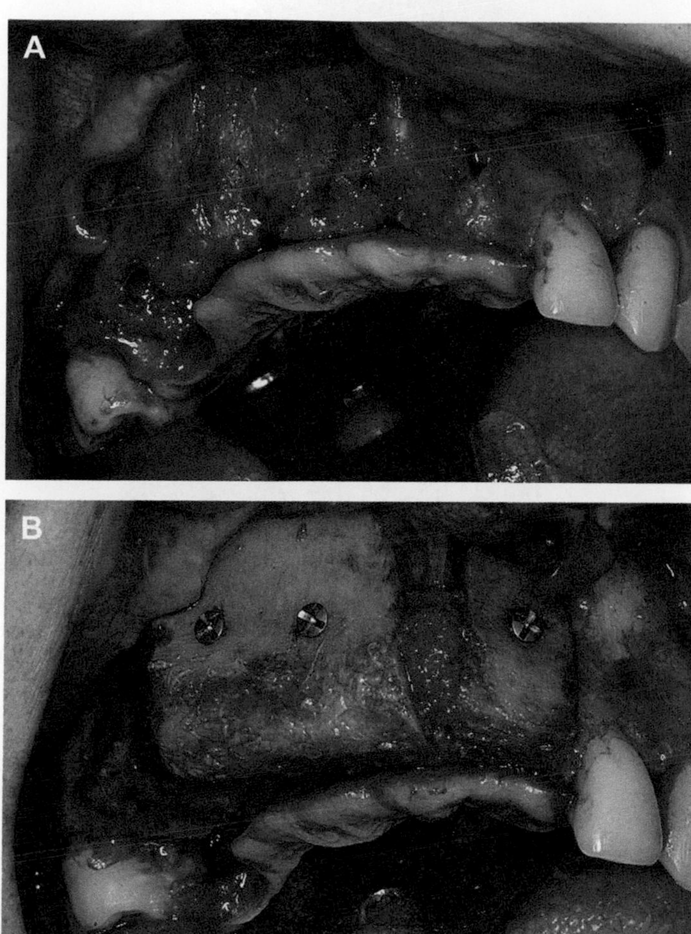

Fig. 2. Maxillary iliac crest bone grafting. Maxillary defect shown with horizontal and vertical deficiencies (*A*). Reconstruction of the maxillary defect with iliac bone graft (*B*). (*From* Misch CM. Maxillary autogenous bone grafting. Oral Maxillofac Surg Clin North Am. 2011;23(2):230; with permission.)

Allogeneic bone comes in different particle sizes, which can influence the degree of osteoconductivity in grafted bone. Among the literature, it is widely accepted that a particle size of 100 to 300 μm has the greatest osteoconductive potential.[12] Less predictable results have been observed with the use of large particle sizes 1000 to 2000 μm and smaller than 1000 μm. Particles with a size less than 100 μm have been suspected to elicit a macrophage response that results in rapid resorption of the graft and loss of desired bone volume. Allogenic bone has several distinct advantages over autogenic bone. The bone does not need to be harvested and thus, eliminates a separate surgical site for the harvest. Current literature shows similar results and predictability when augmenting with allogeneic bone when compared with allograft. Xavier and colleagues[13] conducted a split mouth study to compare volumetric changes after sinus augmentation of completely edentulous maxillae with autogenous and allogenic fresh frozen bone particles. Autograft was harvested from the ramus and

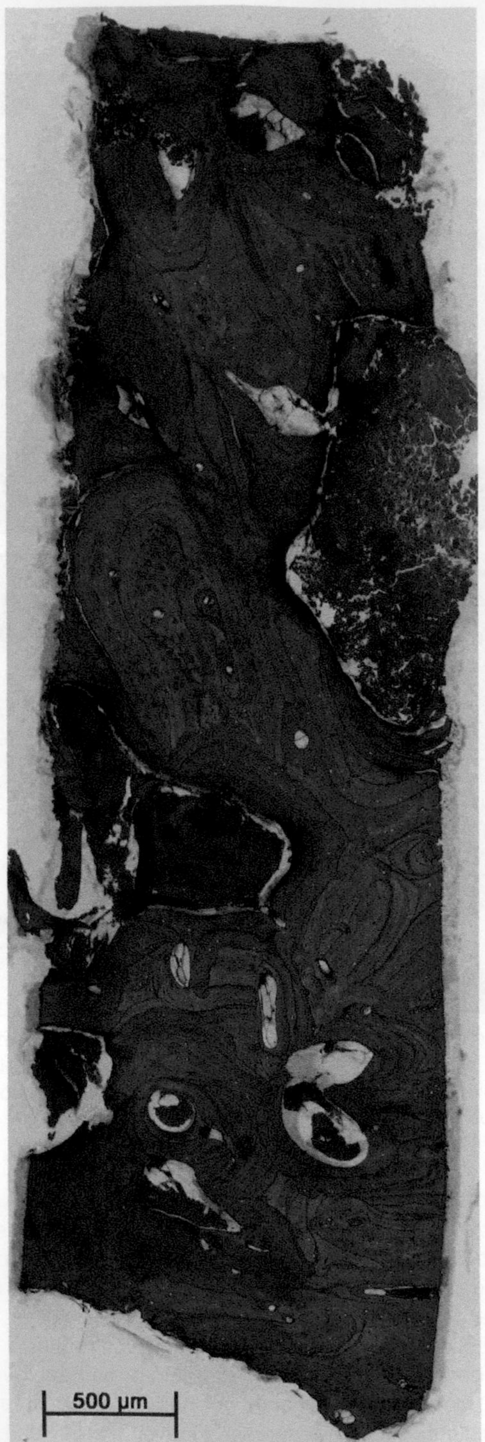

Fig. 3. Histologic specimen of fibular bone 10 years following grafting to the mandible and implant loading. (*From* Duttenhoefer F, Nack C, Doll C, et al. Long-term peri-implant bone level changes of non-vascularized fibula bone grafted edentulous patients. J Craniomaxillofac Surg. 2015;43(5):614; with permission.)

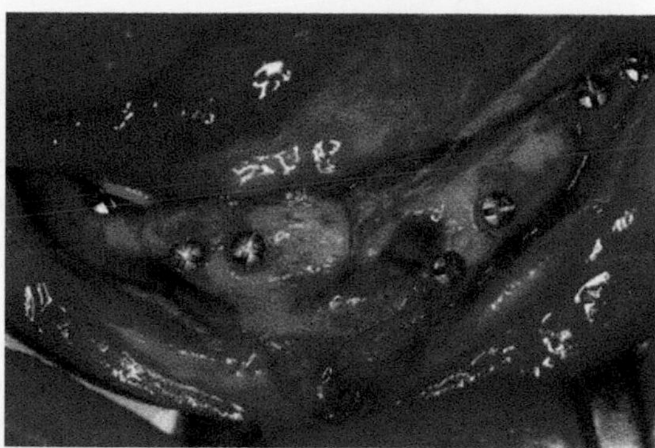

Fig. 4. Intraoperative photograph showing well-vascularized avascular fibular graft 3 months following surgery before implant placement. (*From* Nelson K, Glatzer C, Hildebrand D, et al. Clinical evaluation of endosseous implants in nonvascularized fibula bone grafts for reconstruction of the severely atrophied mandibular bone. J Oral Maxillofac Surg. 2006;64(9):1429; with permission.)

placed concurrently with allogenic bone graft. Radiographic examination was completed using computed tomography scans and the volume was evaluated at 1 week, 6 months, and 12 months following grafting. The study found no statistically different volume of augmentation achieved with autograft or allograft with the added advantage of no harvest site morbidity with allograft alone for sinus augmentation.[13]

Monje and colleagues[14] conducted a systematic review of the stability and predictability of allogenic block grafts in augmenting atrophic maxilla. The article reportedly reviewed 361 cases of allogenic block grafting to the maxilla followed for a mean of 4 to 9 months after surgery. Nine of the 361 cases failed within 1 to 2 months after surgery. A mean of 4.79 mm of horizontal volume gain was reported from 119 grafted sites. The study concluded that block allograft is a predictable and suitable alternative to autogenous bone grafting for horizontal bone augmentation with reduced morbidity to the patient when compared with autografting.[14] Acocella and colleagues[2] conducted a clinical and histologic examination of allogenic bone grafted to restore atrophic maxillary ridges. Sampling procedures were carried out at 4, 6, and 9 months following augmentation. At 4 months the histologic examination showed creeping substitution from vital host bone into the allograft in the beginning stages. Additionally, poor neovasculature and rare presence of osteoclasts was observed. Some specimens showed varying amounts of fibrous tissue mixed with new bone formation. After 6 months cellular activity was still poor and residual graft was slowly being replaced by new bone. Finally, observations at 9 months showed high number of empty osteocyte lacunae with fibrous tissue. Overall, the histology was characterized by vital new bone surrounded by nonvital bone with empty osteocyte lacunae in way of resorbtion.[2]

The disadvantages of allograft include possible transmission of disease and lack of osteoinductive properties. Chaushu and colleagues[15] explored the possible complications with the use of bone allograft for alveolar augmentation. The study investigated the complications and respective rate of complications with allogeneic block grafts. A total of 137 sites were grafted. Grafted sites included the anterior and posterior maxilla and mandible. Partial and total graft failure occurred in 7% of their population. Soft tissue complications included membrane exposure in 30%, failure of wound closure in 30%, and perforation of the mucosa over the grafted bone in 14%. The study reported an infection rate of 13% and more complications were observed in the mandible than in the maxilla. The study attributed their findings to difficulty with soft tissue coverage and graft exposure. Additionally, the study suspected the decreased vascular supply to the mandible, and technique sensitivity also contributed to the complication rates.[15] Similar studies in the literature reported similar complications and rates.[16,17] Barone and colleagues[18] investigated the stability of deep frozen bone allograft and the success rates of implants placed in the augmented ridges. A total of 24 alveolar ridges were augmented with block and corticocancellous allograft secured with screws (**Figs. 5** and **6**). Dehiscence and early exposure were observed in two of the grafted sites. Subsequently the grafted material was removed because of the presence of infection. The remaining grafts were deemed successful at implant placement with evidence of good vascularization. The grafted sites were restored with implant-supported prosthetics. Two of the installed implants failed to integrate and signs of infection were noted. The failed implants were removed and replaced with successful integration of the implants. The study concluded that predictable outcomes are possible with allogeneic grafts to augment the maxilla.

Xenogenic Bone

Xenografts are defined as a tissue transplanted between animals of different species. Xenografts currently are harvested from bovine or equine sources. Because xenografts are sourced from different species the sterilization procedure is more rigorous than that of allogeneic grafts. This results in reduced osteoinductive properties of the bone. A distinctive advantage of this bone graft is that it has an abundance of availability and the material cost is far lower than that of allogenic bone. Evidence in the literature shows that to achieve any robust bone regeneration with xenografts conjunctive signaling molecules, such as BMP, or platelet-rich plasma must be used. Additionally, xenografts may have poor handling properties requiring placement of a membrane to ensure stability of the graft. Xenogenic grafts are processed in a different manner than that of allografts. The xenografts are processed to remove all of the organic constituents of the material. The remaining material is composed of only the mineral constituents. An example of such processes is by temperature deorganification. This process burns away the organic component of the graft material and leaves the mineral substructure.

Lima and colleagues[19] conducted a randomized controlled split mouth trial to investigate the volumetric stability of autologous and xenogenic block grafts. The study

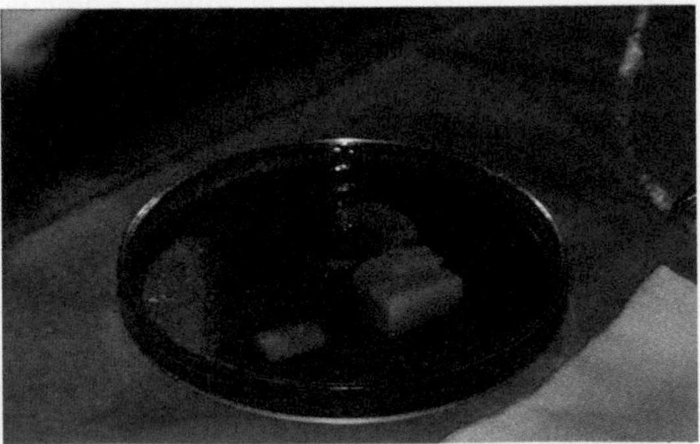

Fig. 5. Corticocancellous block allogenic block allograft restored in rifamycin. (*From* Barone A, Varanini P, Orlando B, et al. Deep-frozen allogeneic onlay bone grafts for reconstruction of atrophic maxillary alveolar ridges: a preliminary study. J Oral Maxillofac Surg. 2009;67(6):1302; with permission.)

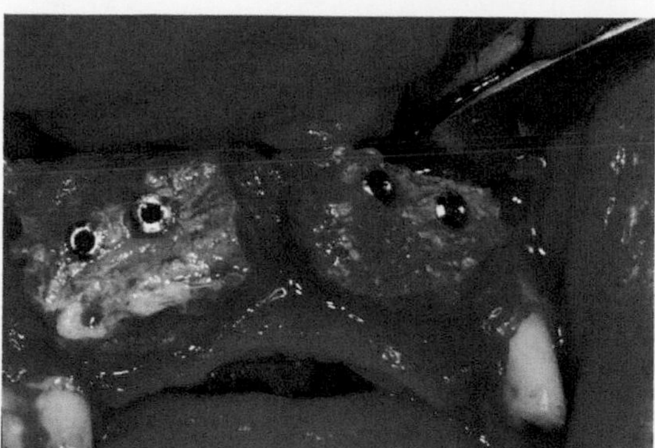

Fig. 6. Horizontal onlay augmentation. (*From* Barone A, Varanini P, Orlando B, et al. Deep-frozen allogeneic onlay bone grafts for reconstruction of atrophic maxillary alveolar ridges: a preliminary study. J Oral Maxillofac Surg. 2009;67(6):1302; with permission.)

additionally investigated the stability of the implants placed in these grafts. The study grafted patients who required grafting of the anterior maxilla. Half of the maxilla was grafted with xenograft and the remaining half was grafted with mandibular ramus graft that was milled with the use of a bone mill. Differences in preoperative thickness of bone were not reported to be statistically significant. Following a healing period of 6 months implants were placed in the grafted bone. The bone thickness achieved with each graft was measured clinically and with the use of three-dimensional imaging. After a healing period of 6 months the bone thickness was not statistically different between the test and control subjects. However, the study did find greater insertion torque achieved with autogenous bone when compared with the test graft. The study concluded that autogenous bone and xenogenic bone for maxillary reconstruction is predictable and reliable.[19] Li and colleagues[20] conducted a study to investigate the effectiveness of xenograft in augmenting atrophied posterior mandible using a tunneling technique. The study grafted the mandibular ramus with block xenograft and examined the histology of the grafted area 9 months postoperatively. The study observed consistent bone formation through the bovine bone block in all samples. The study concluded that xenograft might provide alternatives in grafting materials.[20] Finally, Simion and colleagues[21] investigated the histology of vertically augmented bone with a 1:1 mixture of xenograft with autogenous graft. The autograft was harvested from the mandible with trephine burs. The graft was combined with xenograft and applied to a perforated graft site. A tenting technique with polytetrafluoroethylene membrane and implants that were placed simultaneously was used. When analyzed, the bone histologically showed lamellar bone with direct continuity with the regenerated bone. The core section of the regenerated tissue showed residual autogenous bone and xenogenic bone particles. The study provided evidence of intimate contact of the host bone with the newly regenerated bone. Blood vessel invasion was observed more frequently in the core section of the graft. The study supported the use of xenograft combined with autogenous graft for better bone regeneration. However, this study stated that xenograft undergoes slow resorption and substitution with new regenerated bone.[21]

Alloplastic Bone

When grafting in the oral cavity, such challenges as handling properties, lack of structural support, and pressure from contraction of tissues during healing can make obtaining predictable results difficult. Alloplastic grafting materials have been engineered for improved handling properties and specialized use. Alloplastic bone grafts are defined as grafting materials or bone substitutes made synthetically or derived from coral of algae hydroxyapatite (HA). Examples of alloplastic materials include coralline calcium carbonate, bioceramic alloplasts (β-tricalcium phosphate), and bioactive glass, to name a few. Alloplastic materials are often combined with allogeneic grafts when grafting the maxillary sinus. The grafts have properties of being radiopaque and do not resorb, which provides support to the graft against the contractile forces of the sinus membrane when healing.

The grafting success of HA materials depends on the total surface area that is available for the body to interact with. Porous materials allow penetration of osteoblasts and osteoclasts to invade and allow space for vascular invasion to incorporate the material into the host's tissue. The biologic basis of why coral-based HA works lies in the material's macromolecular structure. The structure of the material is similar to that of the bone macromolecular structure. Coral, which is composed of calcium carbonate, is processed by manufacturers to produce calcium carbonate, which holds a similar structure to HA. Engineers have even developed a subtype of calcium phosphate that allows it to be more resorbable. Resorbable HAs have been synthesized at a particle size that allows the macrophages of the body to remove the particles essentially making the material resorbable. Biphasic calcium phosphate is such a type of alloplast. The material is engineered from a combination of HA and tricalcium phosphate or from pure tricalcium phosphate. Depending on the ratio of HA to tricalcium phosphate, the degree of resorpability of the material changes.

Alloplasts can have the unique ability of allowing bone to bond to its surface. Silica-based materials, also known as bioactive glass, have this property. Bio-gran (Palm Beach, Florida) and PerioGlas (Jacksonville, Florida) are two such examples. The bone creates a chemical bond between the bone and glass interface. Maintaining the particle size within a narrow range allowed for the materials to degrade enough to allow cells to access the particulate and lay down new bone in the material. The glass gets lost through degradation processes over time.

Calcium sulfate was developed as bone void filler. Its excellent handling properties made it useful as a binder with other materials or as a barrier laid on top of bone graft. First the material is synthesized in its hemihydrate form ($CaSO_4$ ½ H_2O). Mixing with water yields a partially hydrated solid form of plaster of Paris.

Engineers have provided clinicians with multiple options when making a selection for reconstructive alloplastic materials. Bechara and colleagues[22] conducted a study comparing the predictability of nonceramic HA when used as a graft against autogenous bone graft. The authors conducted a split mouth study to evaluate the stability of the grafted sites. The study used a sandwich osteotomy technique to reconstruct vertical height of bone by placing graft material between the osteotomized segments. Autogenous bone graft was harvested from the ramus of the host and HA was placed in the contralateral mandible. The segments were stabilized with titanium plates and screws (**Figs. 7** and **8**). The bone was sampled at 6 months and histologic examination revealed residual graft material in the experimental group (**Fig. 9**). Additionally, bone marrow density and marrow spaces were similar between the test and control subjects. The study concluded that the results showed that alloplastic HA graft material is a suitable substitute for grafting the mandible using a sandwich technique. Orsini and colleagues[23] also conducted a split mouth study to regenerate periodontal defects with calcium sulfate and autogenous bone graft. Twelve patients were treated in this study using guided bone regeneration. Autogenous bone graft was harvested from the mandible and coated with a collagen membrane or calcium sulfate. The graft

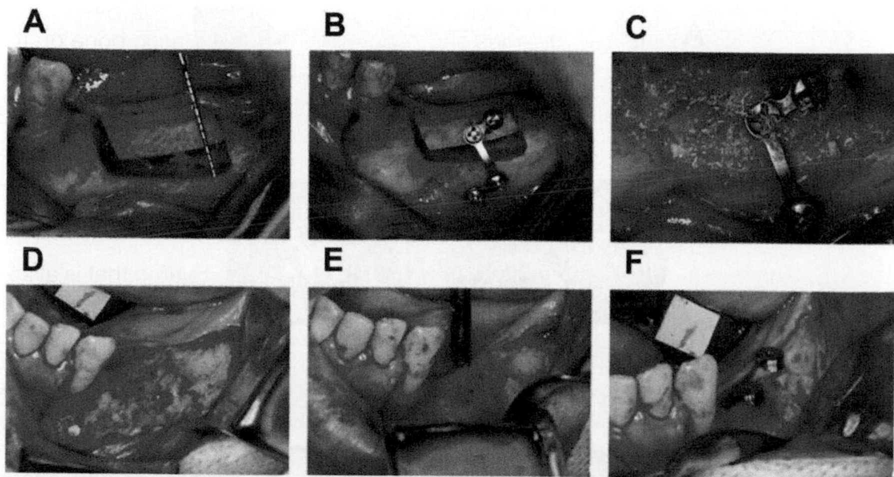

Fig. 7. Clinical view of the posterior mandible (*A*) after osteotomy, showed the vertical gain limited to 4 mm, (*B*) fixed with miniplates, (*C*) grafted with hydroxyapatite, (*D*) after 6 months of healing, (*E*) retrieval of the bone biopsy in the long axis, and (*F*) implant placement. (*From* Bechara K, Dottore AM, Kawakami PY, et al. A histological study of non-ceramic hydroxyapatite as a bone graft substitute material in the vertical bone augmentation of the posterior mandible using an interpositional inlay technique: A split mouth evaluation. Ann Anat. 2015;202:2; with permission.)

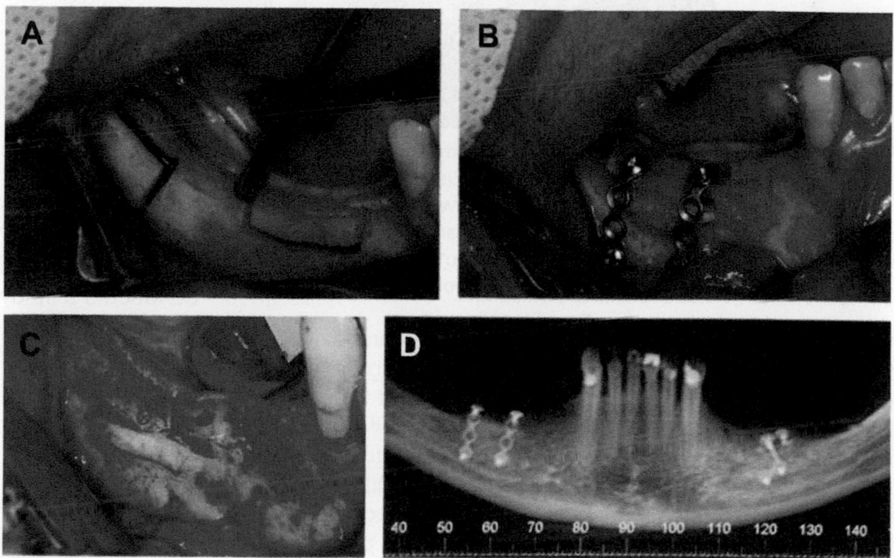

Fig. 8. Clinical view of the autogenous groups (*A*) osteotomy and bone graft performed, (*B*) two miniplates were fixed to stabilize the graft, (*C*) after 6 months of healing, and (*D*) radiographic view of the bilateral case (autogenous and HA group). (*From* Bechara K, Dottore AM, Kawakami PY, et al. A histological study of non-ceramic hydroxyapatite as a bone graft substitute material in the vertical bone augmentation of the posterior mandible using an interpositional inlay technique: A split mouth evaluation. Ann Anat. 2015;202:3; with permission.)

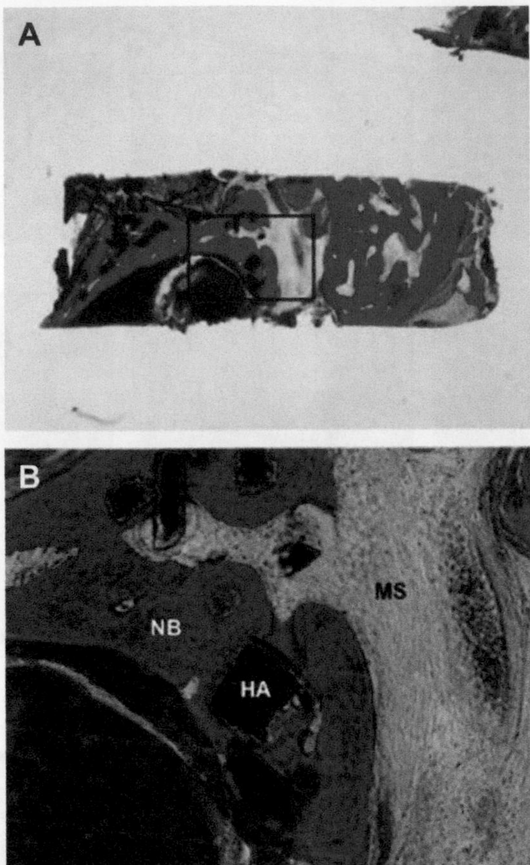

Fig. 9. *(A)* Low- and *(B)* high-power (×100) histophotograph of hydroxyapatite incorporated bone graft material. The hydroxyapatite particles are surrounded by newly formed bone. HA, Hydroxyapetite; MS, Medullary Space; NB, New Bone. (*From* Bechara K, Dottore AM, Kawakami PY, et al. A histological study of non-ceramic hydroxyapatite as a bone graft substitute material in the vertical bone augmentation of the posterior mandible using an interpositional inlay technique: A split mouth evaluation. Ann Anat. 2015;202:5; with permission.)

was exposed in 6 of 12 cases covered with membrane and 4 of 12 cases covered with calcium sulfate. The grafted sites healed following the exposure by secondary intention with good tissue coverage and quality of soft tissue. There was no statistical difference in the regeneration of periodontal defects. This study suggested that alloplastic materials can act as a barrier surface to prevent soft tissue invasion.[23]

The current consensus for grafting with alloplastic materials is for its use as an adjunct used in conjunction with autograft or allograft. The mechanical properties of the alloplastic material make it ideal for handling properties. The predictability of the graft when used alone is suspect.

BONE MORPHOGENIC PROTEIN

Prosthetic rehabilitation with goals of alveolar bone augmentation and regeneration meets considerable clinical, technical, and biologic challenges. Complications are frustrating for not only the clinician, but also the patient. In recent literature bone regenerative agents have emerged as a predictable and dependable method of regenerating bone. A popular and well-studied biologically active agent is BMP. To be specific, interest is directed in BMP 2 and 7.[24] BMPs are a family of osteoinductive proteins that stimulate endochondral and intramembranous bone formation from mesenchymal cells in situ.[25]

Boyne and colleagues[24] investigated the safety and efficacy of BMP 2 in inducing adequate bone for endosseous dental implant rehabilitation. Patients who required maxillary bone augmentation via maxillary sinus augmentation were included in the study. Patients were treated with the use of rhBMP-2 via an absorbable sponge at concentrations of 0.75 mg/mL, which was placed under carefully reflected schneiderian membranes. No additional grafting material was introduced. The control group received bone allograft. Bone induction was assessed by computed tomography scans obtained before, 4 months, and 6 months postoperatively. The mean height of bone induction at 4 months was 11.3 mm. The mean increase in ridge width was 4.7 mm. In the control group the mean height gained was 10.2 mm and 2.0 mm of width. At 4 months the mean height for bone induction did not statistically differ between the control and BMP groups. Furthermore, the study examined histologic samples of bone induced by BMP (**Figs. 10–12**). The study found mature bone formation in grafted sites with no distinguishing features from organic, native bone. The study concluded that BMP can safely induce adequate bone for the placement of functionally loaded implants for oral rehabilitation.

In a similar study Triplett and colleagues[25] compared the effects of bone induction in maxillary sinus lifts. The study prospectively compared patients who received BMP alone against a control group that received autograft. The height and density of the bone was measured with computed tomography scans. The bone was biopsied in a standardized method and compared histologically. The mean bone formation in the BMP group at 6 months was 7.8 mm versus the control group, which showed growth of 9.4 mm. No histologic difference was found by comparing the biopsy samples of both groups. The study reported no complications, which could be solely tied to use of BMP. The study reported complications associated with bone harvesting in the control group (pain, paraesthesia, and gait disturbance). A total of 160 patients were randomized and enrolled; 251 and 241 implants were placed in the BMP and

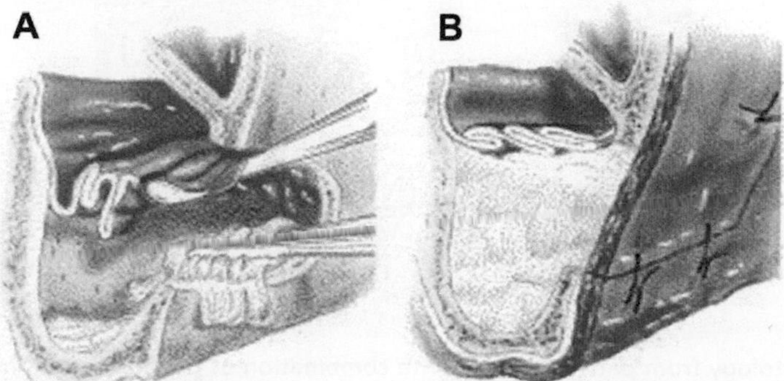

Fig. 10. (*A*) Completed schneiderian membrane elevation with the use of currets. (*B*) Augmented schneiderian membrane with BMP-infused sponge to induce bone formation. (*From* Boyne PJ, Lilly LC, Marx RE, et al. De novo bone induction by recombinant human bone morphogenetic protein-2 (rhBMP-2) in maxillary sinus floor augmentation. J Oral Maxillofac Surg. 2005;63(12):1695; with permission.)

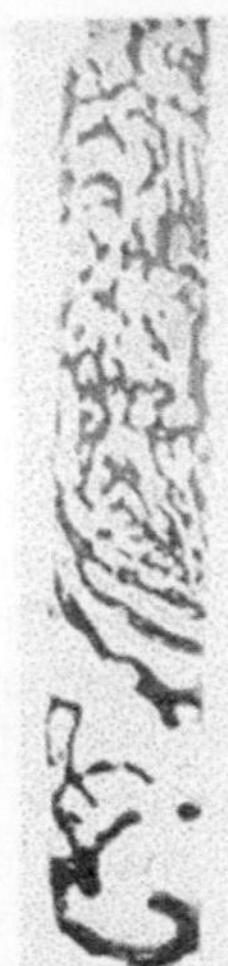

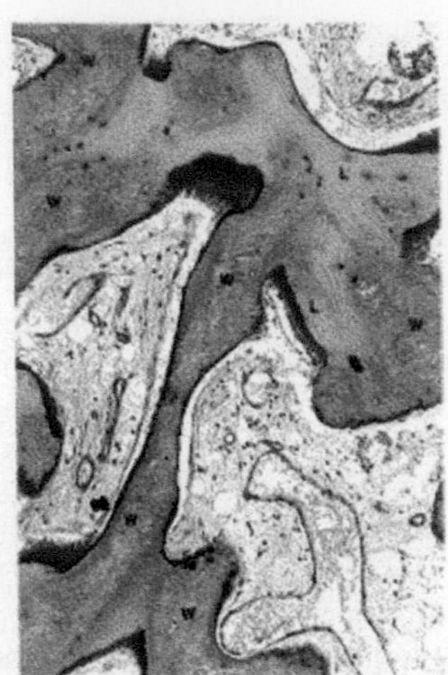

Fig. 11. Histology from patient treated with 0.75 mg/mL rhBMP-2. Twenty-eight weeks postoperative (Goldner stain, original magnification ×10). (*From* Boyne PJ, Lilly LC, Marx RE, et al. De novo bone induction by recombinant human bone morphogenetic protein-2 (rhBMP-2) in maxillary sinus floor augmentation. J Oral Maxillofac Surg. 2005;63(12):1701; with permission.)

control groups, respectively. Implants were rendered failed in 42 of 241 implants in the control and 50 of the 251 implants in the BMP group. The study concluded that there is comparative effectiveness in bone induction and regeneration when BMP is compared with the gold standard of grafting.

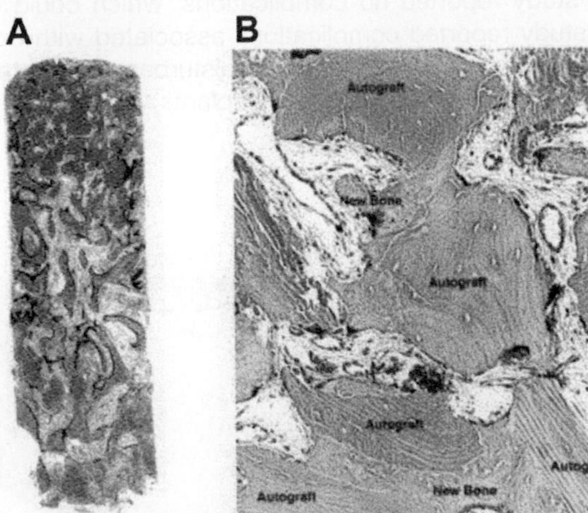

Fig. 12. Histology from patient treated with combination of demineralized, freeze dried allograft and autograft 34 weeks postoperative (Goldner stain, original magnification ×10). (A, B) High- and low-power pictomicrograph of sampled bone from BMP augmented sinus alone. (*From* Boyne PJ, Lilly LC, Marx RE, et al. De novo bone induction by recombinant human bone morphogenetic protein-2 (rhBMP-2) in maxillary sinus floor augmentation. J Oral Maxillofac Surg. 2005;63(12):1701; with permission.)

SUMMARY

Autogenous bone has been the staple and gold standard for grafting purposes. Recent trends in bone grafting practice have seen increased use of allograft combined with growth factors, such as platelet-rich fibrin and BMPs. However, although clinically effective these methods come with risks and complications, such as harvest site morbidity with autogenous grafts and risks of disease transmission with allografts. Recent advances in engineering have showed promise in resorbable synthetic grafting materials. Newer materials show promise of clinically significant volumes of bone augmentation with resorbable membranes, which would eliminate important complications and allow for increased patient comfort and safety. Autogenous bone grafts will most likely remain the gold standard of grafting materials and will continue to be essential in reconstruction of the maxillofacial skeleton. New materials will most likely shift the bone grafting philosophies of clinicians toward synthetic resorbable materials in the future.

DISCLOSURE

The authors have nothing to disclose.

REFERENCES

1. Chiapasco M, Zaniboni M, Boisco M. Augmentation procedures for the rehabilitation of deficient edentulous ridges with oral implants. Clin Oral Implants Res 2006;17(Suppl 2):136–59.
2. Acocella A, Bertolai R, Ellis E 3rd, et al. Maxillary alveolar ridge reconstruction with monocortical fresh-frozen bone blocks: a clinical, histological and histomorphometric study. J Craniomaxillofac Surg 2012;40(6):525–33.
3. Arrington ED, Smith WJ, Chambers HG, et al. Complications of iliac crest bone graft harvesting. Clin Orthop Relat Res 1996;(329):300–9.
4. Banwart JC, Asher MA, Hassanein RS. Iliac crest bone graft harvest donor site morbidity. A statistical evaluation. Spine 1995;20(9):1055–60.
5. Ross N, Tacconi L, Miles JB. Heterotopic bone formation causing recurrent donor site pain following iliac crest bone harvesting. Br J Neurosurg 2000;14(5):476–9.
6. Seiler JG 3rd, Johnson J. Iliac crest autogenous bone grafting: donor site complications. J South Orthop Assoc 2000;9(2):91–7.
7. Skaggs DL, Samuelson MA, Hale JM, et al. Complications of posterior iliac crest bone grafting in spine surgery in children. Spine 2000;25(18):2400–2.
8. Fretwurst T, Nack C, Al-Ghrairi M, et al. Long-term retrospective evaluation of the peri-implant bone level in onlay grafted patients with iliac bone from the anterior superior iliac crest. J Craniomaxillofac Surg 2015;43(6):956–60.
9. Dullenhoeter F, Nack C, Doll C, et al. Long-term peri-implant bone level changes of non-vascularized fibula bone grafted edentulous patients. J Craniomaxillofac Surg 2015;43(5):611–5.
10. Nelson K, Glatzer C, Hildebrand D, et al. Clinical evaluation of endosseous implants in nonvascularized fibula bone grafts for reconstruction of the severely atrophied mandibular bone. J Oral Maxillofac Surg 2006;64(9):1427–32.
11. Boyce T, Edwards J, Scarborough N. Allograft bone. The influence of processing on safety and performance. Orthop Clin North Am 1999;30(4):571–81.
12. Goldberg VM, Stevenson S. The biology of bone grafts. Semin Arthroplasty 1993;4(2):58–63.

13. Xavier SP, Silva ER, Kahn A, et al. Maxillary sinus grafting with autograft versus fresh-frozen allograft: a split-mouth evaluation of bone volume dynamics. Int J Oral Maxillofac Implants 2015;30(5):1137–42.
14. Monje A, Pikos MA, Chan HL, et al. On the feasibility of utilizing allogeneic bone blocks for atrophic maxillary augmentation. Biomed Res Int 2014;2014:814578.
15. Chaushu G, Mardinger O, Peleg M, et al. Analysis of complications following augmentation with cancellous block allografts. J Periodontol 2010;81(12):1759–64.
16. Bahat O, Fontanesi FV. Complications of grafting in the atrophic edentulous or partially edentulous jaw. Int J Periodontics Restorative Dent 2001;21(5):487–95.
17. Keith JD Jr, Petrungaro P, Leonetti JA, et al. Clinical and histologic evaluation of a mineralized block allograft: results from the developmental period (2001-2004). Int J Periodontics Restorative Dent 2006;26(4):321–7.
18. Barone A, Varanini P, Orlando B, et al. Deep Frozen Allogeneic Onlay Bone Grafts for Reconstruction of Atrophic Maxillary Alveolar Ridges. A preliminary study, J oral Maxillofacial Surgery 2009;67(6):1302.
19. Lima RG, Lima TG, Francischone CE, et al. Bone volume dynamics and implant placement torque in horizontal bone defects reconstructed with autologous or xenogeneic block bone: a randomized, controlled, split-mouth, prospective clinical trial. Int J Oral Maxillofac Implants 2018;33(4):888–94.
20. Li J, Xuan F, Choi BH, et al. Minimally invasive ridge augmentation using xenogenous bone blocks in an atrophied posterior mandible: a clinical and histological study. Implant Dent 2013;22(2):112–6.
21. Simion M, Fontana F, Rasperini G, et al. Vertical ridge augmentation by expanded-polytetrafluoroethylene membrane and a combination of intraoral autogenous bone graft and deproteinized anorganic bovine bone (Bio Oss). Clin Oral Implants Res 2007;18(5):620–9.
22. Bechara K, Dottore AM, Kawakami PY, et al. A histological study of non-ceramic hydroxyapatite as a bone graft substitute material in the vertical bone augmentation of the posterior mandible using an interpositional inlay technique: A split mouth evaluation. Ann Anat 2015;202:1–7.
23. Orsini M, Orsini G, Benlloch D, et al. Comparison of calcium sulfate and autogenous bone graft to bioabsorbable membranes plus autogenous bone graft in the treatment of intrabony periodontal defects: a split-mouth study. J Periodontol 2001;72(3):296–302.
24. Boyne PJ, Lilly LC, Marx RE, et al. De novo bone induction by recombinant human bone morphogenetic protein-2 (rhBMP-2) in maxillary sinus floor augmentation. J Oral Maxillofac Surg 2005;63(12):1693–707.
25. Triplett RG, Nevins M, Marx RE, et al. Pivotal, randomized, parallel evaluation of recombinant human bone morphogenetic protein-2/absorbable collagen sponge and autogenous bone graft for maxillary sinus floor augmentation. J Oral Maxillofac Surg 2009;67(9):1947–60.